Unloving Care

Unloving Care

The Nursing Home Tragedy

A TWENTIETH CENTURY FUND STUDY

Bruce C. Vladeck

BASIC BOOKS, INC., PUBLISHERS

NEW YORK

The Twentieth Century Fund is an independent research foundation which undertakes policy studies of economic, political, and social institutions and issues. The Fund was founded in 1919 and endowed by Edward A. Filene.

Board of Trustees of the Twentieth Century Fund

Library of Congress Cataloging in Publication Data

Vladeck, Bruce C.
    Unloving care.

    "A Twentieth Century Fund study."
    Includes bibliographical references and index.
    1. Nursing homes—United States.   2. Nursing home care—United States.   3. Medical policy—United States.
I. Twentieth Century Fund.   II. Title.
[DNLM: 1. Public policy—United States.   WX150.3 V865u]
RA997.V57   362.1′6′0973   79-3076
ISBN: 0-465-08880-5 (cloth)
ISBN: 0-465-08881-3 (paper)

To the memory of my father

CONTENTS

FOREWORD

The shabby treatment accorded the elderly inmates of the nation's nursing homes has been extensively documented, and numerous recommendations to improve conditions have been put forth. Yet when Bruce Vladeck proposed a study of nursing homes and public policy to The Twentieth Century Fund, its Trustees, two of whom have been involved in an official investigation of the scandalous conditions in New York State, recognized that his intention of examining the roots of the problem might be the approach to dealing with the still unsolved problems that could make the difference. The Trustees decided to support his proposal despite the obvious risks attached to dealing with so perplexing and pervasive an issue. Hence, we are particularly proud that Vladeck has succeeded in delivering all that he had originally promised—nothing less than a thorough explanation of how public policy failed and what must be done to correct the errors of the past.

As a foundation engaged in public policy research, the Fund seeks to diversify its risks in terms of both the issues it studies and the scholars it supports. We seek a mix of seasoned minds that have a record of accomplishments in public policy analysis with young and basically untested scholars interested in public policy issues. Vladeck was in the latter category, but from the beginning of his research, it was evident to those of us supervising his work that he had a grasp of the complexity of his subject, that he cared passionately about the effects of the shortcomings he discovered, and that he had the insight and maturity to propose ways in which the industry could be reformed.

Vladeck believes that prevailing conditions are such that we may be able to bring about needed change. Perhaps he is indulging in unwarranted optimism, but his painstaking analysis of the incremental mistakes that led to the misdirection of public policy and to the scandals that accompanied it make clear that he is a hardheaded realist. Certainly, he has demonstrated in a thoroughly balanced and informed manner just what went wrong, so there is reason to believe that his prescriptions point in the direction that public policy ought to go.

Whether or not his recommendations are accepted, Vladeck's review should be of special interest to policymakers and legislators concerned with the reasons why the noble objectives of public policy not only fail to be realized but are often changed in ways that represent a perversion of policy. The real tragedy of nursing home policy is that the result of good intentions was the victimization of people in need and the rewarding of the least deserving.

Our investment in Vladeck has paid off; he has made a notable contribution to the public policy debate on nursing homes and, in fact, to public policy in general. It is a considerable achievement that, I predict, will be reflected in future policy measures.

M. J. Rossant, Director
The Twentieth Century Fund
September, 1979

ACKNOWLEDGMENTS

The truism that any book is the work of many hands applies with particular force to this one. When I began working on it, I knew extremely little about nursing homes; almost everything in the book reflects, however indirectly, the assistance of others.

To put first things first, this book was made possible by the generous financial support of The Twentieth Century Fund. At the fund, I was assisted by Bill Diaz, Carol Barker, and especially Gary Nickerson; Wendy Mercer's level head and good humor provided simple solutions to any number of potential fiscal crises. Pamela Gilfond was an enthusiastic and energetic editor. I remained at The Center for Community Health Systems of Columbia University throughout the study; Dorothy Jones, Randy Humphrey, and Ruth Reich handled administrative details on that end. I owe a special debt of gratitude to Dr. Robert J. Weiss, director of the center, who first encouraged me to seek outside funding for this project and provided moral and administrative support throughout.

The most important things I was able to purchase with the funds provided by The Twentieth Century Fund were the services of Jim Linnane, Marsha Brown, and Carol Stock. Jim worked as research assistant for the first ten months of the project and continued to play an active part, including reading drafts of the manuscript, throughout. Much of what is best in this book, and most of what required the hardest work, is the result of his efforts. Marsha Brown worked as project secretary for a year and a half. In addition to typing innumerable letters and manuscript pages, she held things—and me—together. Carol Stock typed the revised manuscript with awesome speed and efficiency.

The almost two hundred people listed in the Appendix gave generously of their knowledge and their time, and this book is based largely on what they said. I am grateful to all of them, but a few must be singled out for special thanks. Cathy Worley and Cathy Hawes, both of the Ohio Nursing Home Commission, were extraordinarily generous with their time and energy, as was Dr. Wes Whittlesey of the Oklahoma Department of Institutions, Social and Rehabilitative Services.

Mary Adelaide Mendelson, who must spend too much of her time fending off importunate researchers, opened both her home and her files to me. Professor Gerald Grob of Rutgers University undertook to provide this novice with a short course in the history of American social welfare. John Geagan of the Service Employees International Union and Mary Sughrue of the Office of the Special Prosecutor in New York helped, in their radically different areas of concern, to arrange many interviews. Marie Callender, formerly director of the Office of Nursing Home Affairs in the Department of Health, Education, and Welfare, took many hours from more pressing concerns to help me get historical details straight. Milton Dezube, of what is now the Health Care Financing Administration, was similarly generous on matters of reimbursement policies. Through all, my good friend, Monsignor Charles J. Fahey, kept tabs on my temporal if not spiritual progress.

Dave Crowley and especially Larry Lane of the American Association of Homes for the Aging helped in many ways, from arranging interviews to reading a draft of chapter 3. Larry probably received and made more phone calls about this project than anyone not on the payroll; the book has been improved immeasurably by his assistance. Among the most important things he did was put me in touch with Frank Frantz who, among other things, was immensely helpful with chapter 3.

Phoebus Dhrymes and Nick Rango read and commented usefully on chapters 4 and 6, respectively, and Nick was a continual source of stimulation and argument. In addition to their helpful readings of chapter 7, Gene Bardach and Bob Kagan organized a splendid conference on the regulatory process and let me come (on an earlier visit to Berkeley, Bob's hospitality extended to use of his washing machine in the midst of a critical water shortage).

Several people, in addition to Jim Linnane, read the entire manuscript in draft. Paul Thompson and Bruce Spitz provided many helpful comments and substantial additional education, and Bruce and his colleagues at the Urban Institute (notably Jane Weeks, John Holahan, Bill Scanlon, and Burt Dunlop) generously shared much of their own research with me. I am especially grateful to two of my favorite public servants, Andy Fleck and Mildred Shapiro, who were not only my most expeditious readers but who, with their very different personalities and styles, influenced much of my thinking on these issues. At a later stage, Fred Goldman offered useful comments on the revised

Acknowledgments

draft, as did Bob Morris and Ted Marmor, who were engaged as reviewers by The Twentieth Century Fund.

It is customary to acknowledge the assistance of one's family. In this case, my gratitude is more than pro forma. In addition to innumerable instances of concrete advice and assistance, my parents, through a lifetime of example, have shaped the views and attitudes underlying everything I have done here. My wife, Fredda Wellin Vladeck, not only tolerated my frequent absences, whether at home or out-of-town, but also remained my most concerned and thoughtful critic, while shouldering a disproportionate share of familial burdens. My daughter, Elizabeth, was born shortly after this project got underway; while she contributed nothing directly to its completion, she merits mention on grounds of sheer delight.

Given how hard they labored to save me from myself, none of these good people are responsible for any errors, misstatements, misinterpretations, or mistakes in what follows.

Unloving Care

1

Introduction

Each Morning, more than one and a quarter million Americans awaken in nursing homes. Most of them are very old and very feeble. Most will stay in the nursing home for a long time. For most, it will be the last place they ever live.

At any given time, one in twenty elderly Americans resides in a nursing home; of those over seventy-five, the proportion rises to one in ten. Moreover, the best estimates are that for every five people who live past sixty-five, one will spend at least part of his (or more likely, her) life in a nursing home, with the risk of institutionalization increasing with each additional year of life.

There are more than 17,000 nursing homes in the United States—as opposed to roughly 7,000 general hospitals—and their aggregate revenues exceed $12 billion a year. They have been described as "Houses of Death,"[1] "concentration camps,"[2] "warehouses for the dying."[3] It is a documented fact that nursing home residents tend to deteriorate, physically and psychologically, after being placed in what are presumably therapeutic institutions.[4] The overuse of potent medications in nursing homes is a scandal in itself.[5] Thousands of facilities in every state of the nation fail to meet minimal government standards of sanitation, staffing, or patient care.[6] The best governmental estimate is that roughly half the nation's nursing homes are "substandard."[7]

The typical nursing home is a much better place than it was a few years ago. It is far more likely to be at least partially fire-resistant, to be managed by an administrator with some formal training in care of the disabled elderly, to have some system to regulate the dispensing of

3

prescription drugs, and to provide activities that go beyond the parking of residents in front of dayroom television sets.

Still, scandals recur with depressing frequency. The one that occurred in New York in 1975 is, perhaps, the most notorious.[8] This may be because of New York's position as a national media center, because then-Vice-President Rockefeller was implicated and testified in a televised hearing investigating nursing homes, and especially because it was aggressively pursued by a new state administration. But similar scandals were occurring or have since occurred in Illinois, California, Texas, Pennsylvania, and Ohio; and formal governmental investigations were undertaken in all those states, as well as in Connecticut, New Jersey, Minnesota, Wisconsin, Michigan, and Kansas.[9]

Most of the nursing home scandals involved financial chicanery and political influence. But the indifference, neglect, and physical abuse of patients continues: infirm old people are left lying for hours in their own excrement; severely scalded or even drowned in presumably attended bathtubs; illegally restrained in "geriatric chairs"; or attacked, sometimes suffering broken limbs, by nursing home employees. Although the overall quality of nursing homes improved substantially in the preceding decade, there were still, in the United States in 1978, nursing homes with green meat and maggots in the kitchen, narcotics in unlocked cabinets, and disconnected sprinklers in nonfire-resistant structures.[10] The increasingly small proportion of truly horrible nursing homes may be less distressing in the aggregate, though, than the quality of life in the thousands that meet the minimal public standards of adequacy. In these, residents live out the last of their days in an enclosed society without privacy, dignity, or pleasure, subsisting on minimally palatable diets, multiple sedatives, and large doses of television—eventually dying, one suspects, at least partially of boredom.

The existing nursing home industry is almost entirely a creation of public policy. Two-thirds of the total revenue of nursing homes comes from government. The explosive growth in the number and capacity of nursing homes over the past fifteen years was prompted primarily by the increased availability of public funds. Nursing homes are among the most closely regulated of all institutions, at least in theory; everything from the thickness of their walls to the variety of their menus to the qualifications of their personnel falls under the aegis of one or another government agency. If conditions in the nation's nursing homes are scandalous, then there has been a scandalous failure of government. The most comprehensive survey of nursing home problems ever undertaken in this country, that of the Subcommittee on

Introduction

Long-Term Care of the Senate's Special Committee on Aging, bears the title "Nursing Home Care in the United States: Failure in Public Policy." It is impossible to be more succinct than that.

A diagnosis of government failure is, of course, hardly unusual in American public discourse. The attitudes of Americans toward their governments has always ranged from suspicion to hostility. Political insurgents, and even many incumbents, conventionally campaign on a platform of running "against Washington," and the academic study of public policy is dominated by faculty members who devote their professional energies to explaining why government programs don't work.

The old woman residing in a nursing home is supported by public funds because there is no one else to support her. The nursing home is regulated, however well or poorly, by government because no other social institution has the capacity, the will, or the legitimacy to do so. The real issue is not how poor government performance is, but why it is as poor as it is, where it may be better than it looks, how it might be improved, and whether or not there is any alternative. That is what this book is about.

It is increasingly dangerous to attribute the failure of government programs or policies to the inherent incapacities or shortcomings of government, as though failure were somehow genetically programmed into all the misbegotten offspring of executives and legislatures. As long as public discourse remains mired in the rhetoric of bad government and good private action, attempts to concentrate attention on issues of real substance will be too infrequent and too limited.

The life of the elderly nursing home resident is little affected by cosmic, often empty, debate on the inherent virtues or defects of government. But it is affected, daily and intimately, by public policy. The price the resident pays for care and how much money is left over for personal expenses, the size and furnishing of the room, the scheduling of meals, how often the resident is seen by a physician—all these and almost every other aspect of the resident's day-to-day existence are affected by government policies. This book will explore how.

This book will, therefore, try to do two things. First, it will examine public policy toward nursing homes—what it is, how it was made, what its effects are, where it has succeeded and failed, how it might be different. The experience of nursing home policy teaches many useful lessons that can be applied to other areas of public concern. But above all, this study is important because the problems of the infirm elderly are real and immediate, because we are not doing a very good job of dealing with them, and because something must be done to make things better.

At the same time as it looks at nursing homes, this book will explore the causes of government failure. Government performs poorly, at least in part, because it is expected to perform poorly, because failure in that sense has, from the earliest origins of the nation, been designed into government and is the price we pay for values we apparently hold dearer than governmental success. Some of the sources of failure in nursing home policy may be peculiar to the problems of nursing homes or the people they serve; others may just be products of the inherent inferiority of foresight to hindsight. But the roots of failure are deeply seated in American attitudes toward government—as embodied not only in public opinion, but in laws, administrative structures, judicial procedures, and even in the Constitution.

The first three chapters of this book describe what nursing homes are like and what public policy toward them is. They provide a brief topographical look at the American nursing home industry, a description of the people who reside in nursing homes, and an attempt to understand what nursing homes are all about. They also trace the history of public policy and its effect on what actually goes on in individual nursing homes. Separate chapters address reimbursement policies and government concerns with program cost; the relationship among public policy, capital financing, and the growth of the nursing home industry; governmental definitions of "levels of care," and the process by which individual residents end up at individual facilities; regulation of the quality of care; and problems of fraud and abuse in government programs involving nursing homes. A discussion of the politics of nursing home policy follows. Looking at the influence of political factors on specific policy choices will help to define some of the realistic limits on efforts at reform, a subject that will be considered in the last three chapters.

The grand abstractions of public policy must be tied to the concrete needs, problems, and aspirations of individual citizens. At this very minute, there are people with intractable problems, suffering physical and emotional pain, some of which may result from the actions of governments that, at least in theory, are responsive to our wishes and concerns.

2

No Place Like Home

Bricks and Mortar

AT FIRST GLANCE, the interior of a typical nursing home looks like a patient-care floor in a general hospital. Rows of wide doors open off both sides of a long corridor; between the doors, a waist-high railing provides a handhold for those who have difficulty walking or for those who move by wheelchair. The rooms on which those doors open, like hospital rooms, usually have two single beds sitting high off the floor on heavy electromechanical frames, with movable side-rails attached. Next to each bed is a night table; elsewhere in the room are two dressers and a small closet. As often as not, another interior door leads to a bathroom. The walls are painted in institutional colors and the floors are generally tile, although carpeting is not uncommon.

As in a hospital, the center of activity, and often the physical center of the floor, is a nursing station. A high-fronted desk, wide enough to permit two or three people to sit at it, looks out onto the corridor. Behind it and to the sides are books and manuals, miscellaneous supplies, racks filled with patients' charts, a lockable medicine cabinet, and perhaps doors to a supply room and a staff bathroom or lounge. Not infrequently, diplomas or state licenses hang on the wall behind the nursing station, along with other official-looking documents, all neatly framed. Everywhere there are notices, lists, and schedules attached to bulletin boards, taped to walls or to the front of the nursing station.

But nursing homes are profoundly unlike hospitals, and while the most important differences are in the characteristics of their patients and their staff and in what patients and staff do all day, there are also physical differences. The lobby is almost invariably much smaller and more crowded than that of even the most modest general hospitals. With very few exceptions, there are no X-ray rooms or laboratories and no operating or recovery rooms. While there may be a pharmacy, it is unlikely to be manned by a pharmacist. Basic support facilities like the laundry and the kitchen are much more often visible. Connected to the kitchen, in most nursing homes, is something one rarely finds in a hospital—a dining room, with movable furniture and sliding partitions, used for activities as well as dining. It is one of the few physical reminders that nursing homes are places where people live.

From the outside, physical differences are more apparent. If the nursing home is proprietary—that is, operated for profit, as most are—the lot it occupies contains only the building (small compared to most hospitals) and a parking lot. The building may well abut one or more of the boundaries of the property. It may be on a commercial strip highway, surrounded by other small businesses, gas stations, or even, in one famous case, a junkyard.[1] It may be in the middle of an urban street. Real estate speculation and trafficking in land played an important role in the growth of the nursing home industry, and developers were reluctant to waste valuable property.

On the other hand, many voluntary—that is, not-for-profit—homes, especially those outside the inner cities, occupy relatively generous expanses. In warmer climates, these may be lushly landscaped, complete with outdoor furniture; but the grounds are there even in less hospitable climes, set aside, tax free, as the sites of possible expansion programs.

Most American nursing homes, proprietary or voluntary, are obviously new. Even when the exteriors are poorly maintained, as they often are, it is readily apparent that most of the nursing homes standing today have been built since 1965.

A visitor is also likely to be struck by the smell. One-third of nursing home residents are incontinent, so there is always some odor of either urine or disinfectant. In the better nursing homes, this produces a kind of mustiness; in the worst, the stench can be overpowering.

But the "typical" nursing home is an abstraction. There is enormous diversity in American nursing homes.

At the latest count, there are close to 18,000 nursing homes in the United States, using the definition of a residential facility providing some degree of nursing services over and above routine bed and board.[2] The average nursing home has about seventy-five beds, 90 percent of which will be filled on any given night.[3] About three quarters of all nursing homes are proprietary. Between 5 and 10 percent are operated directly by government. The remaining 3,000 or so are operated by charitable organizations, most commonly those under religious or denominational auspices.[4] Voluntary nursing homes tend to be slightly larger than proprietary ones, government homes much larger than either. As a result, just over two-thirds of all beds are in proprietary facilities; almost 10 percent are directly operated by governments, generally counties or localities; and the remaining 22 percent are under voluntary auspices.[5]

These gross figures obscure substantial variation from one part of the country to another. While, on the national average, there is one nursing home bed for every twenty people over the age of sixty-five (the exact number is 51.9 beds for every thousand people sixty-five and over), Minnesota has more than twice that (more than one bed for every ten elderly), and West Virginia, Arizona, Florida, New Jersey, and the District of Columbia all have less than half the national average (only one nursing home bed for every forty or more elderly citizens).[6] A full breakdown of nursing home availability by state appears in table 1.

It might be expected that the highest proportion of nursing home beds to elderly would be in those states that attract large numbers of elderly migrants—the retirement areas of the so-called "Sunbelt." Or, since the numbers being discussed are ratios, it might be expected that the highest ratios would be in areas with the fewest elderly—a statistical necessity if all areas had the same number of nursing homes. Neither supposition is true. In fact, the two states most commonly thought of as having large retirement communities, Arizona and Florida, both rank very low in nursing home availability, while the states with the highest ratio of nursing home beds per elderly are those in the most frigid reaches of the "Snowbelt." As table 1 also shows, there is no systematic relationship between the number of nursing homes and the size of a state's elderly population.

Insofar as there is any pattern at all in the distribution of nursing homes, it is largely a regional one. Table 2 shows that the greatest supply of nursing home beds relative to population is found in the wheat and (to accommodate Wisconsin) dairy states of the upper Midwest and Great Plains, with their heavy concentrations of northern European ethnic groups. Next in line are the fast-growing states of the intermountain region and of what might be called the "petroleum belt" of the Southwest, where nursing home construction may have outpaced the growth in elderly population. With the signal exception of Geor-

TABLE 1
Variations in the Supply of Nursing Home Beds

State	Nursing Home Beds Per 1,000 Elderly (1974-75)	National Rank	National Rank in Elderly as Percent of Total Population (1973)
Minnesota	116.8	1	17
Wisconsin	110.7	2	18
Nebraska	95.1	3	4
Colorado	94.9	4	43
Montana	90.6	5	29
Kansas	82.5	6	6
South Dakota	82.0	7	7
Oklahoma	81.9	8	8
Texas	80.0	9	36
Alaska	78.5	10	51
Washington	76.4	11	25
North Dakota	73.7	12	15
Georgia	73.0	13	41
Iowa	71.0	14	3
Connecticut	69.1	15	28
Utah	68.8	16	48
Idaho	62.6	17	32
Oregon	62.5	18	14
Arkansas	62.4	19	2
Massachusetts	60.0	20	11
Vermont	58.6	21	19
Ohio	56.3	22	30
Maine	56.0	23	9
Rhode Island	55.0	24	12
Missouri	54.7	25	5
Wyoming	53.2	26	37
National Average:	51.9		
Louisiana	50.0	27	38
California	50.0	28	35
Illinois	50.0	29	26
Indiana	50.0	30	31
New Hampshire	48.9	31	21
Michigan	47.7	32	39
Pennsylvania	47.4	33	13
Maryland	41.4	34	45
Delaware	39.3	35	44
Nevada	37.7	36	49
South Carolina	37.5	37	46
New Mexico	37.4	38	47
Alabama	35.8	39	23
New York	34.2	40	16
Hawaii	33.6	41	50
Mississippi	33.3	42	22
Tennessee	31.1	43	24
Virginia	30.6	44	42
Kentucky	28.7	45	20
North Carolina	26.2	46	40
District of Columbia	25.8	47	34
New Jersey	25.7	48	27
Florida	24.5	49	1
Arizona	24.3	50	33
West Virginia	15.9	51	10

SOURCE: Derived from American Health Care Association, *Long Term Care Facts* (Washington, D.C., American Health Care Association, n.d.), pp. 10-11 and 50-51.

TABLE 2
Regional Patterns of Nursing Home Availability

Region	Nursing Home Beds per 1,000 Elderly	National Rank	Region	Nursing Home Beds per 1,000 Elderly	National Rank
UPPER MIDWEST			**PACIFIC**		
Minnesota	116.8	1	Alaska	78.5	10
Wisconsin	110.7	2	Washington	76.4	11
Regional Average	96.5		Oregon	62.5	18
Nebraska	95.1	3	Regional Average	52.1	
Kansas	82.5	6	National Average	51.9	
South Dakota	82.0	7	California	50.0	28
North Dakota	73.7	12	Nevada	37.5	37
Iowa	71.0	14	Hawaii	33.6	41
National Average	51.9		Arizona	24.3	50
			MIDWEST		
			Ohio	56.3	22
INTERMOUNTAIN			Missouri	54.7	25
Colorado	94.9	4	National Average	51.9	
Montana	90.6	5	Regional Average	51.7	
Regional Average	74.7		Illinois	50.0	29
Utah	68.8	16	Indiana	50.0	30
Idaho	62.6	17	Michigan	47.7	32
Wyoming	53.2	26	**MID-ATLANTIC**		
National Average	51.9		National Average	51.9	
New Mexico	37.4	38	Pennsylvania	47.4	33
			Maryland	41.4	34
			Delaware	39.3	35
SOUTHWEST			Regional Average	37.1	
Oklahoma	81.9	8	New York	34.2	40
Texas	80.0	9	District of Columbia	25.8	47
Regional Average	72.9		New Jersey	25.7	48
Arkansas	62.4	19	**SOUTH**		
National Average	51.9		Georgia	73.0	13
Louisiana	50.0	27	National Average	51.9	
			South Carolina	37.5	37
			Alabama	35.8	39
NEW ENGLAND			Mississippi	33.3	42
Connecticut	69.1	15	Regional Average	32.5	
Regional Average	60.6		Tennessee	31.3	43
Massachusetts	60.0	20	Virginia	30.6	44
Vermont	58.6	21	Kentucky	28.7	45
Maine	56.0	23	North Carolina	26.2	46
Rhode Island	55.0	24	Florida	24.5	49
National Average	51.9		West Virginia	15.9	51
New Hampshire	48.9	31			

SOURCE: Derived from American Health Care Association, *Long Term Care Facts* (Washington, D.C.: American Health Care Association, n.d.), pp. 10-11 and 50-51.

gia, the states of the Southeast have the fewest nursing homes, reflecting their continued shortages in social and health services of all kinds, notwithstanding the growing economic prosperity of the region. Surprisingly, the mid-Atlantic region, with its long tradition of high per-capita incomes, high social welfare expenditures, and aggressive state governments, is only one step ahead of the South in terms of nursing home supply.

There is still greater variation in nursing home availability within states. California, for example, is close to the national average in availability of nursing home beds, but the supply in San Francisco is extremely limited, while that in Los Angeles County has traditionally been ample. In New Jersey, there is an extremely low supply in the northern counties of Bergen, Passaic, and Hudson (largely bedroom suburbs of New York City), while supply is much higher in the southern and seafront counties. (The "market" for nursing home services, however, is highly localized. Ideally, persons in nursing homes should be no more than an hour's drive from members of their immediate families or, when there is no immediate family, their former homes and neighborhoods.)

Despite the variation in nursing home availability, the occupancy rate tends to be the same everywhere in the country. Nursing homes are all about full most of the time in New Jersey and New York where there are relatively few beds, but they are also nearly full in Minnesota and Wisconsin. In almost every state, those homes with the best reputation have long waiting lists. In fact, 72 percent of *all* nursing homes report having a waiting list.[7] Average occupancy rates everywhere in the country exceed 85 percent and are generally closer to 95 percent. Since resident turnover makes 100 percent occupancy essentially unobtainable on an annual basis, these figures are very high. By comparison, the national average for acute care hospital occupancy is less than 75 percent, and in many areas it is much lower.

The pattern of high occupancy rates regardless of bed availability suggests that people in nursing homes in areas where there are lots of beds may not be that different from those not in nursing homes in places where supply is tighter. Thus, whether or not an individual is in a nursing home is partially a function of where that person lives.

Flesh and Blood

The typical nursing home resident is an eighty-year-old, white widow or spinster of relatively limited means suffering from three or four chronic ailments.[8] All the dimensions of this characterization (age, race, marital status, income, and health) are important. However, when comparing the nursing home population to the rest of the elderly, age and marital status are crucial. Compared to other elderly people, nursing home residents are older and more isolated socially, but they are not much poorer or more disabled.

The growing recognition of the aged as a social category and a political force tends to obscure the heterogeneity of that part of the population that is more than sixty-five years old. Among the characteristics in which the elderly differ is age itself. Of the 20 million Americans over sixty-five enumerated in the 1970 census, 7 million, or 35 percent, were between sixty-five and sixty-nine years of age; another 5.4 million, or 27 percent, were between seventy and seventy-four. As might be expected, most of the elderly are "young old"— under seventy-five years of age.[9]

In nursing homes, though, fully 84 percent of the residents are seventy-five or older. The average age is over eighty, and the number of residents over ninety exceeds the number between sixty-five and seventy-four. In 1973–74, there were 180,000 nursing home residents in the ninety-and-over category, 163,000 between sixty-five and seventy-four.[10]

Women live longer than men. The older the population, the higher a proportion of women it will have and the more likely it will be that those women are widowed. This logic applies to nursing homes with double force. Fifty-nine percent of the total over-sixty-five population is female; in nursing homes, that figure exceeds 72 percent. While 49 percent of the people over sixty-five are married, only 12 percent of those in nursing homes are. Of the general population over seventy-five, 23 percent are still married, more than twice the number of those in the same age group living in institutions.[11]

Nursing home residents, therefore, are not only old but isolated. Many have lived most of their adult lives with a spouse but are now widowed. Fifteen percent of the nursing home population—compared with about 5 percent of the elderly population as a whole—never married.[12] For those who had children, the children, if they are still alive, are themselves probably of late middle age or elderly; certainly, the surviving children of the 180,000 residents over ninety are mostly over sixty-five. It is widely estimated that roughly one-third of nursing home residents have no surviving immediate families, while about one-half have no immediate family members nearby.[13]

Nursing home residents are poor, even poorer than the elderly in general. Seventy percent (as opposed to less than 50 percent of the entire elderly population[14]) have incomes of less than $3,000 a year. Typically, the sole income of a nursing home resident is a social security retirement or survivor's check, along with a subsidy from her family, when there are other family members. (One of the reasons why there are relatively few nursing homes in Florida and Arizona—although other factors contribute more to the nursing home shortage in Arizona—might be that some of those elderly affluent enough to relocate to retirement areas are also affluent enough to avoid, or at least defer, nursing home placement, presumably by purchasing services, like those of companions or housekeepers.)

Blacks and Hispanics are underrepresented in nursing homes, relative to their proportion of the total elderly population. Nine percent of the elderly are nonwhite, but only 5 percent of nursing home residents are, although elderly blacks suffer more disability than elderly whites. One reason for this may be differing cultural attitudes toward the elderly; this appears to be the case with Hispanic cultures. Another reason may stem from the fact that many elderly blacks reside in the South where nursing home availability is below the national average—although which is cause and which is effect is difficult to unravel. Primarily, the situation reflects the persistent pattern of discrimination in services of all kinds in all parts of American society; in this regard, nursing homes are not very different from other institutions.

There is no question that nursing home residents have serious health problems. The typical resident has between three and four serious chronic conditions, of which one is mental or psychological. Half have been diagnosed as "senile," although considerable controversy surrounds that term and the estimate is undoubtedly too high. Between 30 and 40 percent have arthritis or rheumatism; and an equally large, overlapping proportion suffers from heart disease. Nearly 15 percent are diabetic, and more than one in ten is at least partially paralyzed.[15]

In terms of functional limitations, less than half can walk unassisted; more than 30 percent are incontinent at least part of the time; one-third need assistance with eating; and more than two-thirds need assistance with bathing and dressing.[16]

As striking as this picture of illness and disability may be, the deterioration it reflects afflicts many older people. The elderly population, especially the "old elderly," outside of nursing homes is not very different. The prevalence of arthritis in the total elderly population is roughly the same as that in nursing homes. Heart disease affects approximately 20 percent of the total elderly population, as compared to about 35 percent of those in nursing homes, but in groups of equal age distribution, the proportions are much closer. Much the same can be said for diabetes and impairments of hearing and vision.

The nursing home population does suffer more functional disability than the elderly population as a whole. Nursing home residents are more likely to be crippled.[17] But a number of studies suggest that for every nursing home resident with a functional impairment, there are somewhere between one and two-and-a-half elderly people with similar degrees of impairment living outside institutions.

As a general rule, illness and disability are necessary but not sufficient conditions for nursing home institutionalization. The other necessary condition is the absence of alternative care.[18] Typically, a frail, old woman is supported by a husband, daughter, or sister who does the shopping, helps clean the house, and provides transportation to the doctor, until the caretaker himself or herself becomes ill or dies. Or an elderly couple manages to cope by leaning on one another until one is hospitalized and then the other is no longer able to live alone. Or two old women in adjacent hospital beds recuperating from strokes or fractured hips are discharged at roughly the same time, one to the home of her daughter, the other, who has no surviving family in the community, to a nursing home.

The exception to these generalizations is mental illness, especially "senility." There is no question that, in some individuals, increasing age leads to irreversible deterioration of mental capacity characterized by disorientation, confusion, loss of short-term memory, and perhaps inappropriate behavior. There is also no question that many far less serious, and much more easily reversible, physical and emotional symptoms that affect the elderly, most notably depression, are often mistaken for senility. All too often, inadequate or mistaken responses to those symptoms lead to further deterioration which does become permanent. A primary reason for institutionalization of those who do have social supports and have been receiving care from family members or others is increasing mental disorientation, leading to the need for more constant and skilled supervision. It is largely beyond the capacity of any one individual, no matter how caring or dedicated, to provide adequate care outside an institutional setting to someone who really is extremely senile, or who acts for some other reason as though he is. A high proportion of such people end up in nursing homes.

Nonetheless, it should be clear by now that the commonly accepted belief that growth in nursing home utilization is the result of the "abandonment" of elderly parents by their children, or is yet another symptom of the breakdown of the nuclear family in modern urban society, is simply untrue. To quote Elaine Brody, a leading gerontologist, "the responsible behavior of families towards older people has been so thoroughly documented that it is no longer at issue in gerontological research. The cultural rejection of the aged has not been acted out on the individual or family level, despite the vastly increased pressures created by larger numbers of people for whom the younger generations are responsible."[19] In fact, there is a general consensus in the professional community that families are far more likely to wait too long for outside assistance, particularly institutional assistance, especially in cases of mental or emotional problems, than not to wait long enough.[20]

Thus, while the number of people in nursing homes has tripled over the last two decades, it would be a mistake to attribute even a significant share of that growth to changes in family relationships. The over-seventy-five population has nearly doubled since 1960, and the number of old people in other institutions, especially mental hospitals, has fallen dramatically. A generous estimate would be that one-quarter of the growth in nursing home use is accounted for by changing family patterns. The rest has resulted from demographic change, the greater availability of public subsidy, and the increase in supply.

Finally, most people who enter nursing homes stay a long time. The average length of stay is 2.6 years, the median 1.5. More than a quarter stay more than three years, and another third stay one to three years.[21] In the oxymoronic language favored by health administrators, 30 percent of all nursing home discharges are due to death; most of the others are sent either to general hospitals (often to prevent the embarrassment of having the resident die in the nursing home itself) or to other nursing homes (generally for financial reasons).[22] Some small proportion of nursing home patients receive rehabilitative services of adequate intensity to permit their returning home; another small, but uncounted, proportion simply cannot stand the nursing home and leave.

Most remain until or through the acute episode that eventually kills them. As leading epidemiologist and public health official Andrew C. Fleck has said, "People die someplace. Men and children die in short-stay hospitals. Old men die at home and acute-care hospitals. Women over age eighty die in nursing homes, unless they are black."[23]

The Missing Physician

Nursing home residents are regularly in need of medical attention. Nursing homes are commonly conceived of as medical facilities. No less than two-thirds of nursing home residents have their care subsidized by government programs created to finance medical care. Yet one of the most shocking facts about day-to-day life in nursing homes is the absence of physicians.

Every "skilled" nursing home must, by law, have a "medical director," a physician with overall responsibility for medical care within the facility. "Intermediate" facilities also have responsibility for the medical care of their residents. In both types of facilities, each patient must have a personal "attending" physician who is supposed to see the patient within thirty days of admission and every thirty to ninety days thereafter (depending on whether the patient is classified as needing "skilled" or only "intermediate" care). Physicians are supposed to be responsible for general overseeing of all services to their patients and have sole responsibility for prescribing and monitoring medications.

But physicians in general are not enthusiastic about caring for the elderly, especially the more infirm, nor do nursing homes fit into the contemporary pattern of medical practice revolving exclusively between hospital and office. Thus, the formal requirements for physician involvement in the care of nursing home residents are often met only on paper, if at all. Examinations are superficial, if performed. The fraudulent "gang visit" persists, in which a physician's involvement with the patient may extend to no more than preparation of a claims form. Too much consultation, and even prescribing, takes place over the telephone.[24] Physicians appear to accept, without substantial complaint, the failure of the nursing home to follow their directives for patient care. Orders for follow-up testing, rehabilitative services, dietary changes, or special nursing services are routinely ignored. Physicians would never tolerate such practices in hospitals treating their patients, but they seem to accept them as an unavoidable norm in nursing homes.

And physicians acquiesce in, when they do not create, the terrible problem of overmedication. In a survey of "skilled nursing facilities," those presumably reserved for the most seriously ill patients, federal investigators found an average of 6.1 prescriptions per patient. Fifteen percent of the patients had *ten* or more prescriptions; only 0.1 percent had none. The most commonly prescribed drugs are laxatives and aspirin or aspirin substitutes, and more than half the patients had prescriptions for tranquilizers or sedatives—most often extremely potent psychoactive agents like thioridazine (Mellaril) or chlorpromazine (Thorazine), which have serious and often irreversible side effects and which are medically appropriate for only a small fraction of the nursing home patients receiving them.[25]

Worse, an alarmingly high proportion of these and other prescriptions for dangerous medications are written "p.r.n.," which means, "as needed." The "need" is most often determined by nurses or, illegally, by lower-level nursing personnel. The temptation to employ such drugs for behavior control, when the nursing staff is shorthanded or indifferent or late at night when a resident becomes agitated or awakes confused and "anxious," is too rarely resisted. In facilities that are perpetually short-staffed or otherwise incapable of rendering even basic care, residents may be sedated all the time.

Since the long-term effect of psychoactive drugs tends to be a progressive downward spiral in the patient's mental capacities, this routine is self-perpetuating. It may begin without deliberate intent. But it would not be possible without the acquiescence of the physicians who are writing the orders for the drugs in the first place.

Other kinds of pharmaceuticals are also overprescribed and overused in nursing homes. The federal survey referred to previously also found that far more patients have prescriptions for antihypertensive medications than have hypertension,[26] and it has been suggested that the need for laxatives would not be so great if residents got assistance in going to the bathroom when they asked for it. The use of drugs in nursing homes is clearly more responsive to the economic and administrative needs of the facility than to the medical needs of its residents.

The overprescription of drugs is a general problem in modern American medicine, but in nursing homes it is especially dangerous. In hospital practice, physicians rely heavily on nurses and other professional staff to monitor the condition of patients, to make regular notations of patient status, and to alert them to untoward changes in patient condition. This kind of monitoring is particularly important for patients receiving powerful drugs. To a large extent, it is what nurses are trained to do. But in nursing homes, there are not enough nurses, and those there are heavily burdened with administrative responsibilities. The aides, who are most in touch with the patients, have no formal training in medical matters, although the more experienced do become adept at their work. If a physician were to rely on the nursing home staff for the same degree of support that he receives from a hospital staff, the result would almost necessarily be inferior care.[27] When, on top of that, the physician himself is less concerned and attentive, the level of care may become minimal. This is true not only for drug therapy but for all other forms of care.

Under these circumstances, it should hardly be surprising that nursing home patients tend to get worse after their admission to nursing homes. According to an independent government survey of nursing homes, the most common postadmission diagnoses were urinary tract infections, eye and ear infections, and bedsores.[28] These are diseases, not of age or frailty, but of inadequate institutional care itself.

Nurses and Aides

To care for their residents, nursing homes employ slightly more than 700,000 people, or roughly sixty-six employees for every hundred residents.[29] Most are unskilled, untrained, and low paid. Only 5 percent of all nursing home employees are registered nurses (RNs), and another 6 percent are licensed practical or licensed vocational nurses (LPN).[30] On the average, there are just over three RNs and another four LPNs for every hundred patients. But, since the residents are there twenty-four hours a day, seven days a week, while a full-time employee works, on average, thirty-three hours a week, the numbers are more like 1.5 licensed nursing personnel (RN and LPN) per hundred patients.

Ninety percent of direct patient care in nursing homes is delivered by aides,[31] a category that by law and usage implies no formal training or education. Just under half of all nursing home employees are aides.[32] It is aides who rouse the patients in the mornings, escort them to the bathroom and to meals, assist them in dressing, clean up after them, and as a general rule administer—illegally—at least some of their medication. When residents cannot walk, aides lift them out of bed and push their wheelchairs. When residents are incontinent, aides clean up after them. When residents cannot bathe themselves, aides assist them. When residents cannot speak or make themselves understood, aides must divine their meaning.

Few jobs in this society are worse than those of aides in nursing homes. With the exception of a few large cities where nursing home employees are unionized, the minimum wage prevails universally at entrance. Raises given for length of service, increasing skill, or work at night or on holidays are more the exception than the rule. Fringe benefits are equally limited.[33] The work is often unpleasant. As one union official put it, "It's bad enough to clean your own baby's diaper; think of doing it for some smelly old person who isn't even nice to you, and doing it four or five times a day." It is often physically demanding—120-pound women routinely lift inert old men who weigh at least as much as they do. The rate of workmen's compensation claims among nursing home employees is very high. And it is generally a job without much gratification. Aides bear the brunt of nursing home residents' grievances. Few aides ever see any of their patients get better. Fewer still ever advance up the occupational hierarchy within the nursing home.

As a general rule, aides in nursing homes are overworked. Many states now mandate a minimum number of "nursing hours" (90 percent of which are provided by aides) per patient, per day. But most nursing homes cut corners. Personnel expenses take the largest single chunk out of their budgets and provide the easiest economies. It is routine practice for nursing homes to arrange their staffing patterns as though no one ever called in sick, leaving themselves shorthanded when people do, or to be in no hurry to fill the many vacancies that occur when people quit. Nursing homes are perpetually short of staff on weekends and holidays. The patients obviously suffer most from this understaffing, but the aides also suffer. Not only must they work that much harder, but they tend to be acutely aware of how little they are doing for each patient, and of how inadequate the services are. Demoralization frequently follows.

Lack of gratification is also tied to inadequate training. In most of the country, nurses' aides are hired literally off the street and learn whatever they do learn about their jobs by following another aide around for several hours or days. Several states now enforce the requirement that aides have some formal training before they begin working. Many nursing home administrators undertake such training efforts on their own (a videotaped instructional program prepared by the American Health Care Association, the trade association and lobbying arm of the proprietary institutions, is especially popular). Many other facilities, however, figure that it simply doesn't pay. Aides leave too quickly.

The personnel turnover in nursing homes is phenomenal. The most widely quoted statistic of an estimated annual turnover among nonprofessionals of 75 percent is badly out of date, but the most recent available.[34] If a home employs forty aides on January 1, only ten will be left by Christmas. Many leave for better-paying jobs in hospitals. Others just get fed up and quit, returning to the labor market eventually to work in other nursing homes.

Given the wages and working conditions, nursing homes tend to draw from the very bottom of the labor pool, the least skilled and least educated. In inner cities, the work force is heavily black and Hispanic, often adding another element of potential hostility to the highly charged relationship between residents and aides. In rural and suburban areas, aides are likely to be middle-aged women entering or reentering the work force. In some parts of the country, notably the upper Midwest, high school students are frequently employed on the second shift or as part-timers.

Thirty-two percent of nursing home employees are not engaged in "nursing"; they work in the kitchens and laundries, do the heavy housekeeping, and perform plant maintenance.[35] Except for the rare skilled handyman or maintenance worker, these employees are also low paid and poorly motivated, and they also quit in alarming numbers.

Apart from nurses, skilled and professional employees constitute less than 6 percent of the full-time equivalent employees in nursing homes. Every home must have a full-time administrator, and the larger homes all have other administrative personnel. The balance comprises the physicians, dentists, pharmacists, dietitians, occupational therapists, physical therapists, speech pathologists, activities directors, social workers, and secretaries.[36] In a typical one-hundred-bed nursing home, apart from the administrator, the full-time equivalent professional nonnursing complement is less than five. Few though they are, therefore, nurses are the primary professional providers of care in nursing homes.

Traditionally, nursing homes have been at the bottom of the nursing totem pole. They had the lowest professional status and were largely ignored in nursing education. Because nursing homes also paid lower wages and provided inferior benefits, the nurses who worked in them were widely seen as the least capable—stereotypically, they were those who had failed in the hospital setting or those who, on reentering the labor market, were unable to get hospital jobs. Sometimes they were part-timers supplementing hospital income.

That situation has changed somewhat in the last few years. The wage differential has shrunk—in major cities it is now about 10 percent.[37] The labor market has tightened. And nursing home employment has come to seem more attractive to nurses.

The sources of that attraction tell much about what happens in nursing homes. First, nurses in nursing homes are rarely under the direct supervision of physicians and thus enjoy a great deal of autonomy. Second, a large proportion of these nurses fill essentially administrative positions. By law, each nursing home must have a "nursing director" who has primary responsibility for all patient care in the facility. That is more responsibility and authority than nurses can find almost anywhere else. Finally, nursing homes are much smaller, much less formal and bureaucratic, and much less specialized than hospitals; that, too, is an attraction for many. As a given consequence, and also because of a substantial federal investment in improving the skills of nursing home nurses, the quality of nurse staffing in nursing homes has probably increased substantially over the past seven to ten years.

Even so, more than half the registered nurses in twenty-one major cities surveyed by the Bureau of Labor Statistics were part-timers, although in less urban areas that proportion is probably smaller.[38] Part-time employment is common in nursing, especially for night and weekend shifts, but the figure still suggests that nursing homes cut payroll corners and that nursing homes remain a second job for many of the nurses who work in them. Much of the nurses' time in nursing homes is spent doing paperwork. However qualified they may be, nursing home nurses spend far less time in actual patient care than formal staffing ratios or even common sense would suggest.

Dollars and Cents

Taking the average nursing home of seventy-five beds with an average annual occupancy of 90 percent and taking as a rough ball-park estimate an average charge per patient day of $25, the "typical" nursing home will have annual revenues of just over $600,000. At least half of all nursing homes are owned by individuals or partnerships controlling between one and five facilities. In the multibillion-dollar world of health care, nursing homes are small potatoes. A good-sized urban hospital will generate revenues of $600,000 a week, and a group of half-a-dozen orthopedists or radiologists may bill as much annually as an average nursing home. But there are a great many nursing homes, and the aggregate revenues exceed $12 billion a year.[39] Moreover, that aggregate is growing at least as fast as the revenues of any other part of the health industry.

More than half the $12 billion is public money. The best approximation is that 60 percent of revenues come directly from government, mostly from Medicaid, the program originally designed to provide health services to the poor.[40] (More than 60 percent of nursing home residents have their care paid for by Medicaid, but since Medicaid pays at a lower rate than most other programs, the dollar share for Medicaid is somewhat lower.) In addition, a large, but entirely unknown, proportion of "private" payments to nursing homes must be drawn from individuals' social security benefits and may thus be considered public money. Estimated conservatively, more than 80 percent of nursing home revenues are derived from tax dollars, whether paid out directly by governments or passed through individuals.

For the individual Medicaid beneficiary, government pays the difference between what the beneficiary can pay and what the facility is entitled to, plus $25 a month for a "personal needs allowance" theoretically retained by the resident. (If a nursing home is entitled to $750 a month and an average resident received $230 from social security, Medicaid will pay $545.) Unless there are supplements from family or friends, the nursing home resident whose care is paid for by Medicaid has less than a dollar a day available for personal spending money. In the past, that money was routinely embezzled by many nursing homes. Now, more residents are able to spend it. Among the things it must cover are cigarettes, candy, and food outside of regular meal hours, haircuts, all personal beauty and grooming aids, all discretionary transportation—almost everything over and above simple bed and board. It is no wonder that families supplement these funds or that the 50 percent of residents without family able to provide supplements hoard their meager holdings so carefully.

Many individuals who enter nursing homes as "private" patients soon acquire Medicaid eligibility through what is known as the "spend-down." In many states, Medicaid coverage is available for nursing home care for all those for whom the costs of care exceed income once assets (above a nominal level generally in the range of $1,000 to $3,000) have been liquidated. Essentially, Medicaid requires nursing home residents to exhaust their life's savings before qualifying for public assistance. (Given the costs of nursing homes and the limited assets of most American families, that process can take place very rapidly.) Under Medicaid, children are not financially responsible for the care their parents (a phenomenon that has helped give rise to the mythology of family "dumping" of the elderly) but spouses are; hence, the phenomenon of couples married fifty years divorcing to enable one of them to get a nursing home subsidy without totally impoverishing the other. The spend-down for nursing home care presents many middle-class families with an excruciating dilemma. Either they can violate the law by covertly attempting to transfer the parent's assets before admission to a nursing home (possession of a single savings account accumulated through years of frugality and hard work can cause disqualification) or they can watch passively as an inheritance goes up in smoke. For those families unwilling or unable to transfer assets covertly, nursing home services have thus become the most effective barrier to intergenerational transfer of income ever seen in this country.

Days and Nights

Nursing homes, unavoidably and inescapably, are institutions. Even in those nursing homes making the greatest effort to be "homelike," meals are at scheduled hours and sleeping late means missing breakfast. Although the majority of residents have lived most of their adult lives by themselves or with a spouse for some period, most rooms have two or four beds, and almost everybody has a roommate. Even when a facility encourages residents to bring personal possessions with them, there is just not enough space; a chair, a dresser, and a television set are likely to be all that will fit. And no matter how many pictures go on the walls, the color of those walls and of the drapes and the floor will be identical to that of dozens of other rooms.

The nursing home resident who can bring even one piece of furniture and keep a few private mementos belongs to a fortunate minority. Many facilities forbid nonstandard furniture, and in many places personal belongings are routinely stolen. In most places, nursing home residents are not permitted to keep any form of alcohol in their rooms, or even nonprescription medical items. A jar of skin cream or a bottle of aspirin can become a precious piece of contraband.

Clothing and grooming pose problems for nursing homes. Keeping track of seventy-five to one-hundred individuals' laundry is no small task, and many nursing homes don't bother to make the service available; residents are forced to make other arrangements, if they can, or wear standard-issue hospital supply. Many facilities will do resident laundry, for a fee, which must come out of that meager $25 a month. Only a few do laundry for free. Aides are supposed to assist residents with personal grooming, but there are rarely enough aides to go around, so hair is uncombed, and faces unwashed. For male residents unable to do it for themselves, a shave can be a big event but an infrequent one.

The one exception to this pattern is haircutting. For most nursing homes, this is a moneymaker, and even the smallest and least well-equipped facility will have room for a beauty parlor. The customary arrangement is for a local professional to provide the service on a concession basis, paying a fixed fee or a percentage to the nursing home. While the cost comes out of residents' personal funds, the hairdressers are tightly booked in all but the most demoralized facilities. All too often, residents are clad in dirty, unpressed clothes, with their finger- and toenails unkempt and their faces dirty, but they have the latest coiffures.

Public areas in nursing homes tend to be crowded. Historically, state laws have specified square-footage requirements for bedrooms but not for public areas, and land and construction costs were minimized by keeping the nonbedroom space as small as possible. Dining rooms do double duty as dayrooms and chapels. Nursing homes may be the only American institutions left in which the ancient art of lobby-sitting continues to flourish.

Old, sick people in nursing homes tend to be constantly surrounded by other old, sick people. Nursing homes, after all, are places where people go to live until they die. A leading activist in services to the elderly has coined the term "thanaphobia" (fear of dying) to describe the attitudes of old people toward nursing homes, an attitude not only shared but often held in heightened form by those who live there. While nursing home residents will not infrequently look out for one another, the degree of social interaction and interpersonal solidarity may be distressingly low. The characteristic picture is that of a dozen residents arrayed in front of a television or sitting in a hall, each staring straight ahead. If anyone is talking, it is mostly to herself.

Because so large a proportion of the residents in most nursing homes have difficulty getting around unassisted, the logistics of moving them to a scheduled activity can become extremely complex. When three or four aides have to move thirty or forty wheelchair patients to the dining room for a meal, early arrivals may be parked for an extended period, especially when elevators are involved. As in the army, life in a nursing home is characterized by a lot of hurry up and wait. A dining room or activity room begins to fill up as much as an hour before the scheduled activity, and there is nothing to do to fill all that time. In what can only be described as inadvertent deadpan, two gerontologists have written that "most residents who come to an institution are old women with little or no school, camp, work, or army experience to help them to adjust to regimentation."[41] It is doubtful that those who have had such experience like it any better, even if they "adjust" more smoothly.

Ambulatory patients also get to the dining room early because, as in all institutions, meals are especially weighted with emotional significance. They provide the primary opportunity for sensual gratification. In the drab nursing home world, the rotation of menus is one of the few sources of variety and even excitement. The scheduling of meals is one of the few things to give structure to a resident's time. Eating is something to do.

Most nursing homes in which the administrator is not willfully callous to the needs of the residents devote considerable attention to their food service. For the real corner-cutters, raw food costs are always a source of potential savings, and the food in their facilities is minimal in both quality and quantity. Even in the best institutions, though, the food is unavoidably institutional. Under any kind of cost constraint, cooking three meals a day, day in and day out, for a large number of people of differing tastes is a formidable challenge. It is all the more difficult in nursing homes where a large proportion of residents are on special diets and few have all their teeth. (One of the best ways to assess the overall quality of a nursing home would be to determine the proportion of residents who have properly fitted dentures or the proportion needing them who have dentures at all.) As with all institutional food, in nursing homes starches predominate, fresh vegetables are a rarity, and nothing has any taste. For those who care about food, ice cream is the great salvation.

Apart from meals, the major diversions in nursing homes are "activities." All nursing homes are required by law to provide some; the good ones present their residents with daily schedules that can look like those of the most overorganized summer camps. Residents will be busily engaged in handicrafts or discussion groups in the morning, music and more handicrafts in the afternoon, and lectures, movies, or bingo in the evening. Activities are especially important because of their central role in limiting or even reversing mental, emotional, and physical deterioration in the elderly. The role of volunteers and outside groups counts for a great deal, and high school glee clubs and drama groups have no more appreciative audiences.

Nevertheless, as three researchers from the University of Virginia put it, nursing home residents "spend most of their time (1) in the facility and (2) doing nothing."[42] They describe nursing homes as "good places to watch television, get your hair done, play bingo, or pray."[43] In the public areas of most nursing homes, the televisions are always on. In the course of research for this book, I often asked administrators and others with considerable experience in nursing homes what people did all day before there was television. Most couldn't even begin to answer.

Several years ago, there was quite a fad for "reality orientation" in nursing homes, in recognition that institutional life may aggravate tendencies toward disorientation and confusion in the elderly. Systematic and thorough programs of reality orientation are complex and expensive, and their value is still questionable; so the fad has faded. The major remnant, which can be seen in almost all nursing homes, is the "reality orientation board" (RO board for short) customarily placed near a nursing station. Like a prodigital announcement in a train station or airport, an RO board contains permanently affixed lettering on the left and slots or other provisions for making changes on the right. A hypothetical updated RO board will read:

> TODAY IS: FRIDAY, FEBRUARY 24, 1978
> THE WEATHER OUTSIDE IS: CLOUDY

THE NEXT HOLIDAY IS: GOOD FRIDAY
THE NEXT MEAL IS: LUNCH

For at least this observer, the contents of a typical RO board perfectly illustrates the character of day-to-day life in a nursing home.

The drabness and boredom of nursing home life are exacerbated by the infrequency with which most nursing home residents get off the grounds. Mobility is a problem. Many nursing homes are located in suburban areas with little public transportation; even where buses or taxis are available, funds to pay the fare may not be. Some of the better nursing homes take their residents on trips for entertainment, shopping, or other activities, but transporting the disabled is a difficult and expensive task. In describing transportation problems to me, one resident, active in political and community affairs who routinely attended public meetings and hearings in her wheelchair, repeatedly referred to nursing home residents as "prisoners."

The isolation and immobility of nursing home residents make visitors all the more important. Visits break the routine and assure residents they have not been totally cut off from the rest of the world. They provide many of the amenities, from extra foods to a stroll off the grounds, that residents would otherwise lack. And they provide someone to talk to. Six out of ten nursing home residents report visitors once a week or more, and only 10 percent never have any, although "visitors" is defined to include clergy and other volunteers who may be perfect strangers to the resident. The "typical" resident, the older white woman, receives more visits than the average.[44]

No Place Like Home

There are some nursing homes to which none, or very few, of the generalizations in the preceding pages apply. I have seen some myself. Most are voluntary facilities, receiving heavy subsidies from religious or philanthropic groups. Some are proprietary, managed by skilled and energetic entrepreneur-administrators who concluded that superior service might pay off in the long run, if not the short. A few are governmental. Needless to say, not all the undesirable characteristics generally found in nursing homes are found in all. Still, because the effort here was to describe a typical nursing home, no attention was paid to some of the worse outrages and abuses: the physical beating of helpless patients by aides and attendants; the accumulated filth in kitchens, shower rooms, even patient rooms and public areas; and the serving of spoiled or unwholesome food. These problems are not typical, but they do occur.

Nonetheless, the typical nursing home is a pretty awful place. It is a pretty awful place *even when* it is clean and well lighted, staffed to minimally adequate levels, and provides decent food, adequate medical attention, and a full slate of activities. It is awful because the circumstances, medical and social, of the people living there are extremely difficult to do much about, and because the presence of an adequate supply of individuals motivated, educated, and trained to work effectively in such circumstances is extraordinarily rare. Many nursing homes are no better than they have to be—quite a few are not even that good—and only a small fraction are as good as they can be. But even the best cannot escape the reality that, although for many of their residents there is no other choice, they are institutions housing people with profound problems that are unlikely to get very much better.

Nursing Homes and
Public Policy—A History

IF the great unfinished business of the New Deal was national health insurance, the great illusion of the framers of the Social Security Act, the New Deal's most important social welfare initiative, was that old age assistance (cash benefits for the indigent elderly provided on the basis of need) would wither away with the maturing of contributory retirement and survivors insurance. It is from these two lacunae in the program and politics of the 1930s that public policy toward nursing homes has evolved. Each marginal, incremental step in the movement toward publicly supported health care has had a major effect on the nursing home industry, often much different from the effect policymakers intended. A most important reason why the effects have been what they have is the continued dependence of many older Americans on the welfare system.

The purposiveness in the behavior of those who have made public policy for nursing homes over the past forty years should not be overstated. Only once in that period has Congress ever devoted a significant amount of its time to consideration of legislation dealing primarily with nursing homes. Only rarely have nursing home issues occupied the attention of high officials in the executive branch as anything other than temporary interruptions. By and large, nursing home policy has been made not only with limited foresight, but largely by people who, at the time, were primarily concerned with doing something different. It has been an afterthought, a side effect of decisions directed at other problems—mostly those of health care or of poverty.

Since most of the residents of nursing homes are poor and sick, a policy toward nursing homes compounded from health programs, on the one hand, and welfare programs, on the other, might seem not only appropriate but sensible. But nursing homes do not fit comfortably into the prevailing approaches, methods, standards, or mores of *either* health or welfare policies. There is not, and there has never been, a nursing home policy in the United States, except for that peripherally appended to the complex machinery of the health and welfare titles of the Social Security Act.

The history of public policy toward nursing homes is largely a byproduct of broader social welfare legislation, but in a tangential fashion. Recounting that history is like describing the opening of the American West from the perspective of the mules; they were certainly there, and the epochal events were certainly critical to the mules, but hardly anyone was paying very much attention to them at the time.

Before turning to the details of that history, it may be useful to consider the nature of policy change in the United States. First, political scientists have long agreed on what they call the "incrementalism" of American public policy. Policy change comes slowly and one step at a time, bounded as much by what has been in the past as what will be in the future. Radical innovation is the exception rather than the rule; the empiricist character of American public life prefers trying many small things to one big thing. Even the Social Security Act, radically innovative when enacted in 1935, fits neatly into the incrementalist paradigm, because the Great Depression and New Deal were extraordinary, atypical times in American life, and because the post-1935 history of social security has been one of accretion and modification. Every five to ten years, benefits are added and eligibility eased; once in a generation a major modification like Medicare comes along.

Second, is the entrenchment of fixed interests. If, as the conventional wisdom would have it, old programs and agencies never die, it is because the constituencies supported by these programs and agencies cannot, politically, be deprived. Thus, the original entry of for-profit operators into publicly subsidized nursing home services was largely an accident, but with the passage of time, such accidents tend to become irreversible.

The interplay of incrementalism and the tendency for interests to quickly become entrenched makes it extremely difficult for policymakers to unmake past mistakes. Once a private group has knowledge of government largess, they keep coming back for more—and getting it. Defenders of incremental policymaking point proudly to the Social Security Act as an example of how incrementalism can lead, over time, to policies far more comprehensive than this essentially conservative political system would ever be able to swallow whole. But the obverse holds as well: Small oversights and misjudgments grow, over time, into large dilemmas with which a political system attuned to nibbling around the edges of problems is unable to cope. Just as benefits to the indigent retired have steadily expanded since 1935, so too has the supply of substandard institutions prospering at public expense.

Further, much of the history of the Social Security Act and the policies it embodies can be told in terms of constant pulling and tugging between federal and state governments, each with its own political and budgetary problems. Nowhere has this intergovernmental conflict been more intense than in Medicaid and its predecessor policies— those that have played the largest roles in the development of nursing homes. National laws and directives established the basic framework of nursing home policy, and the role of the federal government gets (incrementally) more directive all the time. But what has been left to the discretion of the states, or even of localities within the states, has often been more significant than what the federal government has preempted.

All ill-defined sharing of powers characterizes all aspects of welfare policy in the United States. But Medicaid and its predecessors are not only welfare policies but also health policies, and health care providers are much more competent at looking out for their interests than are individual welfare recipients. State governments and especially state welfare agencies are often no match for them.

Policy change is also heavily influenced by the old truism that how a problem is solved is largely determined by how it is defined. Nursing homes have only rarely been addressed as a policy problem in and of themselves. In the early stages of their development, the problem was defined as one of income poverty for the elderly and especially of the persistence of public almshouses, the heirs to the tradition of indoor relief dating back to Elizabethan times. Since World War II, the problem has been defined as one of support for, and then regulation of, general acute care hospitals, and more broadly, of the health care needs of the elderly. These preoccupations with what were and are profoundly different kinds of institutions have led to many of the most serious shortcomings in policy toward nursing homes.

Poor Laws and Poor Houses

Prior to the Great Depression, the only form of public support available for the destitute elderly was institutional. Public welfare in the United States revolved around the twin principles of the post-1834 English poor laws: local financial responsibility and exclusive reliance on institutional "indoor relief" for the indigent. In the American system, by the early twentieth century, the states generally assumed responsibility for institutions housing the mentally ill and the blind; the other categories of "deserving poor" (the retarded, the chronically ill, and the feeble elderly) remained wards of the counties or municipalities, housed in country "homes" or "farms" at local expense.

County governments were rarely enthusiastic about meeting the expenses of institutional care for the poor, and much of the rationale for county farms was rooted in the fallacious illusion that they could be self-supporting through the labor of their inmates, even though admission was generally reserved for those incapable of participating in the labor force.[1] Typically, poor farms or poorhouses were managed by a single "matron," generally the wife of the superintendent/proprietor who, in agricultural counties, worked the farm.[2] In urban areas, larger facilities and staffs were often the norm, and both were sources of political patronage for the local party organization. Budgets were always low, and anything along the lines of modern "services" for residents unheard of.[3]

The typical almshouses or poor farms were less than desirable places to live. A 1925 Department of Labor report concluded that, "dilapidation, inadequacy, and even indecency are the outstanding physical features of many of our small almshouses. Ignorance, unfitness, and a complete lack of comprehension of the social element involved in the conduct of a public institution are characteristic of a large part of their managing personnel."[4] While the same report looked more favorably on larger urban facilities, which had more extensive staffing and more varied services, many of the city facilities were equally deplorable.

The unsavory reputation of the poorhouses, rather than an inadvertent by-product of mismanagement, was an accepted element in the overall welfare strategy of indoor relief. The economists and Benthamite social engineers who invented the poorhouse were eager to discourage people from using them, and the stigmatization attached to admission was not only intended but encouraged. Fear of the poor farm was seen as a valuable device for keeping the industrial work force appropriately cowed and submissive. Only those truly incapable of labor were to be admitted. The Puritan suspicion that moral degeneracy was the cause of poverty often held sway. Humane impulses toward improving almshouse care thus warred with moral disapproval and the economic imperatives of laissez faire business enterprise.

The plight of the infirm elderly did not quite jibe with the philosophy underlying the poorhouse system. In 1923, more than half the 78,000 almshouse residents were over sixty-five and another 20 percent were between fifty-five and sixty-five.[5] Most were seriously disabled. Although poverty among the elderly was often depicted as the product of "imprudence" in failing to set aside adequate savings, there seemed to be general agreement that chronic illness constituted a legitimate exception to the strictures of Puritan "deservingness." As a result, a major theme in the growing criticism of the almshouse system was the way it housed frail old people, deserving of sympathy and support, cheek to jowl with the retarded, insane, and immoral. In the words of the Department of Labor, "insanity, feeble-mindedness, depravity, and respectable old age are mingled in haphazard unconcern."[6]

To some extent, the problem of consigning the elderly to share indoor relief with less "deserving" social dependents had always been part of the almshouse system. But the problem increased as the proportion of the elderly in the entire population grew—from 4 percent in 1900 to 5 percent in 1920 and closer to 6 percent in 1940—and as chronic illness in the elderly became, if not more prevalent, at least more visible. Yet as late as the 1930s, only a minority of social reformers distinguished between the poor elderly, in general, and the poor disabled elderly, so many of whom resided in almshouses.

Part of the reason why that distinction was not more clearly made may have been the role played by hostility toward the almshouses in the broad movement for old-age pensions (cash assistance) that flourished after World War I, accelerated after the onset of the depression, and culmintated in the Social Security Act. Pension supporters relied heavily on the argument that it was unjust and inhumane to subject the elderly to poorhouse living. The Department of Labor study cited previously was itself undertaken by sympathizers of the pension movement, and Harry Evans' *The American Poor Farm and Its Inmates,* a muckraking study published in 1926 that contributed significantly to the growing public support for outdoor relief (cash assistance), reported on an investigation undertaken at the urging of the Secretary of Labor.[7]

The furor over poorhouses stirred by pension supporters obscured the fact that comparatively few old people actually lived in them—something on the order of 50,000, or roughly two-thirds of 1 percent of those over sixty-five. Roughly the same number resided in charitable private homes for the aged.[8] These institutions, the forerunners of modern voluntary nursing homes, had been founded, by and large, in the latter years of the nineteenth and early years of the twentieth centuries. The first generation of private homes was largely the product of immigrant self-help organizations, which characteristically began by providing settlement assistance and burial insurance for their fellow immigrants and then diversified into other charitable activities, frequently including the provision of homes for elderly widows. The first generation of facilities reflected an ethnic pattern: Scandinavians and Germans built Lutheran facilities; Jews, Jewish facilities. Other religious groups soon followed suit, frequently beginning with homes for retired clergy and their spouses.[9] All of these facilities were somewhat outside the mainstream of organized charity—perhaps because they were dominated by immigrant groups rather than by middle-class Protestant reformers—and they received relatively little attention in the formulation of the Social Security Act.

In 1930, more people over sixty-five resided in mental hospitals (the number in hospitals was close to seventy thousand) than in alms-houses and private homes combined.[10]

The problems of the fewer than 200,000 people over sixty-five living in institutions were entirely overshadowed, however, by those of the more than 7 million who, by the time of the enactment of Social Security in 1935, were experiencing deprivation and destitution to a degree unmatched in American history. It was to their plight that the Social Security was primarily a response.

The Coming of Social Security

Title I of the Social Security Act of 1935 established a federal program of grants-in-aid to the states for old age assistance (OAA)—a system of noncontributory, means-tested old age pensions. OAA was seen as a temporary transitional measure to meet the income needs of the elderly until the contributory, nonmeans-tested system of old age insurance (what is now popularly called social security) could be fully implemented. OAA built on the pension systems established by twenty-eight states at the time of the Social Security Act's passage by providing for 50 percent federal matching of monthly payments of up to $30 to beneficiaries certified for eligibility by the states, subject to certain minimum federally imposed conditions.[11]

One of those conditions forbade payment of OAA benefits to any "inmate of a public institution."[12] The source of this prohibition was obvious: the Social Security Act would not be used for the maintenance of almshouses. So uncontroversial was this provision that it hardly received any attention in the extensive public debate over the law; the almshouse had no defenders.

Enactment of the Social Security Act was an epochal event in the history of American social welfare. It represented the ascendancy of the principle of cash grants to individuals residing in the community, as opposed to institutional incarceration or the provision of earmarked or "in kind" benefits. It was a victory a hundred years in the making—in a struggle that still continues—for the belief that the primary cause of poverty was not imprudence or immorality but a shortage of income. From that belief flowed the notion that assistance recipients should be permitted to spend their benefits as they saw fit and that direct provision of public services was demeaning and stigmatizing. Outdoor relief through a public pension was assumed to be antithetical to indoor relief in an institution. Thus, it made no sense to provide income maintenance to institutional residents.

Two other characteristics of the original OAA program shaped public programs toward the needy elderly for years to come. First, the provision of federal matching through grants-in-aid to the states provided a ceiling on the federal contribution, but no floor. States were free to supplement the federal maximum to whatever extent they desired, but they were also free to spend as little as they wanted. Second, determination of the eligibility of individual beneficiaries was left to the states, subject only to a few minimal federal standards, which have always been enforced through federal-state negotiations over state compliance, rather than through direct federal intervention on the behalf of beneficiaries.[13]

The Social Security Act did not contain any scheme of health insurance. Provision of some form of health insurance for at least some part of the population was supported in the deliberations of the Committee on Economic Security, which drafted the administration's proposal. But Roosevelt feared that the addition of organized medicine to the ranks of an enemy already well mobilized by business interests would jeopardize the whole social security package. He referred health insurance back for still further study, and formal legislation was not proposed until 1939, when the administration supported it only indifferently.[14]

The absence of health insurance from the social security package quickly became apparent in the case of potential OAA beneficiaries too infirm to be maintained in their own homes. Formal recognition of this problem at the national level came in 1938 when the very first issue of the *Social Security Bulletin*, the official publication of the Social Security Board established to administer the Social Security Act, reported that the advent of OAA had had little impact on the elderly residing in almshouses. While some states moved aggressively, after passage of the Social Security Act, to close their almshouses, most did not. One reason was that, as the bulletin reported, "the majority of the persons 65 or more years of age cared for in almshouses require institutional care and hence cannot be removed."[15] Pensions, it turned out, were *not* a substitute for indoor relief, at least not for the elderly who were infirm as well as poor.

But though most of the infirm elderly already in almshouses remained there, restrictions on OAA payments forced others to turn elsewhere. Public facilities began to be supplanted by proprietary homes for the elderly. Social workers barred from placing the least competent and most needy of their clients in public institutions turned to proprietary ones. Moreover, many OAA recipients who had taken care of themselves or had been maintained by their families now had the purchasing power to obtain institutional care on their own.[16]

The depression years had brought some growth in the provision of residential services for the elderly on a private, profit-making basis. "Rest homes" and "convalescent homes" had in fact always existed. Their history may be traced to the colonial community practice of boarding out the indigent elderly, for a fee, in private households—a practice that the growth of almshouses never entirely replaced. The economic stringency of the depression encouraged entrepreneurs whose only capital was a house to enter the business, especially in those localities that provided emergency cash relief to the elderly. Characteristically, unemployed nurses—either individually or in small, informal partnerships—would establish convalescent homes in their own houses in the hope of being able to pay the rent or meet the mortgage payments.[17] The total number of elderly served was very tiny, as most such facilities were small, providing care for no more than a handful of residents, and because at first there weren't that many facilities. But demand, fueled by OAA payments, grew steadily.

By the late 1930s, the number of residents of proprietary institutions must, at most, have been only in the low tens of thousands (no one bothered to count). But the die had been cast. In attempting to provide income security for the elderly and obviate the need for indoor relief, the framers of the Social Security Act, making no special provision for the infirm elderly, created a demand that existing institutions were unable to fill.[18] The oversight was excusable enough. The elderly in need of institutionalization were, as they are today, only a minute and not very vocal fraction of all those in need. But efforts to solve the problem of inadequate income for the majority of the elderly complicated the problems of that minority.

Even at a very early stage, there was widespread dissatisfaction with proprietary nursing homes. Facilities were often dilapidated and frequently unsafe; medical and nursing care was minimal; reports of exploitation and abuse of residents quickly circulated. Calls for public licensing and inspection soon arose.[19] In response, government officials and social welfare professionals posed a dilemma that was to reappear a thousand times in the history of nursing homes: there was a terrible shortage of facilities, and in any locality many individuals who needed institutional care were unable to obtain it. Licensing would mean the closing of some facilities, aggravating the shortage. Better to wait and to rely on education and exhortation of existing operators in the hope they would upgrade their facilities.[20]

Conditions in the charitable homes remained largely static, but their finances changed radically. When OAA was first adopted, there was considerable doubt as to whether any substantial proportion of the residents of charitable facilities would be eligible. Most of those facilities had charged on a pay-as-you-go basis. But as the depression lengthened, the contributions on which the voluntary homes had always relied for covering the margin between income and outgo dwindled, and more and more residents and their families became unable to contribute their share. OAA saved the day, although its impact was felt only slowly as individual facilities began to catch on to its potential, and as more and more residents came to qualify. By the end of the 1930s, most of the charitable homes were back in the black, but the total number of people they were serving was roughly the same as it had been before the onset of the depression.[21]

By the time of Pearl Harbor, then, the seeds of the current nursing home industry had been planted, although they had barely begun to sprout. Private entrepreneurs were offering nursing and personal care services over and above what boarding homes had traditionally provided. Private homes for the aged began to provide health services for their residents. Those almshouses or public hospitals that remained in business began to redefine their clientele and their services. Behind all of this development was Title I of the Security Act, which had injected a substantial new flow of income into the hands of older people and those who sold services to them.

The Hospital Takes Center Stage

Medical care was one of the first domestic concerns to be addressed after World War II. The supply of services, rather than insurance to pay for them, took priority. Social investment in health care facilities had all but stopped with the stock market crash in 1929, and by the end of the war most of America's hospitals were at least twenty years old. Moreover, a technological revolution in medicine no less great than that in communications or aeronautics had been encouraged by the exigencies of wartime, with the widespread usage of penicillin and sulfa drugs its most immediate manifestation. Draft boards and army physicals had found the prewar health of the population alarmingly poor, especially in rural areas. During the war, either through the military services directly or through the Emergency Mothers, Infants, and Children (EMIC) program for military dependents and war workers, many Americans became accustomed to a level of health services, both in quantity and quality, they had never before received.

Federal intervention in civilian health care seemed appropriate. The logical place to start was with hospital construction, since it was least likely to be threatening to the organized medical community. Thus, in 1946, a conservative, Republican Congress enacted the Hospital Survey and Construction Act, commonly known, after its principal sponsors, as Hill-Burton.

Over the next twenty-five years, Hill-Burton provided more than $2.5 billion to help support the construction of 350,000 beds in almost 6,000 separate hospitals, helping to transform the American health care system.[22] The hospital became the hub. It provided the workplace for the growing proportion of physicians in specialty, rather than general practice. It housed the increasingly esoteric technology that embodied, in the public mind, the miracles of modern medicine. Even as late as the 1920s, hospitals were thought of as places where those too poor to be taken care of at home could go to recuperate or to die. By the 1950s, they were, in the language of hospital propagandists, "houses of hope," and every community vied to have one bigger and better than its neighbors. Hospitals consumed a larger and larger share of all dollars spent for health care, especially public dollars, and were increasingly the focus of public policy concern.

Shortly after Congress embarked on its program of massive subsidization of private, voluntary hospitals, it decisively rejected national health insurance. President Truman's proposal, cosponsored in the Senate by Robert Wagner of New York (a cosponsor of the original Social Security Act), failed even to emerge from committee. The American Medical Association, which had begun during the latter years of the war to gird itself for impending battles over the issue, reached its greatest power and effectiveness, using the issue of "socialized medicine" to ride the wave of postwar reaction and anticommunism. While Truman continued, after his reelection, to ritually call for such a program and reintroduce legislation, the battle had largely been lost.[23]

Though national health insurance floundered, social security flourished. The original act was amended in 1939, 1946, and 1948 to increase coverage, expand eligibility, and move old age insurance (transformed in 1939 to include benefits for survivors and thus into old age and survivors insurance) away from a strict annuity-like system closer to redistributive social insurance. The most important amendments were those of 1950, which added means-tested benefits for the disabled,[24] and contained three provisions of direct importance to nursing homes. The first removed the prohibition on payments to residents of public medical facilities, in recognition of the shortage of institutional beds and the growing dissatisfaction with private nursing homes. It was the clear hope of Congress that counties and municipalities would convert what remained of the almshouse/county hospital system into public facilities providing some level of health care along with custodial services.[25]

The second provision permitted, for the first time, federal matching of direct payments by state and local welfare agencies to parties other than the beneficiaries—to the suppliers of health services. A number of the more progressive states had already been making such payments when beneficiaries faced total impoverishment as a result of overwhelming medical costs. The 1950 amendments gave federal sanction and limited support for these "vendor payments."[26]

The 1950 legislation also contained a requirement that states making payments to residents of public institutions or to vendors establish a program for the licensing of nursing homes. There was no specification of licensing regulations or how they were to be enforced. The requirement was minimal, but it had some effect. Most states did not have such laws before 1950. Within a few years most did, although they varied enormously from one to another, contained only the most minimal requirements, and were totally unenforced.[27]

As the 1950 amendments were being debated in Congress, proponents of national health insurance within the Truman administration began rethinking their strategy. Recognizing that a comprehensive proposal was politically doomed, they sought a more modest program that could be expanded incrementally over time, as social security had been. The obvious first step was limited benefits for a limited group, and the obvious choices were hospital insurance and the elderly. While no serious legislative proposal immediately emerged, that decision was the start of a chain of events that culminated in the passage of Medicare in 1965. Wilbur Cohen and I. S. Falk, originators (along with then Federal Security Administrator Oscar Ewing) of this strategy and firsthand participants in the entire history of social security since the early days of the New Deal, were to be the major figures in the push for health insurance from then on. The original proposal advanced by Falk, Cohen, and their colleagues in 1951 contained, it should be noted, no provision for nursing home benefits.[28]

Nursing Homes Emerge

The general quiescence of the Eisenhower administration in domestic legislation, including health and welfare legislation, did not entirely preclude developments of importance to nursing homes. In fact, a number of apparently minor decisions taken in the 1950s irreversibly shaped the landscape in which the major initiatives of the 1960s took place. First, though not chronologically, was an expansion of vendor payments. The 1956 social security amendments, which increased federal support for OAA and the other cash assistance programs, also established separate matching for vendor payments. States would now be eligible for a federal contribution of up to an *average* of $6 a month for all welfare recipients, above and apart from cash grants. The states still had to pay the other half, which kept a considerable damper on the program. But some of the more affluent and progressive states, such as New York and Massachusetts (which not only had very liberal welfare programs but also continued to require localities to pick up a sizable share of the costs), substantially expanded vendor payments for nursing home care.[29]

On a separate front, Hill-Burton was amended in 1954 to provide grants to public and nonprofit entities to construct nursing homes. That initiative was an unintended consequence of private interest-group lobbying. The recently formed American Nursing Home Association (ANHA), representing proprietary interests, had been pressuring executive and legislative officials for assistance in financing capital costs. Demand continued to outstrip supply, and capital was hard to come by, since banks and other conventional sources of financing were reluctant to become involved. The Eisenhower administration bought the ANHA argument that expansion of nursing home capacity was necessary but sought to limit public subsidization to nonprofit facilities.[30]

Two considerations influenced that decision. There was a reluctance to tamper with the extremely popular and successful Hill-Burton program, which for eight years had thrived by lending money only to nonprofit and public facilities. But there were also officials in the executive branch, especially in the Public Health Service in the newly created Department of Health, Education and Welfare (HEW), who were eager to use Hill-Burton to alter the entire character of the nursing home industry. By expanding nursing home capacity under the auspices of nonprofit and public hospitals, those officials sought to create a pattern of ownership—and thus, they hoped, of quality—parallel to that prevailing in hospitals. So when Congress acceded to the administration's request and authorized $10 million a year in Hill-Burton subsidies for nursing home construction, it added qualifying language conditioning subsidies on the requirement that the nursing homes must be operated "in conjunction with a hospital."[31]

While Hill-Burton never provided that much money for nursing home construction (far less than $10 million a year was actually spent), the significance of incorporating nursing home services into the prevailing hospital-based system of health care should not be underestimated. The typical nursing home resident had long been someone with chronic illnesses and impairments, and the first generation of nursing homes distinguished themselves from boarding houses by their promise of "nursing" care. Nevertheless, most nursing homes in the 1950s were overwhelmingly residential and custodial in character. Only a small fraction employed licensed nursing personnel other than the owner; even fewer had any kind of physician involvement. But incorporation of nursing homes into Hill-Burton—and thus into the jurisdiction of the Public Health Service, which administered the program—transformed them, by definition, into medical facilities. Nursing homes would never again be solely an extension of the welfare system; they now belonged to health policy as well.

Nursing homes under Hill-Burton, and long thereafter, were thus integrated into the prevailing ideology of "progressive patient care," in which patients were moved from one level of service intensity to another as their condition changed. Nursing homes were redefined as the final stage of institutionalization for the chronically ill requiring long-term convalescence. Once the need for acute care services was past, patients could be taken care of in nursing home facilities more appropriately and at lower cost. That, at any rate, was the developing rationale.

Inclusion of nursing homes in Hill-Burton also led to the formulation of the first standards for physical construction, facility design, staffing patterns, and the like, apart from the very minimal requirements in the early state licensing laws. The Public Health Service experts who drew up the requirements were heavily affected by their hospital orientation, which is why, to this day, most nursing homes look so much like mini-hospitals. And the 1954 amendments directed the Public Health Service to undertake the first comprehensive national inventory of nursing homes and related facilities. That inventory distinguished four types of facilities, the first two of which, "skilled nursing homes" and "personal care homes with skilled nursing," bear some relationship to contemporary nomenclature and provided some degree of health services over and above room and board. In those two categories, the Public Health Service identified 9,000 facilities, with a total of 260,000 beds, distributed very unequally across the country. The average size was twenty-five beds in the "skilled nursing homes," forty beds in the "personal care homes with skilled nursing." (The latter was a misleading figure, because that category comprised both small proprietary facilities and large public and private nonprofit homes.)[32]

Other developments were taking place outside the bureaucracy. A foundation-created commission on chronic illness called for expanded public funding for nursing home care. The number of elderly in the population, and thus the number in need of long-term institutional services, continued to grow. The 1950 census enumerated more than 12 million persons over sixty-five, almost 8 percent of the population, compared to nine million and 7 percent in 1940.

The growing political agitation for hospital insurance for the elderly, reflecting the Cohen-Falk strategy, generated increasing public attention on the health problems of old people. In 1957, Representative Aime Forand (D., Rhode Island) introduced a bill to provide hospital insurance for the elderly under social security. The first in an annual series of proposals that were to culminate in Medicare, it included coverage for 120 days of nursing home service[33] (which the Truman administration's original proposal had not). The rationale was primarily economic. Cost considerations were sure to be among the political arguments against the program, and nursing home services appeared to offer the prospect of savings in the latter part of extended hospitalizations for the chronically ill.

A final policy development of the 1950s was the granting of government loans and guarantees to proprietary nursing homes. Bitterly disappointed at having been excluded from the Hill-Burton capital funding provisions in the 1954 amendments, the ANHA redoubled its lobbying efforts for federal subsidization of capital expenditures, increasingly relying on the growing sense of need for an expansion of nursing home capacity. After failing with HEW, the ANHA turned elsewhere and succeeded in obtaining legislative authorization (in 1956) for loans from the Small Business Administration and (in 1959) for federal loan insurance under the housing programs of the Federal Housing Administration (FHA).[34] Subsequently, the FHA was to guarantee almost a billion dollars in mortgage loans to proprietary nursing homes and open the doors of savings banks and other mortgage-granting institutions to the industry.

The Road to Medicare

By 1960, there were, at a guess, some ten to eleven thousand nursing homes in the United States, housing perhaps 400 thousand residents.[35] Fewer than fifty thousand of those residents were being directly supported by vendor payments under OAA.[36] An entirely indeterminate number, probably as large or larger, were supported directly by OAA or by state and local subsidies to health facilities for non-OAA beneficiaries. FHA and Hill-Burton were beginning to pump significant amounts of capital into the industry. Licensing programs existed in almost every state, and in some states, standards had been upgraded and improved. The first major scandals in the "modern" nursing home industry had taken place in New York City, where the Department of Investigations had examined all 127 proprietary homes and found a pervasive pattern of noncompliance with staffing and other code requirements, financial irregularities, and real estate speculation.[37] There were still no coherent plans or policies.

For all the increasing attention health professionals were paying to nursing homes, public policy toward nursing homes, such as it was, remained largely a small and tangential part of more general welfare policy. Publicly supported nursing home care was made available to welfare recipients who had a special need for institutional services, just as welfare programs made provision for special clothing and furniture allowances for clients whose houses had burned down. Welfare agencies negotiated rates of payment with individual facilities or promulgated flat rates based on estimates of available funds. Almost everyone agreed that payment levels were inadequate, and services consequently poor. Most inspection and regulation of facilities were also conducted by welfare agencies as part of their broader role of inspecting all facilities (including homes for the retarded, orphans, and the like), in which their charges resided. There was a considerable market for private nursing home services, about which no one to this day knows anything systematic.

Public support for nursing home care varied enormously from one part of the country to another. OAA eligibility levels, and with them eligibility for assistance in paying for nursing home care, differed from one state to another. More than half the beneficiaries of vendor payments for nursing home care were in New York and Massachusetts. Ten states had no vendor payment programs at all.[38]

The broad outlines of nursing home policy remained fixed until the passage of Medicare in 1965, but a substantial change in magnitude occurred after 1960, with the passage of the Kerr-Mills law. Nineteen-sixty was a presidential election year, and the national Democratic leadership, prodded by its allies in organized labor, clearly intended to make health insurance for the aged a major campaign issue. Shortly after announcing his candidacy, John F. Kennedy reintroduced the Forand bill in the Senate. It was quickly killed by the House Ways and Means Committee in a 17–8 vote,[39] and the American Medical Association opposition remained as implacable as ever. But Wilbur Mills, chairman of the Ways and Means Committee and one of the most skilled and astute politicians of the last generation, sensed the increasing momentum behind the Forand proposal and sought, in a classic conservative tactic, to deflect it with a temporizing measure. In conjunction with Robert Kerr of Oklahoma, whose power in the Senate paralleled that of Mills in the House, he devised a new program of "medical assistance for the aged" (MAA).

MAA was essentially an expansion of the vendor-payment program under OAA, with two critical exceptions. First, the states were permitted to define "medical indigency" separately from need for OAA income assistance, so that the state could pay for medical services for the elderly who were not poor enough to receive OAA. Second, there was no ceiling on the federal matching for MAA, in a share ranging from 50 to 80 percent in inverse proportion to the wealth of the states. States were permitted to cover a wide range of services under Kerr-Mills, of which "skilled nursing home services" were listed second, although without defining what such services entailed.[40] A relatively strict, medically-oriented definition had been contained in the House version of the bill, but not in the Senate's—quite possibly a reflection of Kerr's close ties to the proprietary nursing home industry in his home state—and was dropped in conference.[41]

The expectation, at least as stated for public consumption, was that Kerr-Mills would permit the states, if they so desired, to establish far more comprehensive health insurance programs for the needy aged than the limited hospital/nursing home insurance proposed in the Forand bill, without burdening taxpayers with the expense of insurance for the nonindigent elderly. As predicted by Forand and other opponents, and probably anticipated by Mills as well, Kerr-Mills was largely a flop. All but nine states eventually adopted programs, but some did so only on paper; neither Mississippi nor Georgia, for instance, ever appropriated any money for their programs. Only five states had comprehensive programs, and an overlapping five (New York, California, Massachusetts, Minnesota, and Pennsylvania) received 62 percent of federal MAA funds, although they had only 31 percent of the nation's elderly and were all in the lowest category of federal matching percentage.[42]

But if Kerr-Mills had little impact on the overall system of health care for the elderly, its impact on nursing homes was considerably more substantial. Vendor payments for nursing homes increased almost tenfold in the five years before the passage of Medicare, rising to $449 million, or roughly a third of total program expenditures.[43] Although sound data on the number of people that figure represents are not available, the best approximation is that, by 1965, 300 thousand individuals (more than half of all nursing home residents) were beneficiaries of Kerr-Mills payments for nursing home care.[44]

No one fully understands quite why Kerr-Mills had such a dramatic impact on nursing homes, but three hypotheses can be suggested. First, before there were vendor payments, indigent older persons were receiving some medical services from physicians and hospitals without charge, as charity. Because fees paid to all vendors under Kerr-Mills were very low, in comparison with prevailing charges, it was probably easier to continue to provide free services and save on the paperwork. Proprietary nursing homes, though, had no tradition of providing free care. So it is likely that they sought reimbursement under Kerr-Mills much more vigorously than did any other class of vendors.

Throughout the period from the 1950 amendments until very recently, social welfare administrators and other officials perceived a terrible "shortage" of nursing home beds. A principle manifestation of this "shortage" was the number of elderly beneficiaries occupying beds in general hospitals, at rates several times as high as those for nursing homes, who did not appear to be ill enough to need the higher level of care hospitals provide. At the same time, nursing home capacity was expanding rapidly, especially in those states with large vendor-payment programs under OAA and then Kerr-Mills. This incremental capacity, it is reasonable to speculate, was filled largely by welfare beneficiaries. The increasing supply of nursing home beds provided every welfare and hospital social worker a solution to the problem of what to do with elderly beneficiaries who had problems of any one of a number of kinds (social isolation, mental illness, even chronic disease). But even as nursing homes filled up with welfare patients, more and more were brought to the attention of welfare agencies, sustaining the "shortage." So the vendor-payment totals grew without making a visible dent in the perceived backlog of demand for nursing homes.

Third, the concept of "medical indigency" under Kerr-Mills may have created the "spend-down effect." If eligibility for welfare benefits is tied not only to regular monthly income but to the size of medical expenditures relative to income, then many individuals who otherwise would not qualify become eligible for benefits when they encounter large medical expenses. (Individuals who are not poor may become poor if faced with large medical bills; that is the whole rationale for the notion of medical indigency in the first place.) The costs of services typically involved in the average two-year nursing home stay are likely to exhaust the assets of all but the most affluent, and to exceed, on a monthly basis, their regular recurring income. Individuals in this predicament are said to "spend down" to eligibility.

By the time Medicare was enacted in 1965, then, public funds *under a welfare program* were paying a large, and rapidly increasing, share of the costs of a rapidly expanding nursing home industry, especially in those few states with the largest vendor-payment programs—and the largest number of nursing homes. In the debates over the new legislation, almost no attention was paid to this phenomenon. Instead, in 1965, the welfare-based nursing home system was incorporated, willy-nilly, into new programs designed to finance health services. They didn't fit comfortably then and still don't.

The Watershed

After fifteen years of deliberation, involving hundreds of hearings producing tens of thousands of pages of transcripts, after the expenditure of tens of millions of dollars by lobbying groups, after being a major issue in three presidential and at least that many congressional elections, after millions of words of newspaper print and thousands of letters to the editor, Congress finally enacted a law that was to radically transform the provision of medical care in the United States and substantially improve the lives of millions of citizens: the Social Security Act Amendment of 1965—Medicare and Medicaid.

In all this activity, nursing homes received little attention. While nursing homes had become a sizable industry, they were still largely an invisible one, of concern much more to welfare officials and a small isolated cadre in the Public Health Service than to those involved in the planning of a massive health insurance program.

The framers of Medicare were, indeed, eager to avoid any expansion of governmental coverage for nursing home services. Since the late 1950s, Medicare proposals had included some nursing home benefits, but these had always been strictly circumscribed both in duration and the kinds of facilities to which they would apply. Wilbur Cohen (who reentered the government in 1961 and remained the principal Medicare strategist) and his colleagues were well aware that nursing home services tended to be more custodial than medical in nature; they were afraid that their inclusion would open a bottomless budgetary pit that would destroy the politically delicate budget for health insurance.[45] The reason that nursing home benefits were retained at all was precisely because of budgetary considerations. Daily hospital room rates had been rising rapidly throughout the 1950s and early 1960s, and it was expected, accurately enough, that Medicare would fuel that inflation still further. The illusion still persisted that movement of long-stay patients to less-intensive facilities like nursing homes during the latter stages of their institutionalization could create significant savings. Simple arithmetic demonstrated that a nursing home day cost far less than a hospital day.[46]

By the time the Johnson administration resubmitted its health insurance program in 1965, nursing home benefits thus took the form of coverage for sixty days of "post-hospital extended care."[47] The terminology "extended care" had been invented as a way of distinguishing the services to be covered from those then customarily provided by nursing homes.[48] Moreover, the administration's bill limited the facilities eligible to be reimbursed for extended care to those either formally affiliated, or maintaining a written "transfer agreement" for patients and their records, with a general hospital.[49] In other words, what Medicare would pay for was the last stage of convalescence from a protracted illness, after treatment in a hospital.

Administration proposals in the early 1960s, in keeping with the 1954 Hill-Burton amendment, had been more stringent, seeking to limit extended-care benefits to facilities actually under the direct control or management of a hospital. But in 1964, when Medicare passed the Senate, Senator Edmund Muskie succeeded in amending that provision to allow a transfer agreement, on the argument that fewer than one thousand of the nation's nursing homes would qualify under the administration's definition and that provisions for transfer agreements would encourage facilities without hospital ties to improve services in order to acquire transfer agreements.[50]

As Medicare finally emerged from the House Ways and Means Committee in 1965, extended-care benefits were available only during a spell of illness for which the beneficiary had already spent at least three days in the hospital, in facilities that were to meet relatively high standards, and as part of a process closely linked, through physician supervision, to the hospital stay. The only substantive difference from the administration's proposal was that Ways and Means had extended the length of coverage to 100 days.[51]

The almost universal view at the time was that most nursing homes were inadequate, incapable not only of meeting the objectives of the "extended-care" philosophy but even more modest goals of decent custodial service. But policymakers convinced themselves that by passing a law and making available a benefit, government would be able to induce some nursing homes to provide a completely new kind of service. Recognizing that they were trying to square the circle, the authors of Medicare postponed the effective date of the extended-care benefit to January 1, 1967, six months after all the other provisions of Medicare were to take effect.[52]

The extended-care provision was soon to haunt the framers of Medicare, but it was hardly the most significant nursing home legislation (or the most significant source of nursing home policy problems) to emerge from the Social Security amendments of 1965. That was embodied in a part of the legislation not even contained in the administration's proposal, which, when first suggested by Mills, caught the administration somewhat by surprise: combining an expansion of Kerr-Mills, renamed Medicaid, with Medicare.

Medicaid extended medical coverage to all persons, regardless of age, who received cash welfare benefits from federal programs or met state-established criteria of "medical indigency." It mandated a minimum of five "basic" services, of which "skilled nursing homes" was one. It also increased the financial incentives for state participation. It retained the administrative primacy of the states.

Medicaid was often described as the "sleeper" component of the 1965 Social Security Act amendments. If the law had been read literally and if the states had acted aggressively, it could have provided a framework for policy much closer to national health insurance than anything dreamed of since the early days of Truman's second term. So expansive a program was not in the political cards. But the relative ease with which Mills was able to append Medicaid to the administration's Medicare bill makes it possible to speculate that Medicare might have been more ambitious, especially in regard to nursing homes.

In retrospect, two things are clear. First, Mills recognized early in 1965 that the Johnson landslide had changed the balance of forces in Congress on social legislation, including health insurance. The administration, which had so long championed Medicare, was in the anomalous position of supporting a much more moderate measure than Congress was willing to entertain. Conceivably, Cohen and his associates were so wrapped up in their incrementalist strategy that they failed to grasp the opportunity made available to them by the addition of thirty-six new congressmen to the Democratic majority, although they responded expeditiously enough when Mills broached the idea of what was to become Medicaid.[53]

Second, apart from the highly limited extended-care notion, the administration had no strategy at all on what to do about nursing homes. Its position was essentially defensive; nonrehabilitative nursing home care must not be permitted to bust the politically fragile budget for hospital insurance. Nursing homes couldn't very well be left out of a program extending Kerr-Mills. But as no one really knew what to do about them, they were included without much definition. What resulted, largely by default, was an entirely backward approach to the problem. Everyone agreed that nursing homes were inadequate, but that providing a higher level of care to those primarily in need of "custodial" services would be frightfully expensive. Yet Medicaid contained no qualitative specifications at all, while it essentially took the budgetary lid off the vendor-payment program. Continued federal matching funds were guaranteed to the states, without budgetary ceiling, for vendor payments to "skilled nursing homes" for care of welfare recipients and others that states wished to consider "medically indigent."

The nursing home issue was not confronted directly. Medicaid, hastily created and enacted, was only a sideshow in the health insurance circus. Decisions had been made serially, one at a time: first nursing home coverage under Medicare was limited; then Medicaid was added to Medicare, then nursing homes were included under Medicaid—and then the process stopped. Nursing home coverage under Medicaid appears to be partially contradictory to its limitations under Medicare, but there is no law that the policy process must be internally consistent.

Another inconsistency critical to nursing homes involved the ways in which providers of health services were to be paid under Medicare and Medicaid. By 1965, it was frequently argued that one reason nursing home care was so poor was that welfare rates were too low to permit proprietors to provide anything better. To still fears arising from the prospect of government intervention in the medical care marketplace, Medicare provided that hospitals and other institutions, including "extended-care facilities," were to be reimbursed on the basis of the "reasonable costs" of operation, while physicians were to be paid "reasonable" charges.

The initial Medicaid legislation mandated payment to hospitals on the basis of their costs (those who wrote the law wanted to break down the existing "two-class" hospital care system, in which the poor were largely confined to publicly operated facilities shunned by the affluent) but left other decisions about fee-setting entirely to the discretion of the states, which had always paid much less than the private market rate. There was some discussion of cost-related rates for nursing homes, where the quality problem was much more severe than in hospitals, but Mills and others quickly rejected it. The budgetary implications were fearsome, and there was a reluctance to impose such a liability on the states. It was one thing to mandate cost-related reimbursement for nonprofit hospitals, and quite another for profitmaking nursing homes. Besides, everyone agreed hospitals were crucial; only a few cared about nursing homes. In essence, the issue was simply avoided, although it was soon to reappear.[54]

HEW Makes a Law: Medicare

Congressional passage of a law, of course, is only an intermediate step in the formulation of policy. Administrative decisions about nursing homes made in the early stages of the implementation of Medicare and Medicaid more fully delineated and more specifically determined what nursing home policy would be, but they also revealed the contradictions in the compromises Congress had made and the inherent intractability of some of the basic policy problems.

Medicare and Medicaid were administered by different arms of HEW. Medicare, seen as an insurance-based extension of social security, belonged to a newly established Bureau of Health Insurance (BHI) in the Social Security Administration (SSA). Medicaid was to be handled by the Bureau of Family Services of the Welfare Administration; that bureau's Division of Medical Services had been responsible for Kerr-Mills and retained responsibility for the new program.

To look first, as everyone did at the time, at Medicare, those responsible for its implementation were haunted by a single overriding fear. After years of buildup, the government had promised millions of social security beneficiaries that, come July 1, 1966, they would be able to receive hospital care under government insurance. The fear was that there would be no hospitals for many beneficiaries to go to. According to the law, any hospital approved by the Joint Commission on the Accreditation of Hospitals (JCAH), a private accrediting agency, would be "deemed" adequate for Medicare patients. It also provided for Medicare certification for hospitals that met less stringent standards, established under the Medicare law. Even those standards, however, would have disqualified many hospitals, including many that were sole providers of care in rural areas. BHI administrators had recurrent nightmares about the reaction of congressmen from such districts when their constituents, bearing newly minted Medicare cards, were turned away at the door. This fear was aggravated by anticipation of special problems in the South. There was no getting around the 1964 Civil Rights Act which would not countenance Medicare payments to segregated hospitals. The expectation was that the shortage of Medicare-certified beds would be particularly acute in the South.[55]

In response to this perceived crisis, BHI invented the category, for which there was no legal basis, of "substantial compliance": hospitals would be certified for Medicare participation even if they failed to meet the statutory requirements as long as they came somewhat close and demonstrated an intention to improve.[56]

The concept of "substantial compliance" generated a considerable fuss when applied to hospitals but probably caused no serious long-term damage and may even have spurred improvement in the quality of many American hospitals. When applied to extended-care facilities, however, it directly contravened congressional intent to strictly limit such benefits, which in turn represented a softening of the administration's still harder line toward coverage of nursing homes under Medicare.

The actual task of inspecting facilities for participation in Medicare was delegated to the states; BHI provided central supervision and did the formal certifying on the states' recommendations. The emphasis was on speed and on certifying as many facilities for participation as possible, with conscious intent to err on the side of certifying too many.[57] Because there were so few nursing homes that met the statutory requirements for extended care (the capability of providing intensive posthospitalization rehabilitative services), most of those originally brought into the Medicare program came in under the aegis of "substantial compliance."

Six months after the effective date for extended-care benefits, there were only 740 facilities in the country that were fully qualified under Medicare standards to provide them. No fewer than 3,200 others were found to be in "substantial compliance."[58] This ratio of less than one to four compared with a ratio of more than one to one in hospital certification.[59]

The delicately reached compromise embodied in the Medicare law providing coverage for a very limited amount of nursing home services was simply subverted by the exigencies of the administrative process. It was not possible to make the extended-care notion work throughout the nation. Certifying only the 740 fully-qualified facilities would have denied extended-care benefits to many Medicare beneficiaries. Once the door was opened to "substantial compliance," Medicare became liable for payment for services in facilities that its framers never had intended to support. Subsequently, the Senate Finance Committee bitterly attacked HEW for the use of "substantial compliance" in the case of extended-care facilities, but the initial mistake was made by Congress, which had attempted to legislate an impossibility.[60] The administrative actions that resulted, however unwise, represented a reasoned effort to cope with that impossible contradiction.

Although "substantial compliance" was supposed to be an interim measure, provided until nursing homes could be upgraded, the SSA moved much more slowly to remove facilities from the program than it had to sign them up. By 1971, four years later, fewer than 100 facilities had been removed from the program, despite little evidence that those in "substantial compliance" improved very much. HEW had painted itself into a legal and administrative corner from which it was difficult to get out. Decertifying a facility involved the potential admission of bureaucratic error and thus bureaucratic embarrassment. It also laid HEW open to claims of having acted in an "arbitrary and capricious"—hence, unconstitutional—manner. Again, it is always easier for a government not to give a benefit in the first place than to remove one it has conferred.

More striking, though, is that these 4,000 extended-care facilities certified by HEW constituted only a third of the nation's nursing homes. State officials had solicited applications for Medicare certification from roughly thirteen thousand facilities, and some six thousand applied.[61] Presumably, most of those failing to apply fell so far short of the minimum standards that they did not go through the motions. A third of those that did apply could not meet the elastic standards of "substantial compliance." In short, the quality of the 9,000 non-Medicare certified nursing homes could not have been very high. Most were probably older, smaller facilities, housed in converted dwellings that could not meet safety or fire standards, except under state "grandfather clauses" for those that had been in business before licensing standards were enacted or were too small to provide even minimal nursing services.

One of the standards required by the Medicare law was that extended-care facilities have round-the-clock nursing services and employ at least one RN on a full-time basis. The regulations written by BHI interpreted the law to require that, for those shifts on which an RN was not present, there be at least one LPN "who is a graduate of a state-approved school of practical nursing." That clause was included because many states provided for the "waivered" licensing of practical nurses on the basis of experience. Many LPNs employed by nursing homes were "licensed" merely by virtue of having worked in the facility a certain number of years. Nursing home interests opposed the Medicare standards on the grounds that there was a shortage of trained nurses, but, though BHI permitted a one-year waiver of the nursing requirements for some smaller facilities, it eventually enforced them.[62] So proprietary nursing home groups returned to Congress and, in 1972, succeeded in weakening the law.

Throughout the 1960s, there was widespread agreement that there existed a national shortage of nursing personnel, particularly in the rural areas. Subsequent research strongly suggests that the supply of trained nurses is less a function of the total number of licensed individuals than it is of the willingness of employers to pay them good wages. Nurses leave and reenter the labor market readily. Shortages tend to disappear as wages increase.[63] Even though the quality of nursing service is probably the single most important aspect of care in a nursing home, policymakers confronted with an apparent shortage of skilled nurses reacted by weakening standards, rather than by making nursing home employment more attractive.

The most immediate visible impact of the policy of "substantial compliance" on the implementation of extended-care benefits under Medicare was fiscal. On the basis of an assumption of very strict enforcement of facility standards and of strict application of the notion of posthospital therapeutic services, the chief actuary of the SSA had estimated that first-year costs for extended care would range between $25 million and $50 million. In fact, first-year costs approached $275 million.[64]

There were a number of reasons for this tenfold discrepancy. To begin with, "substantial compliance" had led to the certification of many more extended-care beds than the actuary's assumptions permitted, with consequent increase in utilization. Also, the average daily cost was more than 50 percent higher than projected, which was largely the result of the extreme generosity with which the notion of "reasonable costs" was applied to all Medicare providers. Further, the actuary's original predictions were *net* figures, based on the stubbornly held assumption in SSA that extended-care benefits would reduce hospital utilization. Insurance industry spokesmen had predicted just the opposite. The requirement that a beneficiary be hospitalized for three days prior to an extended-care admission in order to qualify for the benefit would lead, they claimed, to a net increase in hospital utilization.[65] There is little evidence that such an increase took place, but neither is there any evidence that availability of the extended-care option saved money for Medicare. There was no one-for-one substitution of extended-care facility days for hospital days. Instead, for each hospital day saved, several extended-care facility days were used.[66] Hence, the basic assumption for an extended-care benefit—that it would save money—turned out just not to be true.

By the time the Nixon administration took office, extended-care claims under Medicare exceeded $500 million a year and appeared to be in as much of an uncontrollable spiral as the other components of the program. Desperately casting around for devices by which the domestic budget could be quickly and relatively painlessly cut, the new leadership at HEW clamped down on extended care. It found considerable support among holdovers from the early days of Medicare, who had never been happy with what happened to their highly limited concept.[67]

SSA took vigorous action. But instead of clamping down on the thousands of facilities still in "substantial compliance," it imposed its sanctions on its beneficiaries and on facilities at random. For the third time, it revised its instructions on extended care to fiscal intermediaries—private insurance companies given responsibility under Medicare for the actual administration of payment to participating facilities. The famous Intermediary Letter 371, issued in April 1969, contained, for the first time, a listing of those services that must be provided if the qualifications for extended care were to be met. The listing included such services as intravenous feeding and injections, which were rarely administered in nursing homes. Intermediary Letter 371 also made it clear that in the future, intermediaries were to err on the side of denying claims rather than on the side of approving them. Denials of extended-care benefit claims increased almost immediately. In the first six months of 1968, 1.5 percent of extended-care claims had been denied; that number had risen to 2.7 percent by June 1969. In the last six months of 1969, the rate rose to 7.1 percent and it increased still further, to 8.2 percent in the early months of 1970.[68]

Because of the inevitable time lags in claims processing, many families were faced with nursing home bills for thousands of dollars for relatives who had died. They had believed the service was guaranteed by their government but were now confronted with liens and garnishments as the affected facilities sought to collect. Other beneficiaries were simply ejected from nursing homes once claims were denied; left not only without care but with substantial bills they were never able to repay, which in some cases became claims against their estates. Many nursing homes soon gave up trying to collect and wrote off substantial losses. They began voluntarily dropping their Medicare certification. Retroactive claims denial accomplished what "substantial compliance" never had—the removal from Medicare participation of more than five hundred facilities.[69]

Gross numbers tell the story. In 1968, Medicare paid one million eighteen thousand extended-care bills (most stays involved more than one bill; each stay involved at least one) for a total of $348 million. By 1972, it paid fewer than 400 thousand bills, totaling $155.6 million.[70] After 1972, the numbers began to rise again, largely as a result of the Social Security amendments of that year. But the essential damage had been done. From the time of Intermediary Letter 371 on, Medicare was no longer a significant factor in the nursing home industry. At great cost, with great confusion, and not inconsiderable pain to thousands of old people and their families, Medicare was finally doing, relative to nursing homes, what its sponsors had first intended—hardly anything.

HEW Makes a Law: Medicaid

The statute was quite specific on what extended-care benefits were to comprise under Medicare; this was not the case under Medicaid. Government officials, therefore, had more discretion as to the kinds of services for which they would pay.

HEW had to move quickly. While Congress provided the SSA with a year to put Medicare in place, it made the effective date for Medicaid January 1, 1966 (just five months after President Johnson signed the law) for those states that could have by that time an "approved state plan"—the device employed in grant-in-aid programs to ensure state compliance with federal conditions.

It was July 1966 before HEW published its Medicaid regulations, months after it had given conditional approval to some states, such as New York, which were eager to be relieved of part of their Kerr-Mills burden. Its regulations, in effect, ordered that by January 1, 1968 conditions for participation as a skilled nursing home under Medicaid were to be identical to those for an extended-care facility under Medicare.[71]

Wilbur Cohen, who by then was undersecretary of HEW, still did not want to pay for custodial services under a health program. His public position was that health services were health services, and custodial services an income maintenance problem, and never the twain should meet.[72] This attitude was perfectly logical, but it flew in the face of reality. The income of many elderly people was just not enough for decent custodial services; but only under the guise of health care could public dollars be made available for such services, however minimally related to health care they might be. Once there were tens of thousands of people in nursing homes at public expense, there was no way to discontinue paying for their care (a benefit once conferred...) and not much point in requiring those facilities to meet more stringent *medical* standards, which would only add to the expense without much affecting resident well-being.

Howls of protest soon arose from the ANHA, supported by members of Congress who reflected the states' concern that if HEW's initial ruling held, they would be left holding an expensive bag. Thousands of individuals were being supported by Kerr-Mills payments in facilities that could never meet Medicare standards. If those facilities were ineligible for Medicaid matching payments, the states might get stuck with the full amount. Instead of providing fiscal relief, Medicaid would thus actually force the states to increase expenditures.

Under considerable congressional and industry pressure, HEW quickly backed down. The interim Medicaid standards adopted in 1967 essentially accepted existing state standards, but, as opposed to those for Medicare, they permitted the charge nurse on any shift to be a "waivered" LPN (licensed on the basis of experience) as long as she had completed formal training requirements by 1969.[73]

The Moss Amendents

Before the 1969 effective date came to pass, the law was changed again. Those changes were essentially the work of the Subcommittee on Long-Term Care of the Senate Special Committee on Aging and represent the only instance on record of a comprehensive legislative attempt to deal with nursing home problems. Collectively, those changes are known as the "Moss amendments," after the subcommittee's chairman, former Senator Frank Moss of Utah.

The subcommittee was formed in 1963 and held extensive hearings in 1965 on "conditions and problems in the nation's nursing homes." What it found was not encouraging. Welfare rates (Kerr-Mills was then still the controlling legislation) were distressingly low, and welfare departments got what they paid for in terms of food, activities, and sanitary conditions. State licensing laws continued to be vague in important areas, and inspection and enforcement were largely paper enterprises. The major problems, though, were the total absence of knowledge and training among administrators; continued shortages in professional staffing; and, especially, fire safety, since the characteristic nursing home was still a converted dwelling in a frame structure.[74]

In early 1966, Senator Moss introduced legislation mandating much more stringent federal standards under Medicaid in all these areas. A companion measure was introduced by Senator Edward Kennedy to require state licensing of all nursing home administrators. The proposals went nowhere the first year but were reintroduced in 1967 with relatively little open controversy as amendments to an omnibus social security bill. After months of heated backstage activity and prolonged bargaining between Moss's staff and industry representatives, Moss's proposals were incorporated into the social security amendments of 1967, which were signed into law on January 2, 1968.[75]

The Moss amendments required that, by January 1, 1969, Medicaid standards for skilled nursing homes were to compel disclosure of ownership and the identity of those with financial interests in the facility; establish standards for record keeping, dietary services, drug dispensing, medical services, environment and sanitation; require transfer agreements with hospitals (now, as opposed to Medicare, in the other direction—to provide acute services for nursing home residents who needed them); and create a program of medical review, administered by the states, to provide a minimal level of professional peer review of medical services and to ensure that individuals who did not really need institutional care were not in nursing homes. More importantly, requirements were established for nursing services, including employment of at least one full-time RN, and formulation of a quantitative ratio of total nursing hours to patient days was encouraged. In states that did not already have more stringent codes, the Life Safety Code of the National Fire Protection Association, an encyclopedic document compiled by a private clearinghouse of the fire insurance industry, was established as the standard. The Moss amendments, for the first time, also provided a stimulus to state enforcement by assigning HEW specific authority to withhold the federal share of Medicaid funds from a facility not meeting all licensing requirements.[76]

The companion Kennedy amendment, which related to the licensing of administrators, was also approved. But a proposal, bitterly opposed by the Johnson administration, to require a system of cost-related rates, which would have brought reimbursement practices for nursing homes into line with those for hospitals, and which some legislators regarded as the key to improving conditions in the industry, failed to pass. By late 1967, the Johnson administration had become preoccupied with Vietnam-induced budgetary concerns, and so the issue was temporarily dropped.[77]

The Moss amendments required HEW to issue a new set of regulations for skilled nursing homes by January 1, 1969. Wilbur Cohen, who had by then become secretary of HEW, described the decision on the content of the regulations as among the hardest he had ever confronted. The problem, as seen by HEW, was that if standards were drawn stringently enough to satisfy professional groups and those within the government most eager to improve nursing homes, then most facilities would be unable to meet them. There would then be considerable pressure on government, at both state and local levels, to increase reimbursement in order to provide funds for improvement. But there was no way of guaranteeing that the money would go to improved services, and, in the meantime, many government beneficiaries would end up out on the street. The alternate course was to sanction weaker standards, which would mean that government would be abetting the continued maltreatment of helpless older citizens, and would be paying for that maltreatment.[78]

As the last days of the Johnson administration drew to a close, there was a frenzy of activity in the top levels of HEW as officials tried to conclude as much business as possible. But though nursing home standards remained a priority issue throughout this period, no final decisions were made. The dilemma was irresoluble.

Nursing standards were again the sticking point. The Moss amendments required only that an RN direct the nursing service and that the staff have "sufficient nursing and auxiliary personnel to provide adequate and properly supervised nursing services . . . during all hours of each day and all days of each week."[79] The original HEW draft regulations were written primarily by Frank Frantz, who had been staff director of the Long-Term Care Subcommittee, midwife to the birth of the Moss amendments, and who was brought into HEW precisely to oversee their implementation. The Frantz provisions required that a nonwaivered LPN be in charge of each shift in facilities with fewer than ninety patients and that two licensed nurses, one of them an RN, be on each shift in homes with more than ninety beds.[80]

The president of the American College of Nursing Home Administrators described these standards as reflecting "precisely" the intent of the Moss amendments. The standards were also endorsed by the American Association of Homes for the Aging, representing nonprofit facilities. But the ANHA was vehemently opposed. (The ANHA was apparently privy to inside information, since one of those employed by HEW to draft the regulations, Harold G. Smith, was, at the same time, a paid consultant to the ANHA.[81] Ever since it became known, Smith's role in the process has been a source of considerable controversy. Whatever his actual influence, it seems reasonable to infer that the ANHA had fairly good "access" to the entire regulation-drafting process.)

In any event, the regulations Frantz proposed were rejected, at least partly because they exceeded the Medicare standards, which made them potentially embarrassing to SSA and to HEW. The draft regulations finally issued on June 24, 1969, dropped all references to a ratio of charge nurses to patients and required only that afternoon and night shifts have nonwaivered LPNs for charge nurses after an effective date of July 1, 1970; until that time, "waivered" LPNs would suffice.[82]

Senator Moss reacted bitterly, convening hearings aimed at putting the blame on HEW. According to Moss, the regulations said, "in effect, that a single, untrained practical nurse on duty in a home with two hundred or three hundred patients or more constitutes 'properly supervised nursing services' on the afternoon and night shifts." A parade of witnesses agreed, pointing out that these standards were weaker than those required by Medicaid before passage of the Moss amendments, that many states already had higher standards, and that there was no substance to the allegation that skilled nurses were in short supply. In response, HEW established an extraordinary ad hoc task force, chaired by the Colorado director of public welfare. Its recommendations largely supported Frantz's original proposal. Nonetheless, when final regulations were issued in April 1970, they were weaker still than those criticized by the task force.[83]

Just why HEW took the position it did on the Moss amendments remains a mystery. Conspiracy theories abound, but hard evidence for them is lacking. Moss publicly confessed that he was mystified. It is reasonable to speculate that there was an unconscious alliance of several state officials and United States senators from the "Sunbelt," all of whom had close political and financial ties to the nursing home industry. That coalition was relatively influential in the early years of the Nixon administration because of that administration's fantasy of building a "new Republican majority," incorporating conservative Democrats around a southern and western base. The fact that proprietary nursing homes were the major for-profit interest in the health sector could not have hurt them in the eyes of an administration permeated with a commitment to free enterprise. Industry complaints over the alleged "stringency" of the regulations thus fell on sympathetic ears at high levels of the administration. Because the major advocates of stronger standards were holdovers from the Democratic administration, viewed with hostility and suspicion in the White House, the industry's pressure carried the day. But that is only an informed guess.

Inventing the ICF

It has already been mentioned that the majority of the nation's nursing homes were unable to meet Medicare standards for extended-care facilities. But some homes were even having difficulty meeting Medicaid's relatively lax interim skilled nursing home regulations. As the Moss amendments moved toward enactment, the higher standards they embodied threatened to drive many smaller facilities, especially those in converted dwellings, out of business. Nursing home interests in Iowa, later supported by their national association, responded to this impending threat with a plan to create a new category of "intermediate-care facility" (ICF), a nursing home with just enough nursing to justify public support as a health-care facility. To sell the ICF, supporters employed budgetary arguments. They began with the incontrovertible evidence that many residents of skilled nursing homes did not really need round-the-clock nursing and then contended that the lower level of service required by such residents could be provided more cheaply in specialized facilities with limiting staffing. The entire Medicaid program was plagued with budgetary problems, and the thrust of the 1967 social security amendments was a series of cutbacks in eligibility and benefits, primarily unrelated to nursing homes. The argument was seductive to administration officials trying to finance the war in Vietnam.[84]

The proposal establishing ICFs is commonly known as the "Miller amendment," after Jack Miller (R-Iowa), a senior member of the Senate Finance Committee. It encountered little opposition, partly because of its promise of budgetary savings and partly because backers of the Moss amendments acceded to it in return for support of their proposals.[85]

ICFs were recognized as eligible for vendor payments under the Social Security Act. However, ICFs were not to be covered under Medicaid, but under the cash assistance titles of the Social Security Act (although the federal matching share was to be computed under the more generous Medicaid formula). That decision appeared to reflect a recognition that ICF care would not and should not be primarily medical in orientation. But there was considerable ambiguity in congressional feelings about the issue.

Some of the more liberal members of Congress saw the ICF as a means of providing vendor payments for nonmedical residential facilities, especially charitable homes for the aging. Others in Congress saw it as a means of shifting the costs of care for nonelderly wards of the state, such as the mentally retarded, to the more generous Medicaid formula for federal matching. Representatives from states with many older, noncompliant facilities, or where the nursing home industry was especially influential, sought to locate ICF statutorily in a place where stringent regulation would be unlikely. But the House Ways and Means Committee insisted on a requirement that services in ICFs not be "merely custodial." Individuals eligible for ICF reimbursement were to be those who needed medical services less intensive than those provided by skilled nursing homes but more intensive than nothing.[86]

The Senate left the Miller amendment entirely open on the issue of standards, but the House insisted on language suggesting that ICFs be held to the same life-safety and sanitation requirements as skilled nursing homes. Its language was sufficiently ambiguous, however, to allow the states to argue that HEW's standards were only advisory and to eventually prevail on the Nixon administration to accept that position. So for more than four years, the law on ICF standards remained uncertain.[87]

Given that curious legislative mandate, it is not surprising that the ICF program immediately became a shambles. Many states, in an attempt to save money, reclassified patients and facilities wholesale, reducing reimbursement in the process. Overnight, people who had been certified as needing "skilled care" in "skilled nursing homes" were found to need only "intermediate" care; but by some amazing coincidence, the nursing homes in which they lived were found to be defined as "intermediate-care facilities." Oregon and Ohio simply reclassified all their substandard facilities as ICFs, saving them the prospect of having to comply with the Moss amendments. In many states, ICF classification was reserved for older facilities incapable of meeting the life-safety requirements of the Moss amendments. Federal ICF standards were not formally promulgated until 1971.[88] By 1973, in many states, the principal determinant of whether a facility was classified as "skilled" or "intermediate" was its ability to provide a modicum of fire safety. Remarkably, some of the same states were found to be paying more per patient day to ICFs than to skilled nursing homes in the same area.

In an effort to save the ICF, Congress amended the law in 1971 to further define "intermediate care," to make explicit HEW's authority to prescribe standards, to move ICF into Title XIX, and to require states to establish a cost differential between ICFs and skilled nursing homes.[89] Subsequent developments fleshed out the ICF definition to the point where it is now substantially identical, in many important areas, to that of skilled facilities. Roughly half the nation's nursing homes are now ICFs. Though the original objectives of the ICF's inventors were largely met (substandard facilities got an extra five to ten years ride on the federal gravy train), it is impossible to find any redeeming virtues in the entire episode.

Nixon's Initiative

The pro-nursing home approach of the Nixon administration that determined the final form of the regulations growing out of the Moss amendments did not last very long.

In June 1970, Elliot Richardson replaced Robert Finch as secretary of HEW. Shortly after Richardson arrived, a reexamination of nursing home policy began, accelerated in 1970 by a series of nursing home scandals. David Pryor (D-Arkansas), a freshman congressman, undertook an investigation on his own by taking, without identifying himself, a job as an orderly in a Maryland nursing home. He reported his experience in a series of vivid speeches on the floor of the House.[90] Thirty-two residents died in a fire in a relatively new nursing home in Marietta, Ohio on January 1.[91] In July, thirty-six patients in a Baltimore home died in an epidemic of salmonella (food poisoning).[92] Ralph Nader issued a report critical of nursing homes and the government agencies charged with regulating them.[93] For the first time, nursing homes became a major national issue, covered on the evening network news shows and making front-page headlines in the newspapers.

As plans for a 1971 White House conference on aging began to take shape, administration officials began to hear rumblings suggesting they would be vulnerable on nursing home issues.[94] But apart from continued hearings held by the Senate's Long-Term Care Subcommittee, nothing concrete happened until the following June, when Nixon, in a major speech in Chicago to the national convention of the American Association of Retired Persons/National Association of Retired Teachers (the largest organized interest group of elderly Americans) inserted remarks about the disgraceful conditions in nursing homes and the commitment of his administration to do something about them. This commitment had been kept secret from HEW leadership, but the audience responded enthusiastically, and a decision was made to follow up.[95]

On August 6, 1971, at a nursing home in Nashua, New Hampshire, the president announced an eight-part program. It was focused on standards enforcement, through a centralization of HEW Medicare and Medicaid enforcement activities; expansion of HEW enforcement staff; expansion of federal training for state inspectors; proposed legislation to permit federal reimbursement for the full costs of the states' inspection efforts; and creation of an Office of Nursing Home Affairs (ONHA) within HEW to coordinate these activities and undertake a "comprehensive study" of long-term care and long-term care policy. It also called for training programs for nurses and other nursing home personnel, and experimental funding for state nursing home "ombudsmen," and promised to use the Moss amendments' created power to withhold federal funds from substandard facilities.

Richardson, who supported those proposals, also recommended that the president give consideration to increasing Medicaid reimbursement for skilled nursing homes on the theory that, in some states, Medicaid rates were too low to permit decent service. But the president had been seeking to cut federal payments to the states for Medicaid (including nursing home payments) for more than a year.[96] No mention of reimbursement issues was made in either of the president's speeches on the subject.

Marie Callender, a professor at the University of Connecticut and one of the nation's few nursing home authorities without ties to the industry, was chosen to head the ONHA. She made enforcement her first priority. She prodded the states into completing inspection of all Medicaid and Medicare certified facilities by the following July; the first time, in many cases, that such surveys had been undertaken following the changes in standards under the Moss amendments. Even though such things are very hard to measure, the qualitative impact of this enforcement effort was probably substantial, despite the failure of most states to follow up either through reinspection or the imposition of sanctions.[97] Subsequently, ONHA pressed for enforcement of the Life-Safety Code, but by late 1973, it had faded from view.

There is some question as to how seriously committed Nixon was to real nursing home reform; internal memoranda strongly suggest that the nursing home issue was regarded largely as a political symbol. The big enforcement push in the spring of 1972 trod on some politically sensitive toes, especially in several states where Republican politicians had financial interests in less than superior nursing homes.[96] The administration's attention turned elsewhere: to China, to the Paris peace talks, to Watergate. After the election, Richardson left HEW for Defense, and shortly thereafter the ONHA was demoted several notches on the HEW organization chart. But the Nixon initiative marked a major turning point in nursing home politics. Where once the only people paying attention had been those with an interest in the industry, the brief spasm of media attention and public applause for reform efforts established the fact that there was political capital in a tough posture toward nursing homes.

P.L. 92-603

By October 1972, the action in nursing home policy shifted back to Congress with the enactment of comprehensive changes in the Social Security Act through Public Law 92-603. It is one of the largest and most complex pieces of legislation ever passed, and in its genesis one of the most curious. It began life as H.R. 1, the Nixon administration's proposal for comprehensive welfare reform. Along the way, it picked up hundreds of incremental changes in the social security system and dozens of amendments to Medicare and Medicaid. As finally passed, it contained over three hundred separate provisions. Social security benefits were increased, and eligibility requirements eased. Medicare coverage was extended to kidney transplantation and dialysis for patients with chronic kidney failure. The first federal controls on capital expenditures by health-care institutions were enacted. A nationwide system of "Professional Standards Review Organizations" (PSROs) was created to monitor the quality of medical care rendered under Medicare and Medicaid. Even more significant, in the context of social security legislation, old age assistance, aid to the blind, and aid to the disabled were consolidated and federalized into the new system of Supplemental Security Income (SSI). It embodied the basic principles of Nixon's original welfare proposal (uniform national standards, a uniform national benefit floor, complete federal funding of minimum benefits) while ignoring the category of aid to families of dependent children (AFDC) to which that proposal was primarily addressed.[99]

P.L. 92–603 contained no fewer than nineteen separate provisions related to nursing home care under Medicare and Medicaid. Among the most important, the classification of nursing homes was consolidated; both Medicare extended-care facilities and Medicaid skilled nursing homes were redefined as "skilled nursing facilities" (SNFs) with a new, more sensible definition of what constituted "skilled care" and with instructions to HEW to develop a single set of standards. These standards were to contain a much more limited and narrow provision for waiver of RN staffing requirements in rural areas.[100]

P.L. 92–603 addressed the problem of retroactive denials of Medicare nursing home claims by establishing "presumptive eligibility" for beneficiaries discharged from hospitals with certain diagnoses. This was supposed to tie into an elaborate system of "utilization review," eventually to be integrated into the PSRO system, in all SNFs and ICFs, to ensure that patients were receiving the "appropriate level" of care.[101]

Nixon's proposal for full federal funding of state enforcement activities was enacted into law. Previously, when those activities had been lumped into Medicaid's administrative overhead, of which the federal government pays half, the states had been reluctant to provide anything close to adequate enforcement staff. Also, provisions for disclosure of ICF ownership and for "independent professional review" of ICF quality of care were added.[102]

Perhaps the most significant change was Section 249 of the law, which required the states, effective July 1, 1974 (later postponed to July 1976), to reimburse both SNFs and ICFs under Medicaid on a "reasonable cost-related basis." It was the expectation of the Senate Finance Committee, which added this section to the bill, that cost-related reimbursement would once and for all remove from nursing home operators the excuse that their income was too low to permit them to provide adequate care. The language of the committee's report also made plain that, while the "reasonable cost" reimbursement methods of Medicare would qualify under the statutory definition, they were not required. It was hoped that the states would experiment with alternative reimbursement systems.[103]

Despite its sweeping scope, P.L. 92–603 had almost no immediate effect on nursing homes. By mid-1973, as the White House became increasingly paralyzed by Watergate, the executive branch had largely ceased to function on domestic issues. It has been argued that the Nixon administration began its second term with the intention of totally remaking the federal bureaucracy, with HEW the most important target.[104] By the time H. R. Haldeman and John D. Ehrlichman resigned in mid-1973, much of the dismantling, but hardly any reconstruction, had been accomplished. It was not until some time in the first full year of the Ford administration that the bureaucracy began functioning again.

The upshot was that the regulations to implement the SNF category were not issued until mid-1974. New ICF standards were issued at the same time but not made immediately effective.[105] After several postponements, implementing regulations for cost-related reimbursement were issued on the last legally allowable day, July 1, 1976, and their effective date was then unilaterally, and probably illegally, postponed by the secretary of HEW until January 1, 1978.[106]

Dollars and Detectives

P.L. 92-603 was the last major legislative initiative at the national level relating to nursing homes. But two subsequent developments are also significant. First, after Phase IV price controls on health facilities were lifted in 1974, Medicaid expenditures went out of control. Between 1974 and 1975, total Medicaid costs, of which the states collectively pay 45 percent, increased more than 25 percent from slightly over $10 billion to almost $13 billion. By 1976, they had increased another 18 percent. Nursing homes accounted for the largest source of these increases. In 1974, Medicaid (counting both federal and state shares) spent $3.5 billion for nursing homes; by 1976, it was spending $5.3 billion—an increase of more than 50 percent in just two years.[107] The states alone were spending $900 million more for nursing homes in 1976 than in 1974.

States struggled to get nursing home expenditures under control. Studies and investigations were undertaken. Implementation of cost-related reimbursement was postponed; the states were in enough trouble already. States could no longer ignore questions of nursing home policy or relegate nursing home decisions to the back reaches of the welfare bureaucracy.

At roughly the same time, nursing home scandals broke in New York and began surfacing in other states. Mary Adelaide Mendelson's *Tender Loving Greed*, the first exposé that attempted to define a direct link between provider fraud and poor care, generated intense national publicity.[108] The notion of "welfare fraud" had always been connected in the public mind with the stereotype of the Cadillac-driving, mink-clad, black welfare mother of ten. Now, people began to realize that the really large-scale stealing was being done by health-care "providers."

The congressional reaction to this growing perception that provider fraud and theft were the real problems was H.R. 3, the Medicare and Medicaid Antifraud and Abuse Amendments of 1977, which incorporated a whole laundry list of legislative proposals. Of the twenty-seven sections of H.R. 3, all but a handful applied to nursing homes, either exclusively or as "providers" of Medicare and Medicaid services. One influential congressional aide estimated that between 10 and 20 percent of all Medicare and Medicaid funds were being stolen or wasted in the bureaucracy. That estimate, which was widely accepted, was a delusion. Hundreds of millions of dollars had been stolen. H.R. 3 would plug the major legal and administrative leaks in health care programs, but no one outside of Congress seriously entertained the notion that fraud and waste were the principal causes of the explosion in program costs. The fundamental flaws were much deeper, and more basic.

4

Paying the Piper

"Follow the Money"
—Deep Throat

THE MARKET for nursing home services is extraordinarily complex for several reasons. First, it is dominated, but not exclusively, by a single buyer (government) that behaves ambivalently. Second, government is the primary *buyer*, but it is not itself a consumer; it buys *for* program beneficiaries.[1] At the same time, the industry is regulated by the government. Third, the consumers of service—whether government buys for them or they buy for themselves—are unable to evaluate the quality of what they are buying, and governments aren't much better at it. Fourth, nursing homes are like hospitals in some ways and very unlike them in others; and no one knows a very satisfactory way of paying hospitals either.

If the only concern of buyers and sellers was the price at which nursing home services were sold, the market could be described as a sophisticated political game, and these complexities would not matter much. But the nursing home market's complexities are tied to *methods* of payment, widely believed to matter as much as gross amounts—as levels of payment, as prices.

The method of payment matters because it provides incentives and disincentives to the sellers and will affect the mix of highly variable goods and services lumped into a "nursing home day." If a special bonus is added for employing a French chef in the kitchen, nursing homes will begin to claim that they employ French chefs; as the bonus increases, so will the number of chefs. If governments were to specifically refuse to pay for toilet paper, nursing homes would search for a substitute or provide none.

There is increasing sympathy for the notion that governments should seek to influence the behavior of private citizens and firms through economic incentives rather than through legal regulation. In this view (popularized most notably by Charles Schultze, chairman of the Council of Economic Advisers) regulation is inherently cumbersome, inefficient, and subject to political abuse, while "incentives" capture all the virtues of ideal markets even when those markets don't exist.[2] This chapter will look at how incentives work, or don't work, in paying for nursing home services.

The Nursing Home Market

In the fiscal year ending September 30, 1977, $12.6 billion was expended on nursing home care. Of that total, almost $7.2 billion, or 57 percent, was spent directly by governments, with $6.4 billion, or 89 percent of the government share, spent under the Medicaid program; of the balance, Medicare paid $360 million, and the Veterans Administration just over $200 million. The costs of Medicaid are shared by federal and state governments, and in nine states (although to a considerable extent only in New York, California, and Nebraska) by localities. Of the $6.4 billion in Medicaid expenditures, just over $3.6 billion, or about 56 percent, came from federal funds, as did all the Medicare and Veterans Administration expenditures.[3]

While governments paid for only 57 percent of the dollar total, those payments bought care for a substantially higher proportion of all residents. A reasonable estimate is that, at any given time, somewhere around three quarters of all residents are being cared for at public expense.[4]

The discrepancy between the proportion of publicly supported residents and the proportion of public dollars is accounted for mainly by the fact that the share of costs borne by the social security or other pension benefits of Medicaid recipients is not included in the Medicaid total. There are very few residents for whom Medicaid itself pays the full cost, and somewhere around 30 percent of "private" expenditures are made by Medicaid recipients.[5] In addition, the law—in this instance usually observed—requires that private charges must be at least as high as Medicaid rates, so Medicaid always pays the lowest unit price. Finally, for those facilities that accept Medicare payments, charges to private patients must be at least as high as the Medicare rate, which is invariably as high, or higher, than Medicaid's—often by as much as 50 percent.

The price of nursing home care, even for comparable levels of service, varies enormously from state to state, and to a lesser but still considerable extent within any given state. Rates vary so much from one state to another because states have been willing to pay very different amounts; they vary so much within states because state payment policies have either encouraged variation among facilities or have kept rates uniformly low, accelerating the development of a "dual market" in which private and Medicaid rates diverge substantially.

Rates in New York are the highest in the country. The better skilled nursing facilities in metropolitan New York City generally charge Medicaid in excess of $60 per patient day, which works out to more than $1,800 a month, or $21,600 a year; the statewide average for skilled facilities exceeds $40 a day ($1,200 a month, $14,600 a year). In contrast, Medicaid in California permits less than $30 per patient day, and most residents are Medicaid beneficiaries; private patients pay anywhere from $10 to $15 more per day. In Illinois, Medicaid rates average less than $20, but there are relatively more private patients. The lowest Medicaid rates have traditionally been those in the South and the less urban midwestern states, with the highest proportion of non-Medicaid nursing home residents.[6]

Variation in rates between states, combined with variation in bed supply and the differing proportion of nursing home residents receiving Medicaid from state to state, produces enormous differences in what state Medicaid programs spend for nursing homes. In fiscal year 1976, New York's Medicaid program spent just over $1.1 billion on nursing homes—more than 20 percent of all Medicaid nursing home expenditures and almost three times as much as California, the state with the second largest Medicaid expenditures. Illinois and Pennsylvania have about the same number of people, but Pennsylvania spends 40 percent more for nursing homes under Medicaid than Illinois. Kentucky has 10 percent more people than Connecticut, but spends only half as much; Wisconsin has slightly fewer people than Missouri, but spends more than five times as much.[7] The full range of state expenditures is presented in table 3.

Roughly 37 percent of all Medicaid expenditures are for nursing

TABLE 3
State Nursing Home Expenditures Under Medicaid

State	Medicaid Nursing Home Expenditure FY 1976 (in millions of dollars)	Rank	State Population Rank	Nursing Home Expenditures as Percent of All State Medicaid Expenditures
New York	1,108	1	2	33.0
California	370	2	1	23.1
Pennsylvania	302	3	4	38.3
Texas	282	4	3	49.6
Michigan	221	5	7	31.3
Illinois	214	6	5	26.9
Massachusetts	183	7	10	30.3
Wisconsin	179	8	16	43.7
Ohio	147	9	6	33.0
Minnesota	128	10	19	40.3
New Jersey	122	11	9	30.2
Georgia	105	12	14	41.1
Indiana	104	13	12	50.5
Connecticut	87	14	24	44.8
Alabama	76	15	21	47.5
Washington	75	16	22	41.9
Oklahoma	74	17	27	46.0
Florida	69	18	8	45.0
Louisiana	63	19	20	30.8
Tennessee	61	20	17	34.9
Iowa	60	21	25	49.2
Virginia	58	22	13	30.9
Maryland	57	23	18	25.1
Arkansas	54	24	33	46.2
North Carolina	50	25	11	24.8
Colorado	47	26	28	43.9
Kentucky	43	27	23	28.7
Kansas	38	28	31	30.4
Mississippi	37	29	29	33.3
South Carolina	36	30	26	34.9
Missouri	32	31	15	25.6
Oregon	32	32	30	33.7
Maine	29	33	38	34.2
Nebraska	26	34	35	43.3
Rhode Island	22	35	39	24.4
New Hampshire	21	36	42	61.8
Hawaii	17	37	40	32.0
District of Columbia	17	37	—	16.4
Utah	16	39	36	40.0
Montana	15	40	43	48.4
South Dakota	14	41	44	58.3
North Dakota	14	41	45	60.8
Idaho	13	43	41	41.9
West Virginia	10	44	34	17.2
Vermont	10	44	48	32.2
New Mexico	8	46	37	22.2
Nevada	6	47	46	28.5
Alaska	6	47	50	54.6
Delaware	4	49	47	23.5
Wyoming	4	49	49	66.6

NOTE: Arizona has no Medicaid Program.

SOURCE: Medicaid Data derived from U.S. Department of Health, Education, and Welfare, Health Care Financing Administration, Medicaid Bureau, *Data on the Medicaid Program: Eligibility Services, Expenditures Fiscal Years 1966-77* (Washington: Institute for Medicaid Management), 1977, Table 23, pages 42-43, and Table 24, pages 44-45. Population ranks from U.S. Department of Commerce, Bureau of the Census, *Statistical Abstract of the United States 1976* (Washington: Government Printing Office), 1976, Table 10, p. 11.

homes, which are the single greatest recipients of Medicaid funds. There also is substantial variation in the proportion of states' Medicaid budgets going to nursing homes (see table 3).[8]

The Medicaid Mill

Medicaid basically involves a system of federal grants to the states for part of the cost of purchasing services for defined beneficiaries from defined classes of health care providers. It imposes a number of program requirements on states but gives the federal government only limited tools with which to enforce them. Medicaid originated as a welfare program and is still characterized by the stigmatization of its beneficiaries and an absence of broad-based political support—even though, because of nursing home costs, a disproportionate share of Medicaid dollars goes for services to the white elderly.

Like other welfare programs, Medicaid obligates the federal government to pay a fixed proportion of state expenditures for defined benefits. Unlike almost any other grant-in-aid federal program, however, Medicaid provides service benefits to individuals with *entitlements* to them. Rather than a cash grant or a standardized commodity like food or clothing, what Medicaid pays for is literally whatever the doctor orders (subject to reams of bureaucratic regulation). The amount of nursing home expenditure is determined not by how many budget dollars there are to go around, but by how many people with entitlements to Medicaid benefits find themselves in nursing homes at any time—a matter over which the states have only indirect control. From a budgetary perspective, Medicaid thus creates uniquely severe problems.

In conventional cash assistance welfare programs, states can exercise some control over expenditures by tying the level of benefits to the number of recipients. If the number of recipients increases unexpectedly, benefits can be frozen or even cut back. Eligibility standards can be "fine-tuned" to reduce the number of beneficiaries, or bureaucratic obstacles imposed to discourage eligible applicants. In noncash domestic assistance programs, such as those in public health or housing, governments can limit expenditures by deciding to allocate a given fixed sum and then serve only as many people as that amount can provide for. But under Medicaid, states are required to pay for all "medically necessary" services for all recipients of cash welfare assistance and all whom they have deemed "medically indigent," regardless of how many services those beneficiaries consume, or at what cost. States can cut back on eligibility for Medicaid only by cutting back on eligibility for cash assistance; but doing so involves depriving a large number of people of basic subsistence in order to reduce the medical expenditures incurred by a small proportion of them. From the viewpoint of state policymakers, Medicaid is thus a particularly "uncontrollable" program.[9]

This description is something of an overstatement in that federal Medicaid policy has provided the states with more and more ways in which to restrict the number of services beneficiaries receive or the number of beneficiaries they recognize. But it is essentially correct, especially for nursing homes. Since coverage of skilled nursing facilities is a required service, every state with a Medicaid program must pay for all the nursing home services received by all individuals whose income is low enough to qualify—a large proportion of all those in nursing homes. The federal government shares this fiscal risk on at least a fifty-fifty basis since it is obligated to pay its share of Medicaid expenditures. But it can resort to printing money; the states must balance their budgets.

This problem has been complicated by the very rapid increase in the supply of nursing home beds and the apparently inexhaustible supply of potential Medicaid beneficiaries to fill them. The states' fiscal obligation is not only open-ended but is particularly vulnerable to rapid increase, because utilization has increased so quickly.

The total units of service the state is obligated to purchase under Medicaid is, of course, only one of two factors involved in determining the total cost to state treasuries. The other is price. Total expenditure equals quantity times price. As a result, the states (with a few exceptions) have been intent upon keeping down the prices they must pay.

The states' desire to keep nursing home prices low is further reinforced by a peculiarity of the Medicaid program. Since Medicaid eligibility is a function of the relationship between an individual's income and his or her medical expenditures, the higher the prevailing price of care, the more people will become eligible for Medicaid. An elderly person who could afford to pay out-of-pocket for nursing home care at $20 a day will quickly become impoverished at $30 a day, and while recurring income will continue to be applied to nursing home expenses, the state will have to make up the differences. Increasing Medicaid rates has the dual effect of increasing costs for those already eligible for benefits and expanding the number of people who are eligible.

Until recently, however, political and practical considerations have tempered the states' determination to pay as little as possible for nursing home services. Very low prices are obviously connected with very poor services. Nursing home residents may be invisible to the general public most of the time, but they have their advocates. Whatever the motives of public officials, they have been reluctant to risk the political embarrassment of extremely substandard care.

Moreover, Medicaid has constantly encountered difficulty in eliciting adequate participation from providers other than hospitals. Nothing obligates a physician or pharmacist or nursing home to provide services to Medicaid beneficiaries, and when Medicaid payments are extremely low, providers refuse to give care to Medicaid recipients. So the states have had to pay higher rates to provide an adequate supply of nursing home services under Medicaid. The impetus to ensure nursing home participation has partly arisen from the continued belief that nursing home services may be substituted for more expensive—to Medicaid—hospital care. As with the framers of the ECF benefit, Medicaid officials, hearing reports of elderly beneficiaries kept in hospital beds at more than $100 a day after the need for acute care has passed, have been eager to be able to move those patients to nursing homes at $20 a day.

The objectives of the states relative to the pricing of nursing home services might well be, then, summarized as the lowest price consistent with minimally adequate quality and adequate provider participation in the program.[10]

The Price of Quality

Like love, a notoriously qualitative phenomenon, "quality" is hard to define and hard to measure—although in nursing homes, one is often acutely aware of whether or not it is there. Yet governments are often critically concerned with the quality of what they are buying and have to make some effort to link the quality of services with their price.

The problems are particularly acute when the commodity is a relatively intangible service like "health care" or "custodial" or "social" care. Money is necessary but not sufficient for the production of quality. Suppliers of health or nursing home services cannot improve quality, in many instances, without additional expenditures. But there is no guarantee that those additional expenditures will improve quality. They may go to enrich the suppliers or simply be wasted.

Consumers are poorly equipped to evaluate the quality of health care or nursing home services. The 50 percent of nursing home residents adjudged senile may be assumed to be undiscriminating consumers. Families and friends don't do much better; nursing home services are complex, and decisions about nursing home placements are often made under traumatic stress.

Even when consumers can make rough qualitative judgments, it may be difficult for governments to do so in the health services market. The individual consumer is presumably capable of deciding for himself whether a price differential is "worth it" in terms of his own income and tastes. But governments, held to strict standards of public accountability, need more precise measures of value, which may be unattainable. If private individuals "overconsume" medical services by paying a substantial premium for marginal qualitative superiority, that simply transfers income from buyer to seller. But if governments overconsume by paying too much more to facilities they think are superior, they are transferring taxpayers' dollars. Unless they can make a good case that the facilities receiving higher payments are *demonstrably* superior, they lay themselves open to charges of political favoritism and illegally arbitrary conduct.

Moreover, the quality of health and social services varies, often in unpredictable ways. The third floor of Harry's nursing home may run like a clock with one particular charge nurse and then go to pieces on the night shift, or when the particular nurse retires. A qualitative evaluation made at any one time may only be accurate for that time, yet decisions to "consume" services generally involve long-term commitments.

The "discipline" of the market is missing; good facilities do not drive poor ones out of business, nor is there a direct correlation between quality and price. In case of hospitals, it is presumed that physicians can make qualitative judgments. At least for their own patients, physicians have incentives to provide a high level of quality, if for no

other reason than to reduce their malpractice liability. Society dele-
gates to the profession the task of assuring at least minimal quality.
But there is not much professionalism in nursing homes. Registered
nurses are the only professionals who spend lots of time in nursing
homes, and their administrative responsibilities and professional isolation make it extremely difficult for them to fulfill a quality-assurance
function. Since nursing homes are places where people live more than
places where they are treated, the only professionals who take responsibility for the overall quality of life are the administrators. But when
a nursing home administrator is not the owner of the facility, his continued employment is contingent on maximizing the facility's profit
or, in the case of nonprofit facilities, the trustees' sense of doing good.

Even were more nursing home administrators governed by norms of
professional responsibility, the role of professionals in quality assurance raises problems of cost. In medical care, professionals have felt an
ethical obligation to provide the highest level of quality. But quality is
governed by the law of diminishing returns. Added spending beyond
a certain point will provide progressively less and less improvement.
(Adding an extra aide to the third floor of Harry's nursing home during the night shift will probably improve the quality of nursing services there, but forty aides for forty patients would undoubtedly be
wasteful.) This is a critical preoccupation of governments when they
buy health or nursing home services.

Paying Hospitals

When, after the adoption of Medicare and Medicaid, the federal
government first began paying for hospital care in a big way, it refused to grapple with these problems. Instead, it agreed to pay the
"reasonable costs" of producing care for its beneficiaries, and "reasonable" entailed only two qualifications. In order to be reimbursable,
costs had to be related to patient care; Medicare would not pay for presents to trustees' wives or the construction of staff parking lots. Also,
Medicare would only pay for costs attributable to its patients; it refused to pay for maternity and pediatric services, since those over sixty-five consume so little of both. Medicare pays "cost," rather than
"charges" (the prices hospitals post), because the system of charges

had been used to perpetuate cross-subsidization among different categories of hospital users, and Medicare proposed to pay the full cost of services for its users and nothing else. Most of the endless squabbling and litigation over Medicare reimbursement to hospitals has revolved around the issue of just which costs are attributable to its patients and which are not.

The original philosophy of Medicare payment was to let physicians and professional accrediting agencies provide whatever level of quality they deemed appropriate, and accept the obligation to pay whatever costs those decisions generated. Since almost everyone else paying for hospital care (essentially Blue Cross) was governed by the same philosophy or simply accepted whatever hospitals charged, there was no incentive for hospitals to behave efficiently, especially since Medicare guaranteed a substantial growth in demand. The "explosion" in hospital costs was thus set off. Between 1965 and 1976, the average daily cost of a hospital day increased from $40 to $156.[11]

There has been a substantial improvement in the quality of hospital care since 1965. Just how much of the cost increases are attributable to qualitative improvement, and how much to inefficient spending of new revenues or windfall gains to providers, is a subject of considerable dispute. The major attempts to cope with Medicare cost inflation over the past few years have sought to improve efficiency without addressing the quality issue. Medicare now puts limits on "routine inpatient service costs" within a geographic area, on the assumption that the most expensive hospitals *must* be inefficient and should not be rewarded for being so.

Another complication is that of "incentives." If the price a seller receives is a function of his costs—if he is paid either just his costs, or costs plus a fixed or flat percentage profit—then reduction in the costs of production achieved through improved efficiency will *reduce* the seller's revenue. Under conventional reimbursement, hospitals have had little incentive to reduce costs and a definite incentive to increase them, since it is a rare institution that does not desire to see its total revenues grow.

A system of payment based on a "retrospective" cost basis is inherently inflationary, since it rewards inefficiency. But when qualitative improvement is important, and not easily measured, it is far from clear how else it might be obtained.

The currently popular thinking on hospital reimbursement is that this problem can be resolved by setting rates on a "prospective" basis. That is, a calculation should be made as to what a hospital's costs will be if its efficiency does not improve, and those costs should become its rate for the coming year. The hospital is then permitted to keep at least part of any cost savings but risks losing money if its costs rise more quickly than projected. One can, as hospitals have feared, go a step further and establish a prospective rate that will cover future costs only if the hospital economizes.

Prospective cost-based reimbursement appears to offer a partial solution to the problem of cost control, but it has shortcomings of its own. Prospective reimbursement offers no guarantee that the economies achieved will not reduce quality. The experience with prospective hospital reimbursement in New York has been that hospitals have been just as likely to reduce direct services to patients as to cut waste or eliminate unnecessary expenditures. In the absence of better quality measures, that kind of behavior is extraordinarily difficult to police or prevent.

Also, prospective cost-based reimbursement takes the "historical" costs of any given institution as the "base" from which future rates are projected. Institutions that have been more efficient in the past are penalized, while those that were wasteful are rewarded. Students of hospital reimbursement have become increasingly uncomfortable with institution-specific rates, although, because hospitals do differ so substantially from one another in the kinds of services they provide and the kinds of patients they treat, no adequate criteria for uniform rates across different hospitals have yet been devised.

Another shortcoming of prospective reimbursement is its focus on an inadequate measure of hospital "output." The unit of service upon which hospital payment has been based has been the "average patient day" or the "average per diem." The costs of providing basic services, including nursing, to everyone in the hospital not in intensive care or the nursery are summed and then divided by the total number of patient-days experienced or projected.

In hospitals, this system creates terrible distortions and perverse incentives. There is enormous variation in what it actually costs hospitals to provide services to different patients, and even to provide services to the same patient at different points in his hospital stay. If a patient is hospitalized for ten days, most of the costs of medical records, admissions testing, and even nursing are incurred in the first three or four days, and the last two days generate less than 20 percent of the total costs. Besides, some patients are sicker, and more expensive to care for, than others throughout their stay. As a general rule, hospitals lose money on the first few days for most patients and on the entire stay of the most seriously ill; they recoup at the tail end of most stays and on the least-ill patients. As a result, they have a powerful incentive to keep people in longer than they otherwise would or than might be good for the patients. If most hospitals behave this way, then society is paying for the support and upkeep of many more hospital beds than it needs.

The tendency to keep patients hospitalized longer than medically necessary is also related to the fact that a high proportion of hospital costs appear, in the short run, to be fixed, so that the incremental cost of caring for an additional patient is very much lower than the average cost for all patients. Because of capital expenses and basic personnel costs—and the inflexibility of hospital staffing patterns in the face of highly variable demand—it costs much more than half as much to run a hospital at 45 percent occupancy than it does at 90 percent occupancy. Low occupancy rates, in an uncontrolled cost-based system, lead to higher average per diems. Aware of this phenomenon, those who concoct systems of hospital reimbursement have built occupancy "targets" into their calculations; it is assumed that hospitals operate at x occupancy, and per diem reimbursement rates are set accordingly. Hospitals, penalized for low occupancies and rewarded for high ones, respond by keeping their patients longer.

These considerations throw considerable light on the notion of saving on hospital costs by increasing the use of nursing homes. Compared to the spectrum of all hospital patients, it costs the hospital far less than average to provide care for old people no longer ill enough to need hospitalization but incapable of being sent home. If they are all moved to nursing homes, the average cost for all other patients must increase. Moreover, relative to other nursing home patients, those recently discharged from hospitals are somewhat more expensive to care for, since they are likely to require more services than those admitted from the community. Pushing people out of hospitals into nursing homes increases the average cost of nursing home care. The savings to society of such a discharge are thus largely illusory, although the savings to a particular payer—such as Medicare, which often stops paying when a beneficiary is discharged from a hospital to a nursing home—may be much greater.

In addition, there are a lot of empty hospital beds and very few empty nursing home beds. The marginal cost of keeping in hospitals a sizable number of patients who need something less than hospital care is very low, since they are occupying beds that otherwise would lie empty. But pushing them out of hospitals, when nursing home supply is tight, generates a demand to construct more nursing homes, which is very expensive. When hospital beds are empty and nursing home supply tight, there is no money to be saved by moving patients from hospitals to nursing homes.[12]

Paying Nursing Homes — An Introduction

Until very recently, most states reimbursed nursing homes on what was essentially a flat-rate basis, although those rates were arrived at in a variety of ways. In Pennsylvania, the Budget Department took the Welfare Department's projection of nursing home utilization for the coming year, determined what funds would be available, and divided by the projected number of residents. Connecticut classified facilities into six groups on the basis of the quality of services they provided, or at least were capable of providing, and established a system of graduated rates with a single, flat rate for each category. Many states, including California in the early 1970s, ostensibly reimbursed nursing homes the costs of providing services but imposed a ceiling on per diem payments so stringent as to become a de facto flat rate. Louisiana, Oklahoma, and Nebraska negotiated rates, the former two on a statewide basis, the latter on a per-patient basis through country welfare departments. Many states used a cost-based system like that employed for hospitals for SNFs but promulgated flat rates for ICFs.[13] Medicare, though, has always used the hospital system of retrospective cost-reimbursement in its payments for skilled care. (That is one of the reasons states paid costs for skilled care but not for ICFs; for SNFs, they were able to piggyback on Medicare cost reports and rate determinations, substantially reducing their administrative overhead.)

The flat-rate system was continually attacked because it was believed that flat rates tended to be set below the costs of providing care of adequate quality. Much of the impetus for cost-related rates arose from the assumption that they would necessarily be higher than what the states were paying under flat rates. In other words, it was not cost-relatedness per se, but a desire for defensibly higher rates that at least partially motivated the trend to cost-related rates.

Tying the rate a facility receives to its costs for providing services should ensure that most of its revenues are being devoted to patient care. Another telling criticism of the flat-rate system has been that those homes that, for whatever reasons, were providing services most cheaply received the greatest profits on operating revenues. At any given fixed price, there is always a direct one-for-one trade-off between expenditures for patient care and profit to the operators; any additional dollars spent on the patients must come out of the operators' profits. Reimbursing operators the full costs of expenditures on patient care, and separately for profits, presumably removes this disincentive to improving service.

Using the flat-rate system in health care also presents a political problem. If price incentives work, efficient operators might reap substantial short-run profits. But the prospect of such profits, while economically attractive for entrepreneurs, is terrifying to custodians of the public purse, especially in an area where quality is so problematic. For all the rhetoric about efficiency in government and maintenance of the free enterprise system, voters tend not to look kindly on officials who permit substantial profits among those who are selling services to government—especially when the recipients of those services are public charges—even though it may be cheaper to pay high profits to efficient producers than costs to inefficient producers. When experience suggests that those making the greatest profits are likely not to be the most efficient producers, but rather those most indifferent to quality, the mistrust of flat-rate prices becomes still greater.

Profits and quality might be less mutually antagonistic if private, nongovernmental demand played a more important role in the nursing home market. Economists who study nursing home reimbursement repeatedly contend that nursing homes will seek to attract more lucrative private patients by improving services. But private patients are only more profitable when whatever qualitative improvements are made to attract them are less expensive than the price differential they are willing to pay. Their demand will increase quality (as opposed to the appearance of quality) only if they are, in fact, discriminating consumers.

Nursing home operators so vigorously seek private patients precisely because they are willing to pay more for the trappings of high quality than it costs the operators to provide them. Conversely, facilities with a high proportion of private patients tend to be superior not because they have more revenue, but because private consumers have affluent families that are *demanding* consumers and exert noneconomic pressure on the facility. Nonetheless, the conflict between quality and profitability still prevails in the private market for nursing home services.

Other criticisms of the flat-rate system have been commonly made—although they cut two ways, describing strengths as well as weaknesses. Because they do not require the reporting of costs to governmental payers, flat-rate systems limit the amount of information available to governments about the economics of the industry they are supporting. Cost reporting, when backed up by systematic audit, can permit governments to oversee rather closely what is going on in facilities—what services are being provided and by whom. When correlated with legal requirements for care standards—a theoretical possibility that has almost never been implemented—such audit information can become a useful quality-control tool. But there are disadvantages to cost reporting: most obvious and unavoidable is the burden of paperwork; less obvious, but frequently encountered, is the incentive to report dishonestly.

Rates that are uniform for all facilities are also uniform for all patients, but it costs more to care for some patients than others. Under a flat-rate system, nursing homes are reluctant to admit those who need, or who are likely to eventually need, the most intensive care. At its extreme, this practice means that the likelihood of being admitted to a nursing home is directly inverse to a potential resident's need for admission. Nursing homes that attempt to care for the most seriously ill operate under a financial penalty, while there is profit to be made in discriminating against them. A retrospective-cost-plus system does not create this incentive to discriminate. On the other hand, an attempt to solve the problem through reimbursement is likely to create other undesirable incentives. When facilities receive extra payment for treating the more seriously ill, the incentive is to classify residents as being more in need of services than in fact they are. This process, which fosters dependency, is widely agreed to have deleterious consequences for the residents. The narrow pre-1972 definition of "extended care" in the Medicare program was believed to have just this perverse effect.

Finally, to the extent that flat rates are significantly lower than costs, their use by the states requires non-Medicaid residents and, by extension, the government itself to subsidize public charges. But this criticism becomes circular since whatever government pays, *however* it sets its price, private rates will be higher.

As a practical matter, these criticisms would appear to be moot, since states are no longer permitted to use flat-rate systems of reimbursement under Medicaid. But the line between the flat-rate system and one based on a "reasonable cost-related" method can be extremely thin. And, whatever their disadvantages, flat rates unquestionably provide the most effective price controls. When quality standards are enforced outside the reimbursement system, and flat rates set at a sensible level, they provide both the strongest incentives for efficiency on the part of operators (since a penny of expenditures saved by a nursing home then literally becomes a penny earned) and the most effective budgetary control for the state.

Cost and Its Relations

Since the inception of Medicaid, New York State has reimbursed nursing homes on the basis of their costs. At first, reimbursement was based on retrospective "reasonable" costs, essentially equivalent to the method employed for hospitals. Subsequently, prospective rates on the basis of "historical" costs "trended" forward to account for inflation were adopted. In 1975, in response to its severe budget crisis and the growing scandals over nursing homes, New York State froze all rates. Before the freeze was lifted in 1977, a variety of new limitations and controls, mostly similar to those now employed for hospitals by Medicare, were tacked onto the basic prospective system.[14]

New York State's cost reimbursement system has imposed an inordinate economic burden on its taxpayers. New York's best facilities, encouraged by what was essentially a blank check, offered, at least until the 1975 freeze, a range and degree of services unmatched by all but a handful of the nation's nursing homes. The average level of care in the state may be slightly higher than the national average—especially in terms of the provision of professional services like social work and physical therapy—and somewhat higher still than it is in the very low-rate states. But, as the 1975 scandals revealed, it is entirely possible for facilities in a cost-reimbursement system to be just as awful as those in a flat-rate system.

The principal beneficiaries of New York State's reimbursement system have been nursing home employees and owners. Wages for entry-level positions in New York City nursing homes are more than twice the national average, and fringe benefits are more than twice as good.[15] New York City nursing home employees are represented by ef fective unions, but so are nursing home employees in major cities in other states, and their contracts are not even close to comparable. Un ionization itself is not the cause. Rather, in the late 1960s and early 1970s, the state government made an effective, if not explicit, policy decision to transfer substantial income to hospital and nursing home employees through the mechanism of reimbursement, by permitting a direct "pass-through" of all labor costs into facility rates. The assump tion was that the federal government, through Medicare and its 50 percent share of Medicaid, would bear a large part of these costs, while the benefits would all accrue to state residents. This made much more sense for hospital care, in which the state's market share, through Medicaid, is relatively small, than it did for nursing homes, but hospital and nursing home employees belong to the same unions.

The enormous profits made by nursing home operators in New York State stemmed largely from manipulation of cost-based reimbursement (fraudulent inflating or misreporting of costs) and property expenses. Apart from the property-cost issue, the widespread stealing in New York was a product of the state's total failure to police the system or enforce its requirements. Before the 1975 scandals, New York em ployed only fourteen auditors to examine the detailed reports of more than 800 facilities.[16] Because *rates* were so much higher in New York, a level of fraudulent activity that may have been no greater than that elsewhere provided much more enrichment for the malfeasors. Yet a cost-related system permitted some facilities to offer relatively good care even when their operators were involved in significant misappro priation. The extremely tight link between poor care and high profits, characteristic of flat-rate systems, is broken in a cost-based system.

The experience of the nursing home industry in New York served as a lesson to other states as they began moving to cost-based reimburse ment system. Assisted by HEW's rather generous interpretation of what "reasonable cost-related" meant, states have concocted complex systems that attempt to meet simultaneously the objectives of quality improvement, compliance with federal requirements, and control of cost increases. The principal devices they have used to meet these con tradictory objectives are ceilings, groupings, prospective reimburse ment, and profit limitations. Ceilings are just what the name implies; states will pay costs up to some limit. Groupings are an attempt to es tablish a uniform rate for similar facilities, by breaking the industry down into relatively homogenous groups; geographical location and the range of services provided are the most common bases for those groupings.

Prospective reimbursement, discussed in connection with hospitals, has particular disadvantages when applied to nursing homes. Existing cost structures in nursing homes do not reflect what professionals would provide in the absence of cost constraints so much as what states have been willing to pay on a flat-rate basis in the past. Many nursing homes, in order to remain in business, have developed cost structures to maximize profits under flat rates. Many proprietary facilities have artificially high property costs while shaving costs for nursing or residents' meals. Whether those cost structures constitute an appropriate base on which to build prospective rates is a serious question, not yet addressed by policymakers.

In terms of incentives to enhance quality, moreover, it is not clear that prospective rates, no matter how cost-related they may be, really differ from flat rates; expenditures on quality improvement must come out of that year's profit. From a long-range perspective, it may be rational for a nursing home to boost patient-care costs as high as possible, accepting a smaller profit, to ensure the highest prospective rate for the coming year and greater profits in the future. But that logic can put operators on a treadmill from which they may never escape and presumes that nursing home operators are much more concerned with the long run than they have ever shown any evidence of being.

The functional similarity between prospective rates and flat rates is increased when cost ceilings are imposed. If the ceiling is uniform throughout the state, it is difficult to see how a prospective rate differs from a flat rate at all. For example, between 1973 and 1977, California paid very low rates on a flat-rate basis. Those rates were determined by a statewide survey of the costs of a scientifically selected sample of nursing homes. A rather stringently defined average cost then became the rate. It was increased each year to account for inflation, although substantially more slowly than the actual inflation experienced by nursing home operators as purchasers of goods and services. Yet HEW agreed to accept that system as meeting the requirements for being "reasonable cost-related," so long as the cost survey is regularly updated and the inflation factor made more realistic.[17] Whether or not that interpretation complies with congressional intent is now being litigated, although given the scanty legislative history, it is hard to see how California can lose. But if it does, it can come into compliance with the law, as it is uniformly interpreted throughout the country, by simply redefining its rate as a "ceiling"—paying less than the ceiling to those facilities whose actual costs are less and only the ceiling amount to those whose costs are greater.

Even though ceilings appear to be inherently inimical to reimbursement on the basis of cost, there is no way to assure cost control without ceilings. California is an extreme case. Cost-related ceilings set at a relatively higher level can serve to create a reimbursement system that retains some of the efficiency incentives and cost-control characteristics of flat rates, while providing some of the quality-enhancement incentives of uncontrolled cost reimbursement.

Logically, the determination of the ceiling should be based on an explicit trade-off between the state's willingness to pay and the desire for quality enhancement. But considerable uncertainty surrounds that trade-off because, at any given ceiling, it is unclear whether those who exceed the ceiling do so because they are especially inefficient or because they are especially generous in the quality of services they provide. Each dollar the ceiling is raised produces something less than a dollar's worth of service improvement, but how much less can never be confidently predicted. Increasing the ceiling can mean the difference between hamburger and filet mignon, but it can also mean the difference between reusing edible leftovers and throwing them out.

So ceilings are set by statistical mumbo jumbo. The method used draws on the system that Medicare has been using to control what it will pay for physicians' fees—a method that was apparently adopted more for its simplicity and its failure to present an explicit political threat to physicians than anything else. The method, known as "profiling," consists of listing, in rank order, all physicians' fees for a given service in a geographic area, finding the 75th percentile, the point below which 75 percent of all fees fall, and calling that the "prevailing" charge. In theory, the "prevailing" level could be set at any percentile level about the 50th, arithmetical median.

There are two ways of constructing profiles to establish cost ceilings in nursing homes. Either the total "routine service costs" of all facilities can be profiled, with the ceiling then set at some percentile, or separate profiles can be constructed for each standard "cost center." In nursing homes, the customary centers are: nursing, dietary, housekeeping, laundry, administration, property cost, and "other."

The logic of profiling is that if 75 or 85 or 65 percent of facilities (however many are below the ceiling) can provide adequate services at those costs, then there should be no reason why others can't, and nothing unreasonable about penalizing those who do. The percentile ceiling becomes a norm, based to some degree on the actual performance of comparable facilities. How accurate a norm it is can be subject to question, especially when separate profiles are established for each cost center. If separate profiles are used, state ratemakers are forced to give credence not only to the total costs reported by facilities but also to the methods those facilities used to allocate costs among cost centers. Since there is no standardized system of accounting for nursing homes, that means that the entire rate structure is planted in a foundation of thin air. A facility may well exceed the norm for a given cost center, not because it is inefficient, but because its accountants use a more rational method for allocating costs than those employed by other facilities.

States can take a given percentile for each cost center, determine the dollar amount to which it is equivalent, and sum across cost centers, producing a single uniform cost ceiling, or they can take a given percentile as the cost ceiling for that cost center. The latter is a far more stringent limitation. Under a single facility rate, a nursing home with high costs in one cost center can remain under the limit by keeping costs down in another, while under individual cost-center ceilings, low costs in one area are not rewarded, while high costs in another are still penalized. Both methods require the same extent of reporting by facilities and the same degree of computation by the state, but the latter is more stringent.

As "reasonable cost-related" is now interpreted by HEW, states can also use the profiling system to set what are, for all intents and purposes, flat rates. Oklahoma, for example, profiles cost centers for all its nursing homes of a given type, sets its limits at the 60th percentile, sums the 60th percentile for all cost centers, rounds to the nearest convenient number, and produces a "cost-related" flat rate.[18] That rate provides a much greater cost-minimization incentive than an identically equivalent *ceiling* that does not permit operators to keep all savings below the ceiling.

However detailed the cost data or sophisticated the states' computations, the critical determinant of how high rates will be under a profiling system is where the percentile cutoff is set. That decision is left largely to the states' discretion, subject to negotiations with budget officials and industry representatives. The notion of a reimbursement "system" might imply that the percentile level is determined on some rational criterion and is kept fixed over time, but there is no effective way of ensuring that states will not monkey with the level whenever they feel budgetary pressure.

In some states, the system of profile-generated ceilings is further complicated by the groupings of facilities into separate classes. Costs tend to vary depending on the size of the facility and particularly as a function of geographical location: doing business in inner cities is often more expensive than in rural areas. Grouping methods attempt to comply with the Aristotelian dictum that like cases be treated alike and unlike cases unlike. But it is often far from certain which cases are like and which are unlike. So when grouping systems do not serve to simply ratify what are essentially uncontrolled full-cost rates (as they do for hospitals under Medicare), they are inherently somewhat arbitrary. For example, facilities in the suburban fringes of metropolitan areas might be classified as either urban or rural, and there is not that much cost difference between a 99-bed and a 101-bed nursing home. One particularly ingenious device, adopted in some states and urged on others by the American Association of Homes for the Aging (AAHA) (the trade association of nonprofit homes) is to group non-profit homes separately, so as not to penalize them for their tradition-ally higher costs and in order to finesse some of the problems raised for them by reimbursement for profits.

The original regulations issued by HEW permitted profit only as a return on net invested equity in the facility.[19] That definition reflected an almost ritualistic commitment to the application of theoretical mar-ket economics in the regulation of public utilities, where allowable profit has always been defined as a return on capital sufficient to per-mit the utility to attract investment from the private money market.[20] HEW's attempt to apply this principle to nursing homes raised a major political storm, and extensive litigation quickly ensued.[21]

Proprietary interests strongly objected to limiting profit to a return on net equity because the industry is very highly leveraged, and many operators have little, or no, equity in their facilities. Many of those op-erators made very nice profits under flat-rate systems and were under-standably upset at the prospect of seeing their profits evaporate.

In addition, serious questions were raised as to whether nonprofit facilities could be permitted profits under such a system. Many states appeared unwilling to pay nonprofit facilities any return on capital, following the Medicare system, which, since its inception, has reim-bursed proprietary facilities for foregone earnings on invested capital but has not permitted a return on capital for voluntary facilities. Vol-untary nursing homes and their representatives complained that due to inflation, philanthropic contributions pay for only a diminishing fraction of construction costs, and that failure to permit them a return on investment would make it increasingly difficult for them to generate funds for new construction. At a minimum, they sought redefinition to profit as a "growth allowance" in which they would be permitted to share.

Limiting profit to a return on equity would appear to vitiate the ability of rate mechanisms to provide incentives for efficiency. In classical market theory, this problem does not arise because competition among producers spurs them to the most efficient production. In public utility theory, a somewhat similar role is served by the availability of, and potential shift of customers to, substitute services. Because government is the primary consumer in the market for nursing home services and does not make its consumption decisions on the basis of comparative prices, such competitive forces are almost entirely absent. Some other incentive for efficiency is needed.

HEW quickly backed down and now permits profits as an efficiency reward under quasi-flat rates or prospective-cost rates.[22]

The Costs of Costs

For a decade, policymakers and analysts have refined, legislated, and regulated nursing home reimbursement. But they have had little success, either in controlling the rate of cost inflation or in inducing institutions to behave more in the way they want them to behave. Cost-based reimbursement has led to higher rates, but whether it has attained any of the qualitative objectives that provided its original rationale remains in question.

The apparent failure of reimbursement mechanisms to achieve their objectives is particularly puzzling because two phenomena on which they are based appear to have validity. Costs rise to the level of reimbursement. And health care institutions tend not to do things for which they are not reimbursed. The logic of reimbursement incentives is impeccable. But in practice, the improvements in efficiency or service that the reimbursement mechanisms are supposed to induce aren't realized. Much of the reason for this failure lies in the process of reimbursement itself.

Ratemaking is cumbersome and complicated and becomes even

more so with each new set of incentives built as "refinements" into the reimbursement system. Cost reports must be checked, audited, then keypunched; computer programs must be written; and statistical analyses performed. Provision must be made for appeals and revisions. Cost-reporting is expensive, especially for enterprises as small as nursing homes. Prior to the adoption of cost-based reimbursement, most facilities did not employ standardized accounting practices and most states had no detailed cost information from nursing homes. Basic reporting and accounting conventions had to be defined largely from scratch.

There is also an important time dimension to reimbursement systems, especially when the rates are set prospectively. Rates for, say, 1978, are generally based on costs for 1976, as reported in 1977. But if the auditing of 1976 cost reports has not been completed, or an appeal has been filed about 1977 rates, then the 1978 rate may be provisional—if it is issued before the beginning of the year at all. The "prospective" rate may not be known until the year is part over. Further, it may well be mid–1978 before final determination of all the appeals and disputes from 1975 are concluded, and those decisions affect the 1976 cost "base," and in turn the 1978 rates. And so on and so on, ad infinitum.

It is dubious whether incentives so deeply mired in complexity and uncertainty can even work. Prices are supposed to be "signals" to sellers. But in cost-based reimbursement, the signals get distorted by the system's own static. Health care reimbursement systems provide extensive employment for lawyers, accountants, and consultants, while confusing the hell out of everyone. Ratemaking becomes a kind of baroque dance in which each new accounting step concocted by the industry is countered by the issuance of new, deliberately opaque regulations by state ratemakers, which must often be interpreted by courts or appeals boards. While that process is going on, the state may autonomously decide to change the rules.

So the dream that cost-based reimbursement could reduce the "political" content of rate-setting decisions has been thoroughly disappointed. Lacking objective criteria for such critical issues as where cost ceilings should be set or how facilities should be grouped, or even what "costs" are for the purposes of cost reimbursement, decisions must be made arbitrarily. In conditions of such uncertainty, the state will attempt to make those arbitrary decisions in ways that limit its budgetary liability while keeping as many facilities in the program as possible; nursing homes will use the threat of withdrawing from the program to influence those decisions to increase their profits or otherwise make their lives easier. When budgetary problems become acute, states will simply change the system to save themselves money. At all times, nursing homes will behave in accordance with the dictum that any system can be beat and devote much of their managerial effort, not to patient care, but to beating the system.

The difficulty of defining quality remains a critical element. Since they can't specify precisely what they are seeking to buy, states specify surrogates, like hours of nursing time, for which they are willing to pay. Some nursing homes then shift administrative or dietary duties onto nursing personnel, while others expand their nursing services and reduce other professional services. Overall rates increase, but no one knows whether overall quality is increasing as well.

As part of the process of adopting new rate systems to comply with the 1972 Social Security amendments, many states sought to more directly incorporate quality "incentives" in their reimbursement systems. Because of the difficulties of measurement and definition, most failed to get past the talking stage. Those devices that have been adopted by some states are either merely symbolic or grounded in dubious logic. New York has separate groupings with separate cost ceilings for each of four classes of nursing homes as determined by quality ratings, but those ratings are so crude that something like 80 percent of all facilities fall into the second highest class. Michigan attaches specific rate penalties to specified violations of state regulatory standards, but that process really constitutes only the incorporation of fines into rates. Illinois now ties rates to an elaborate system of patient assessment, with higher rates for facilities with sicker residents, but lacks the resources to ensure either that patients are being classified accurately or that extra funds are really spent on those with the greatest needs.[23]

Because no one can adequately define quality, no one knows what high quality services should cost. Similarly, the precise incentives that will induce qualitative improvement remain unknown, along with the appropriate *level* of rates. To some degree, this ignorance is not accidental. States have avoided learning the costs of high quality service since they were afraid that those costs would be substantially higher than they were accustomed to paying. If a figure were ascertained at which high quality could be provided efficiently, the states would be pressured to pay those rates, even when they had no way of assuring that the money would be efficiently spent on patient care. The arbitrariness of cost-based reimbursement systems is substantially aggravated by the absence of a target at which the states could shoot. Without a target, it is impossible to tell how plausible the figures cranked out of the computers are. The only standard of comparison is last year's rate, but no one knows how realistic that was.

The Utility of Utilities

Given the increasing complexities of the rate-setting process, the extent to which it is tied to the ostensible costs of production and the degree of borrowing from public utility economics it employs, the argument is often made that nursing homes have de facto become public utilities and that phenomenon should be legitimated by the creation of a formal system of utility regulation for them. This argument coincides with the development of utility-style regulation for hospitals, in which nursing homes have often been lumped willy-nilly. In both Maryland and Massachusetts, independent state rate-setting commissions, modeled closely on those that regulate gas and electricity, set Medicaid and other rates for both hospitals and nursing homes, as would also be the case under legislation pending in California. In Connecticut, an independent hospital rate commission sets private rates for nursing homes, while the state retains control over Medicaid.

The soundest reason for imposing utility-style regulation on nursing homes has received relatively little attention. Utilities are customarily required to act as "common carriers," that is, to provide service to all comers. A common-carrier requirement would strike directly at the problem of provider participation, which is serious for nursing homes. But it would do so at a price—higher rates for public charges. Only Minnesota, which sets rates administratively, not through a utility commission, has adopted such a common-carrier requirement.

One of the curious aspects of the movement for utility-style regulation of health facilities is that it coincides with a period of intense criticism of traditional utility regulation and the movement for "deregulation" of airline fares, railroads, and natural gas. But a far more serious criticism can be made of the application of the utility model to nursing homes. In no industry regulated through independent commissions does government have anything approaching a 75 pecent market share. Permitting such commissions to establish rates that states would then be obligated to pay would constitute a substantial cession of governmental sovereignty. When states are legally obligated, as under Medicaid, to provide certain services to certain citizens, assignment of a rate-setting function to an independent body gives that body a right to create claims on the public budget.

The rationale for utility regulation has always been the need to protect the public from the potentially excessive market power of the suppliers of essential commodities. But governments occupy a potentially dominant position in the nursing home market and are presumably there in the first place to fulfill their duty to serve the public interest. Of course, governments do not always behave in the best interests of the "public." Still, it is doubtful that public responsibility can be assured by diffusing it through the rate-setting process.

To some extent, this logic can be applied to rate-setting methodologies even when they are employed by administrative arms of the state executive. Promulgation of a formal reimbursement system, under the constitutions and administrative procedure acts of most states, obligates those states to follow the methodology regardless of budgetary consequences and to leave some important budgetary decisions to judicial interpretations of ratemaking rules. Sellers should be entitled to protection against arbitrary or capricious behavior by governmental buyers, but sovereignty must be lodged somewhere, and in this country there is a long tradition of requiring a direct chain of responsibility between the use of tax revenues and publicly elected representatives.

Governments rarely effectively exercise their enormous potential power in the nursing home services market. One reason is that government as buyer needs sellers and must commit itself to certain terms and practices in order to establish enough predictability and regularity in the market. It cannot be a totally arbitrary sovereign and still find people willing to do business with it, and it is constrained by rules and regulations about competitive bidding, equal treatment of sellers, and the provision of appeals and arbitration procedures when sellers feel aggrieved. But in other ways, governments may often constrain their market power more than they really need to, or should.

Governments as buyers often make themselves excessively dependent, for example, on too small a number of suppliers. If there is a single buyer, it is to that buyer's advantage to have excess capacity among suppliers, since that will motivate competition for the buyer's business. When monopsony (a market with a single buyer) deteriorates to bilateral monopoly (one buyer, one seller), the buyer is no better off than it would be in a competitive marketplace. But excess capacity among suppliers may be expensive in the short run, and governments often act shortsightedly. So when Lockheed faced bankruptcy, the government had nowhere else to go to buy extremely large jet cargo planes, which it believed it couldn't live without, and thus had to bail out Lockheed.

If there were excess capacity in the nursing home industry, governments could penalize the lowest quality, or most expensive, by cutting off their flow of Medicaid patients. It could experiment with competitive bidding, in which facilities would agree to offer a specified level of services and bid against one another on the basis of price.[24] These ideas are now being experimented with in the hospital sector, where there is considerable excess capacity, but they run afoul of the provisions in both Medicare and Medicaid that those programs not constrain the "freedom of choice" of beneficiaries to pick their suppliers of service. The "freedom of choice" requirements can be waived, or legislatively changed, but governments will have to incur marginally higher costs in the short run to reduce their long-run liability. But governments budget and plan in one- or four-year cycles, so it is likely that reimbursement systems will continue to penalize low occupancy rates in order to save money in the short run, even when low occupancy leads sellers to be much more compliant with the interests of the buyer.

The other possible market response to excessive reliance on a single seller is vertical integration. Rather than permitting themselves to become too dependent on the supplier of a single essential product or service, private firms, to the extent they are permitted by the Antitrust Division of the Justice Department, will seek a merger to bring the supplier more fully under control. But vertical integration in government-purchased services would mean "nationalization" and would run afoul of the ideological and political enmity to public enterprise in the United States.

It would be greatly to the advantage of governments, in their role as buyers of nursing home services, to "nationalize" a small fraction of the industry. These facilities could then serve as "yardsticks" against which private-sector performance could be evaluated. In light of the general ignorance of governments about what it really costs to provide decent nursing home services, the availability of such yardsticks could be particularly important.

There are a number of publicly operated nursing homes, but they are invariably run by agencies and programs different from those that pay for services in private facilities. Something like 600 counties and municipalities still operate nursing homes (many the descendants of county poor farms), many states have veterans' homes, and the Veterans Administration (VA) has its own nursing home system. But because of continued prejudices against publicly operated facilities, most service a very different market from that of the private nursing homes and have only limited utility as yardsticks. Except for the VA system, government-operated nursing homes exist primarily as providers of last resort, serving those clients no private facility will accept. This role precludes public-private competition and does nothing to loosen government dependence on sellers.

Uncle Sam the Buying Man

Governments are only just beginning to recognize that they are buyers of nursing home services. Payments to nursing homes under Medicare and Medicaid are recorded as "in-kind transfer payments" to program beneficiaries. Vendor payments have been regarded as a form of social insurance.

The vendor-payment system originated in reaction to the inferior services provided directly by governments (in public almshouses or hospitals) and to the stigma attached to those institutions. Medicare or Medicaid beneficiaries were to receive the same services as those who had private means. Payment to the facility would be made by the government, on behalf of the beneficiary, at a price negotiated in advance.

But when 75 percent of the consumers are beneficiaries, the logic behind vendor payments falls apart. Even when a smaller percentage of services is paid for by government, the availability of government funds expended on behalf of those whose resources would otherwise be substantially limited increases demand and changes the market.

Yet governments have not yet begun to buy nursing home (or hospital) services in the way they buy paper clips or jet planes. There is no comparison between a typical government procurement contract and a typical "provider agreement" between a state Medicaid agency and a nursing home. The contract obligates the supplier to specific performance standards, whereas a provider agreement, almost without exception, contains neither performance standards nor penalties for nonfulfillment. The state has the option not to renew the provider agreement, but there is little in the way of intermediate sanctions available. In theory, the nursing home is required to meet all the requirements of the state's licensing and health codes, but the separation of the enforcement from the purchasing function seriously limits their enforceability.

In most government bureaucracies, the purchasing function is separated from program activities to provide an internal check on program officials who look too kindly on those selling goods or services to them. But Medicaid, reflecting its welfare origins, has been organized around beneficiaries and treats provider reimbursement as a claims-processing operation, which focuses on the validity of the individual claim rather than the overall performance of the "contractor." Until recently, most Medicaid agencies maintained their data-processing systems in such a way as to make information on providers literally irretrievable. Yet it has been the providers who have cashed the checks.

This failure to recognize the government as a buyer has resulted in increased irresponsibility in the expenditure of public funds not only for nursing homes and Medicaid but in the increasing provision of "in-kind" benefits ranging from day-care services to job-training subsidies.

Private Uses of the Public Interest

Of the three objectives for nursing home payment systems listed earlier (cost control, minimal quality assurance, and adequate provider participation) cost-based vendor-payment reimbursement systems can accomplish only the last. The reasons are clear. There is the difficulty of specifying the components of quality, or the relationship between quality and expenditures, in sufficient detail to be incorporated into reimbursement incentives. There is the failure of governments to take advantage of their potential monopsony power. And there is the inherent weakness of "incentives" in a market dominated by an ineffective monopsonist.

When the "discipline" of the market is lacking, as it is in the market for nursing homes, the response to reimbursement incentives may not produce the results desired. Bonuses for caring for sicker residents may induce operators to make residents sicker, either on paper or in fact. Penalties for low occupancy rates may cause administrators to admit people who don't need to be institutionalized. Higher rates for extra nursing services may turn nurses into tray-passers. If consumers were more discriminating, or quality more easily measured, market forces would make those sorts of responses counterproductive for nursing homes, but neither of those conditions hold.

Theoretically, greater "market" competition could be introduced into the nursing home industry. States could remove restrictions on "entry" created by licensing laws and code requirements. States could forbid facilities to have more than, say, 80 percent Medicaid residents and set Medicaid rates so that attracting private patients was necessary in order to break even—presumably, facilities would then compete on the basis of quality.[25] Or states could distribute Medicaid provider agreements through competitive bidding. The first two solutions founder on the shoals of quality assessment, the third on "freedom of choice" for beneficiaries. To make any of these three proposals work, it would be necessary to create a system of incentives just as complicated, arbitrary, and cumbersome as regulatory processes are now. The problems of quality and consumer choice remain.

Champions of incentives over regulation claim that incentives involve "automatic" and "spontaneous" market adjustments while regulation entails red tape and bureaucracy. But the attempt to induce desired performance by reimbursement incentives results in all the complications and distortions attributed to regulation. It is also ineffective.

While quality cannot be readily defined or measured, it can to some degree be regulated. It just cannot be regulated through reimbursement. That, in turn, would seem to imply that much of the effort devoted to even more complicated systems of reimbursement has, at best, been wasted.

Prior to 1978, California, Connecticut, and Oklahoma all employed something like flat rates to reimburse nursing homes under Medicaid. The California and Connecticut systems have been briefly described. Oklahoma's was even simpler; each year, the head of the state's Medicaid agency would sit down with industry representatives and negotiate a rate. Connecticut's rates under the pre-1978 system were relatively high, though much lower than in neighboring New York or Massachusetts. California's were relatively low, and Oklahoma's still lower (costs in Oklahoma are especially low). None of those states had a provider participation problem. In all three, nursing homes made comfortable profits. And the quality of services was at least comparable to national norms. (Connecticut has long had a reputation for having some of the best nursing homes in the nation.) In terms of the objectives of reimbursement systems, those three states had systems that worked relatively well.

The conclusion speaks for itself. Government should seek the best deals it can bargain for—which might look strikingly like flat rates—armed with good information on what costs would be, and reinforced by stringent regulation. The fact that a reimbursement system embodies a set of incentives does not mean that "ideal" incentives can be designed or made to work. We might be better served if government policy was made and implemented not by Ph.Ds in economics, but by grandmothers employing the skills they practice at the butcher's.

5

Building Capacity

IN 1963, there were just over half a million nursing home beds in the United States. There are now more than a million and a quarter, a net increase of almost 800,000. The total number of new beds constructed over the past fifteen years is probably more than a million, as it can be estimated that half of the beds in place in 1963 have since been closed.

Although detailed financial data are unavailable, it can also be estimated that construction of those million beds cost between $8 billion and $10 billion. Ten billion dollars is a relatively small percentage of the total volume of contract construction in that period, but it is still a sizable sum. Most of that investment has been repaid—in at least some instances many times over—by public funds, but almost all of it was raised initially from private sources of capital influenced strongly by government policy.

In one sense, this construction of nursing home capacity constitutes the most dramatic and impressive success of public policy toward nursing homes. Public officials throughout the last two decades have sought to increase the supply and to improve the quality of nursing homes. If nothing else, the United States now has a substantial number of relatively new, modern, fire-resistant nursing homes. Figure 1 depicts that rapidity with which this change was accomplished.

This construction was not wrought without substantial costs, of which the dollar expenditures were only a part. Methods of capital formation and capital financing have had a substantial impact on the character of the nursing home industry: on the kinds of people who

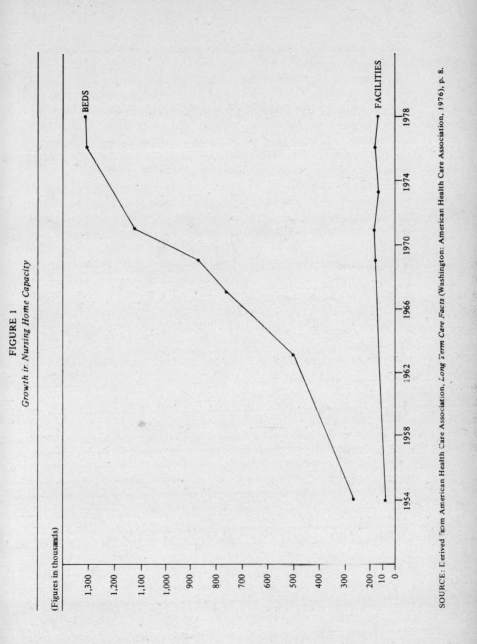

FIGURE 1

Growth in Nursing Home Capacity

(Figures in thousands)

SOURCE: Derived from American Health Care Association, *Long Term Care Facts* (Washington: American Health Care Association, 1976), p. 8.

own and manage nursing homes, on the services they provide, on the substance as well as the structure of day-to-day life in nursing homes. Put most simply, real estate speculation and the provision of services to the dependent elderly do not mix well.

Government involvement in private capital formation in the nursing home industry has taken three forms: reimbursement of capital expenses as part of the general process of Medicaid/Medicare reimbursement; indirect money-market policies, primarily loan or mortgage guarantees; and, more recently, controls on entry through limitations on the construction of new facilities. That mixture of policy tools has produced less than desirable effects.

Americans are hostile to notions of economic planning by governments, and there is substantially less formal economic planning in this nation than in most other industrial societies. But somewhere along the line, people who did not think of themselves as being engaged in economic planning at all made decisions that rechanneled at least some fraction of the nation's economic growth into the construction of nursing homes. Much of the American landscape is now occupied by hospitals, universities, nursing homes, and other institutions owned by private entities but constructed in response to public "investment" decisions. Whether for good or ill, those decisions have preempted at least a part of the nation's economic future.

Moms and Pops

The earliest proprietary nursing homes were almost all small enterprises founded with the personal capital—more in the form of housing than of cash—of the operators. Typically, a woman, sometimes with nursing or similar training, would provide "nursing home" services within her own residence. As demand increased, profits were often reinvested into the construction or acquisition of additional space. In the waning years of the depression, housing was cheap, and there was a plentiful supply of older dwellings with many rooms.

Up until World War II, most proprietary nursing homes provided for no more than a handful of residents (a big nursing home was one with more than a dozen beds) and were staffed by the immediate family of the operator. The capital stock of these "mom and pop" enterprises had been purchased almost entirely from the savings, and then the profits, of those families and could not have amounted to very much. External financing was almost totally unavailable.[1]

The postwar economic boom, combined with the continued growth of the elderly population in need of specialized long-term care and the continued expansion of OAA, permitted many of these family enterprises to expand, a substantial number using GI bill benefits for loans to purchase additional housing which was immediately converted into new nursing home capacity. But sometime in the immediate postwar period, newcomers, whose primary initial concern was real estate speculation, entered the industry. Not much is known in detail about how they entered, but a plausible description can be provided.

The process worked roughly as follows: speculators found themselves holding white elephants (houses bought in the expectation of urban renewal that could not be rented to meet short-term expenses, or houses that were simply unsalable because of their size or deterioration) or they bought abandoned institutional buildings on the cheap in the expectation that they could always figure out something to do with them. Nursing homes, which required very little additional investment to convert to income-generating properties, and which promised a reliable and predictable cash flow, became an attractive proposition. Local welfare agencies were desperate to find beds for disabled OAA recipients and were relatively undiscriminating about the condition of those beds. No special skill or professional training was needed to establish a nursing home.[2]

This kind of speculative activity appeared more or less spontaneously in a number of cities and remained on a very small scale into the early 1950s. Among the first speculators were the Bergmans, Hollanders, Kossows, and others most responsible for giving the industry a bad name.[3] The development of such speculative activity in nursing homes began to open up avenues for more substantial flows of risk capital, and, because real estate speculation is so highly leveraged a process, the first large-scale infusion of borrowed funds.

After 1950, this process accelerated. The initiation of vendor payments increased the funds available to pay for nursing home care and meant that welfare agencies were paying providers directly, assuring the regularity of payment and giving the providers an identifiable political entity with which to bargain for rates and on which to exert pressure, increasing opportunities for legal and illegal graft. The boom in hospital construction meant the abandonment of many outmoded hospital buildings, which were available cheap and readily convertible to nursing home use.[4] And the economic prosperity of the Korean War era provided a lot of small businessmen with surplus funds they were eager to invest.

Meanwhile, the first wave of increased government regulation following the enactment of state licensing laws in response to the 1950 Social Security amendments began to drive some of the "moms and pops" out of business. Compliance with these laws often required capital outlays, for improvement, say, in sanitation or ventilation, or increased managerial skills, which older operators were unable to supply. Other entrepreneurs offered those services in exchange for part-ownership or bought the original proprietors out entirely. The pattern of interlocking ownership (full and partial) dominated by a few individuals that would eventually characterize the industry in some areas began to take shape.[5]

Among those supplying capital in this period were individuals associated with organized crime. For obvious reasons, no one has very much concrete information about the role of organized crime in the industry, but some things are clear. When potentially profitable industries need capital that cannot be obtained from more conventional sources, loan-sharking tends to flourish, and loan sharks have a way of moving in on borrowers and taking over their businesses. Over the past several decades, organized crime interests have eagerly sought to invest surplus cash in "legitimate" business enterprises. Nursing homes would have been an obvious avenue. There is some documented evidence of nursing home ownership by individuals with relationships to organized crime;[6] although the pattern cannot be regarded as pervasive, structural conditions in the industry were attractive to organized crime interests and individuals with similar economic motivation. Most of the criminals in the nursing home industry have, however, been independents.

By the mid-1950s, the predominant pattern of ownership of the proprietary nursing home industry was still very small and fragmented, capitalization was extremely thin, and margins were very low. Most facilities had originally been built to serve some other purpose, and their owners had little background or formal training in anything related to health services or care of geriatric patients. Yet the demand for nursing home care was very great and growing rapidly.

In contrast to the proprietary sector, voluntary and public facilities played a passive role. Had they worked at it, voluntary agencies could have captured a far larger share of the growing market for nursing home services. But they weren't very interested. Sources of capital probably played a central role, since debt financing was largely unavailable and philanthropy tended to be directed to other places. Most charitable homes for the aged remained very small, independent enterprises, disinclined to merge with or cooperate with one another.

Hill-Burton funds for nursing home construction became available to hospitals after 1954, but the voluntary hospitals were indifferent. There wasn't that much money to begin with, and the physicians and trustees who controlled hospital affairs were not interested in long-term care. Many more chronic-disease hospitals used public funds to convert to acute-care hospitals than acute-care hospitals built long-term facilities. It is widely believed that much of the money that was provided to hospitals under the Hill-Burton program for construction of nursing home beds was eventually subverted to acute-care use.[7]

There was some hope in the early 1950s that local governments, which were eligible for Hill-Burton funds, would reenter the long-term care market in a significant way, either by converting what was left of county almshouses or hospitals into nursing homes or by building new ones. In a few states, notably Minnesota, the counties took up the challenge, but there was substantial, general hostility to publicly owned enterprise, and local governments had far more pressing priorities for capital spending. With voluntary homes for the aged too small and too poorly managed to respond, and hospitals and local governments uninterested, filling the growing demand for nursing home services was left largely to the proprietary sector.

Opening the Gates

The real boom in nursing home construction did not begin until the late 1950s and early 1960s, with the opening up of conventional capital markets to private entrepreneurs. The first step in that process was the 1956 legislation authorizing the Small Business Administration (SBA) to make either direct or "participation" loans to proprietary nursing homes. An even more important stimulus was the availability, after 1959, of FHA mortgage insurance for the purchase of new nursing home facilities.

While SBA loans were initially limited to only $100,000, they could be used for renovation and working capital as well as for new construction, and in the late 1950s they were readily available in much of the country. Since many of the SBA loans were "participation" loans in which local banks or other financial institutions took a share, they constituted the first nursing home industry access to those institutions.[8] Banks show remarkable inertia: they are reluctant to lend money to new borrowers; but so long as accepted borrowers repay their loans, banks are likely to keep lending to them, regardless of how much their ability to repay may change. Moreover, while it was not supposed to happen, some enterprising entrepreneurs were able to use the proceeds of SBA loans as down payments to obtain additional mortgages. In 1959, $100,000 could but a twenty-five-bed nursing home; when leveraged, it could permit the purchase of a fifty- or sixty-bed facility.

SBA loans were limited to "small businesses," with annual revenues of less than $1 million. The program thus encouraged new operators to enter the business—and old operators to form dummy corporations—and perpetuated a pattern of small and independent nursing homes.

Because of the stringent dollar limitations and their applicability to improvements on existing facilities, SBA loans had nowhere near the impact of the FHA program, which insured mortgages from conventional lenders for the construction and purchase of *new* facilities.[9] Since its beginning, the FHA has insured more than $1.2 billion in nursing home mortgages, accounting for more than 120,000 beds, roughly 10 percent of the national total.[10] Moreover, the impact of the FHA nursing home program is substantially understated by the volume of mortgages directly guaranteed since the availability of guarantees encouraged lenders to write mortgages even when the insurance was not provided. The FHA mortgage insurance programs set inertial lenders into motion, and they tend to remain in motion, even without additional impetus.[11]

Because FHA mortgages were available for up to 90 percent of project cost, they reinforced the pattern of extremely thin capitalization in the nursing home industry. They also encouraged another new class of entrepreneurs to enter the industry. These were builders who quickly caught on to the large profits that could be made from owning nursing homes. In addition, those "mom and pop" operations that had managed to hold on until the early 1960s were able, for the first time, to get mortgage money to replace or expand their old facilities. Once mortgages were more freely available, nursing home investments also became an attractive tax shelter for physicians, who could readily qualify for nursing home licenses, provide the facilities with an assured flow of patients, write off interest and depreciation as a tax loss, and bury the profits.[12]

Appreciating Depreciation

The availability of 90 percent low-cost mortgages, along with generous tax treatment of commercial property investment, high occupancy rates, limited regulatory stringency, and expectations of future growth, all combined in the early 1960s to create a boom in nursing home construction. That boom accelerated with the reimbursement principles adopted by Medicare after 1965. Although Medicare never paid for that large a proportion of nursing home days, it was widely expected that it would, and its principles set the tone for all other reimbursement systems and the setting of private charges for self-pay patients.

As already noted, Congress required Medicare to pay health facilities their reasonable costs and then left the process of defining "reasonable" to a series of committees organized by the Bureau of Health Insurance. Within those committees, the most hotly debated issue was the definition of capital costs.

Traditional, pre-Medicare methods of cost-based reimbursement for hospitals had allowed inclusion of interest payments as a cost but had never recognized depreciation. In conventional accounting practices, depreciation (the "consumption" of tangible assets) has long been considered a cost of doing business. But third-party payers in the hospital sector contended that the physical plant of nonprofit hospitals was a community resource, built with the philanthropic contributions of the community. Since the assets "belonged," in some sense, to the community, it would not be justifiable to compensate the hospital for the using up of those assets. The American Hospital Association pushed very hard for inclusion of depreciation in the Medicare cost formula; it also pushed for inclusion of accelerated depreciation. It succeeded on both counts.[13]

Under the original Medicare regulations, a hospital or nursing home that built a new facility with an expected life of forty years could be reimbursed in the first year of operation for 3.75 percent (150 percent of straight-line depreciation) of the total cost of the facility as depreciation, plus the entire interest cost of whatever bonds or mortgages had been used to finance the construction. Because, under most conventional mortgages, payments in the early years are mostly interest, with little amortization, this meant that the reimbursement could well exceed what the institution had to pay out on its mortgage. Even more important, it meant that construction of new facilities could essentially be paid for through reimbursement. Lenders were not unaware of this phenomenon, and so the credit markets opened wide to health care facilities.

Reimbursement of depreciation for voluntary hospitals was justified on the grounds that depreciation funds would permit hospitals to reproduce themselves as they became obsolete, thus perpetuating vital social institutions, but it had different implications for proprietary nursing homes. Through reimbursement for depreciation, profit-seeking nursing home investors would be repaid the entire cost of their investment plus a return on actual invested equity, while retaining ownership of the facility, and the right to resell it for a capital gain. In short, the government would gradually buy the nursing home from the lender—and then give it to the investor. And that worked for even the most naive and scrupulous investors; with a little larceny, the investor could arrange to have the government buy the facility two or three times over.

Still, Medicare's reimbursement principles were also successful in encouraging growth in nonprofit nursing homes. The market share of voluntary nursing homes had fallen throughout the 1950s and 1960s. Since the onset of Medicare, the number and capacity of nonprofit nursing homes have grown steadily, and the proportion of nonprofit beds in the industry as a whole has also increased. Philanthropy no longer had to raise the total construction cost for a new facility; with banks, bond underwriters, and insurance companies willing to provide debt capital, all that was needed was the down payment.

Speculation and Peculation

The sources of debt capital for profit and nonprofit nursing homes have differed somewhat: proprietaries have relied more heavily on mortgages from conventional mortgage lenders such as savings and loans or savings banks, while many of the nonprofits have used the private placement of bonds or notes. Both have relied on private markets.[14] But if the sources of financing for nursing homes construction have been essentially conventional, little else has been. In the proprietary sector, capital development has been dominated by real estate speculation.

When a family or a firm invests in buildings and real estate, it makes a long-term commitment. Land and buildings last a long time and produce whatever economic "benefits" they offer over time. Acquisition of a house or a factory entails foregoing the use of liquid assets (cash) at the present time (by using them for down payment, front-end interests costs, and so forth) in the expectation that the fixed asset (the building) will produce value (housing, productive capacity) in the future.

The essence of real estate speculation is a desire to capture profits sooner, not later. The speculator is less concerned with the life of the property than with the income it can generate in the short term. Typically, he seeks to *withdraw* value from fixed assets and turn them into cash. The vital ingredient is the availability of debt, because his concern is not with a "bottom line" surplus of assets over liabilities but with cash flow.

In the simplest case, picture a speculator who constructs a 100-bed nursing home at a total cost of $1 million. He invests $100,000 of his own in cash and obtains mortgage financing for the remaining 90 percent, on a twenty-five-year (flat payment, amortizing) mortgage at 9 percent. The first year's mortgage payments come to $90,633, of which 89 percent is interest and the rest amortization. All interest payments are tax deductible. So is depreciation, on an accelerated schedule, because since 1954 the Internal Revenue Code has sheltered real estate investment for commercial property. To encourage such investment, it permits a tax deduction greater than actual outlays. Under existing law, assuming a forty-year useful life for the facility, 3.75 percent of its entire value, or $37,500, is deductible depreciation expense under the tax code. The first year's tax deduction ($80,600 interest plus $37,500 depreciation) equals $118,100, $27,500 more than the mortgage payment. In a 50 percent tax bracket, that is a gain of $13,750—the "shelter" aspect of the investment.

If the nursing home operates under cost-related reimbursement or its equivalent, both the interest and the depreciation are returned through Medicare and Medicaid payments. A conservative, nonspeculative owner, concerned with the long-term well-being of the nursing home as an income-producing asset, might put these depreciation payments and the tax savings from the deduction of depreciation into a special savings account, since some day he may have to start amortizing the facility or begin making repairs or saving to build a new one. A more conventional investor might reinvest the cash in the facility or a new one. But the speculative owner will take the $37,500 in reimbursed depreciation expense and put it in his personal bank account while sheltering an equal amount of his other income with the depreciation tax deduction. In other words, he will withdraw value from the property. Still, another way of describing that process is to say that the speculator has reduced his equity in the property from $100,000 to $62,500 or that his cash flow (assuming that the original $100,000 investment was the previous year) is $37,500 depreciation plus (assuming a 50 percent tax bracket) $18,750 in tax savings, minus the $10,000 in amortization of the mortgage, for a total of $46,250.[15]

This cannot last. Before very long, generally five to seven years, amortization of a mortgage exceeds depreciation, so that the speculator would have to put more cash into the facility than he is taking out; unless he sells or refinances. Conventionally, when real property changes hands, depreciation begins all over again, with the price at which it was sold determining the amount to be depreciated. The trick for the speculator is never to put cash *into* the facility, to withdraw as much as possible in the early years of a mortgage, and to sell it as soon as the cash flow threatens to turn negative. In some fundamental economic sense, the facility has less value than when he bought it since he has withdrawn the depreciation. But in a period of inflation, with increasing demand for nursing homes and a market artificially inflated by phony transactions, he will probably get far more than he paid, adding a substantial capital gain to the positive cash flow he has experienced for five to seven years.

Nursing homes change hands, or appear to change hands, with alarming rapidity. In California and Texas, to take two examples, it is estimated that 10 percent of all homes are sold or resold each year.[16] Medicare and Medicaid will no longer reimburse accelerated depreciation, and regulators have become increasingly picky about assuring that sales prices reflect real market values, rather than artificially inflated prices, but the tax advantages for accelerated depreciation remain, and the unwillingness of operators to put cash into their facilities by amortizing mortgages appears still to be strong.

This discussion has assumed a totally unsophisticated speculator. The real fun comes with a few simple refinements. The first involves the question of valuation. To return to the hypothetical nursing home constructed at a cost of $1 million, assume that the builder finances it with a construction loan which he repays by selling the completed facility to himself for $1.5 million. Banks do not assess the value of commercial property on the basis of construction cost but on a combination of market price and earning potential. ("Market price" assumes a true market transaction, so if the builder sells the facility to himself he will do so through a dummy corporation.)

In such a transaction, the builder can pocket an immediate profit of $500,000 while obtaining a mortgage of 90 percent of the inflated value, with its correspondingly inflated depreciation. Five to seven years later, he resells—with any luck, for $2 to $2.5 million. If he wishes to continue operating the facility, he will sell it to a friend seeking a tax shelter and lease it back on a net lease that converts all his capital expenses to (deductible, reimbursable) operating expenses. Or instead of selling he can refinance, using a second mortgage to cash in on any appreciation in the "market" value of the facility.

This process of selling, reselling, leasing, and refinancing was, for a while, limited only by entrepreneurial imagination and legal and accounting ingenuity.[17] At this writing, after four years of intensive effort, the special prosecutor for nursing homes in New York is still trying to disentangle nursing home ownership patterns, and there is no reason to believe that the pattern in New York is radically different from anywhere else. The apparent guarantees of an assured market, through Medicaid more than Medicare, made lending institutions more than happy to continue to provide the financing and less than rigorous about the assessment of valuation. Both individual entrepreneurs and corporate chains engage in this kind of trafficking, and both have taken their profits, not on the balance sheet but in after-tax cash flow.

A principal result has been that there is very little investment equity left in the proprietary side of the industry. In many instances, there is substantial *negative* net equity (more is owed on a facility than it is worth at a true market price). That negative net equity represents a part of the enormous profits that have been extracted from the real estate side of the nursing home industry over the past two decades. It also explains why much of the industry has been so bitterly opposed to limiting profit under reimbursement formulas to a return on net equity and why some parts of the industry have fought bitterly for a flat property reimbursement of $1 to $3 per bed per day.

This kind of speculation requires a steady increase in the market price for facilities (ultimately a function of the amount of revenue they can generate and thus of reimbursement practices). It also requires lenders that are prepared to finance sales and second mortgages. In just the past few years, things have begun to change in the nursing home industry, and real estate profits are increasingly hard to come by. The big money has been made, and many of the first generation of speculators are leaving.

These changes have come about as a result of New York nursing home scandals, in which real estate manipulation was a central focus of investigation. Reimbursement systems have been altered. Most state Medicaid plans are far more stringent in their treatment of depreciation than the IRS, and it is becoming increasingly difficult for owners of facilities whose market value, and concomitant mortgage load, was inflated by a decade of manipulation to find buyers. Many of those selling out are taking (tax deductible) paper losses.

The increasing stringency in regulation of all aspects of the nursing home industry has made it more difficult for operators to meet high mortgage payments and still maintain levels of service high enough to dissuade regulators from bringing sanctions against them. It is less possible than before to skimp on operating expenses. In many facilities, therefore, the cash flow has turned negative as operators are forced to put cash back into their facilities or risk defaulting on their mortgages.

While the windfall profits were nowhere near as great, substantial real estate speculation was still profitable in states employing flat-rate reimbursement systems and flourished to an extent nearly comparable to that in states employing cost-related reimbursement systems. Both the tax code and the failure to enforce qualitative standards (which permitted diversion of revenues from care to inflated mortgage payments) made this possible.

In New York State, in 1977, about a third of all proprietary nursing homes with mortgages held by savings banks or savings and loans were at least technically in default on their mortgage payments.[18] The simultaneous squeeze from regulatory and reimbursement mechanisms had gotten too great, and the resales market had dried up. News travels fast through the investment community, and mortgage money is now essentially unavailable for proprietary nursing homes in New York and surrounding states. Unless cost-related reimbursement turns out to be much more generous than anticipated, the drying up of mortgage money may well spread.

The Costs of Speculation

Enormous profits were made by many entrepreneurs in the nursing home industry, especially before the 1969-70 Medicare cutbacks. No data are available, but testimony before the New York State Moreland Act Commission, which investigated nursing homes, suggested that it was possible, under cost-related reimbursement, to generate a return on actual investment of 10 percent per *quarter* without doing anything at all illegal.[19] Anecdotal evidence describes entrepreneurs in almost every state who became millionaires on initial investments of only tens of thousands of dollars. No doubt there were many "moms and pops" who eschewed, or failed to understand, such fancy real estate techniques and who never made more than a comfortable living, and no one knows what typical profits for individual operators have been. But the money was there for the taking.

Lenders have also been well served by this process. Speculative activities involve risks for banks as well as for borrowers, but there is good reason to believe that the risks in lending to nursing homes were relatively low. There have been few bankruptcies in the nursing home industry, and while there have been some mortgage foreclosures, until recently banks have had no serious difficulty reselling foreclosed properties. Yet lenders charged interest rates to nursing homes comparable to those for riskier investments and financed a high proportion of total investment. Here, too, there was money to be made.

Profits are supposed to accrue to those who successfully meet public demand, and there is no question that the growth of the nursing home industry was highly responsive to a perceived need for facilities, backed by government dollars. When markets expand rapidly to meet rapidly increased demand, speculation is unavoidable and may even be desirable. In that sense, speculative profits are the premium consumers collectively pay for rapid growth. But other aspects of speculation are less easy to defend.

To begin with, there is the divergence between assessed valuation and actual construction cost. Given that reimbursement systems have been relatively indifferent to the quality of physical facilities and that regulatory codes have stressed fire safety and minimum square footage requirements for patient rooms, those investing in nursing homes have had a strong incentive to economize on public areas and land requirements. A facility can generate $22 in total Medicaid reimbursement per bed day, which produces $1.50 of revenue after operating costs have been subtracted, whether or not it has adequate dayrooms, lobby space, or outdoor recreation areas. When assessment for purposes of writing a mortgage is on the basis of potential for generating income, a facility without those public areas is considered just as valuable as one with them. Yet it has obviously cost less to construct. Initial profits to the original owner are thus greater in the more cheaply constructed facility, while property tax liability is lower. That is probably why most public areas in nursing homes are so small and why design decisions routinely work against resident comfort and convenience in favor of low costs. It may also explain why construction costs for nonprofit facilities have generally been so much greater.

The belief is widespread that the dominance of the nursing home industry by individuals whose backgrounds were in real estate or construction contributed significantly to the poor level of care. It is clear that many of those who entered the industry over the past fifteen years or so had no background in health care or geriatrics. It is also clear that many nursing home administrators tended to see quality as secondary to the most petty kinds of cost considerations (the price of disposable diapers, the savings in buying day-old bread, the skimping on inventories of cleaning materials). There have also been a large number of out-and-out crooks in the nursing home business. And there has been an increasing prevalence of absentee ownership. There is some limited evidence that nursing homes with owners regularly on the premises provide better care than those whose owners only cash the checks.[20] There is also more turnover with absentee owners, and that has to be disconcerting to nursing home residents.

Nursing homes are in a highly leveraged industry. Because equities are small and cash surpluses quickly withdrawn, working capital is always very tight, and operating margins small. Maintenance is skimped, corners are cut in staffing, and a delay in the Medicaid check to a facility can mean a week's diet of starches and canned goods. Small nursing homes are always running out of critical supplies because they cannot, or will not, tie up cash in inventories. Apart from its immediate consequences on the quality of life within the facility, this kind of skimping has a demoralizing impact on staff, who are sometimes unsure of how secure their next paychecks are.

At another level, the extent of leveraging in the nursing home industry means that a disproportionately high share of industry revenues goes to interest cost, rather than for expenditures of more direct

benefit to residents. Over time, government reimbursement systems
have paid out enough to buy the capital plant of the nursing home industry several times over, but that plant is still owned largely by the
banks that hold the mortgages. The roughly 10 percent of all reimbursement dollars going to capital expenditures in the nursing home
sector do not appear to be excessive until it is recognized that a large
part of those funds are not for maintenance of the industry's capital
stock—through depreciation reserves and increased equity—but for
interest premiums and personal profits.

The high degree of leveraging also creates a kind of perpetual instability in the nursing home industry as a whole and within the life of
any given institution. Nursing homes are always changing hands or
changing financial structure; skimping and corner-cutting fluctuate
with financing cycles and shifts in reimbursement methods or levels.
The one economic certainty in the typical nursing home is that the
monthly mortgage payment must be met. Expenditures on staff and
supplies can wait, if necessary, but capital financing costs must be
covered.

Consequently, real estate speculation in the nursing home industry
has meant that purchasers of nursing home services—primarily government—pay a premium for an inferior commodity. The price of rapid expansion has been high, in economic and noneconomic terms.
Since governments can borrow money more cheaply than anyone else,
the wisdom of encouraging so much speculative borrowing, at higher
interest rates, in pursuit of the public goal of expanding nursing home
capacity is questionable, especially in light of the kinds of profits, and
the sort of people who have made those profits, such speculation has
engendered.

Links and Chains

Approximately fifty publicly owned corporate chains control about
20 percent of all proprietary beds (or 12 percent of all nursing home
beds) with aggregate annual revenues comfortably over $1 billion.[21] In
states west of the Rockies, their market share is considerably larger,
and everywhere they are a source of public and regulatory concern.

The chains originated in the immediate post-Medicare period, which coincided with one of the longest sustained booms in the history of the stock market. Hundreds of enterprises that had previously been closely held, or had not even existed, entered public capital markets. For a brief period, at the peak of the boom, the hottest class of such stocks was that of nursing homes. In 1968 and 1969, more than fifty nursing home chains issued stock, the value of which appreciated very rapidly. Typically, chains went public when their entire assets were only a handful of facilities completed or in construction, along with grandiose plans for further expansion. Some began without any assets at all.[22]

In 1968 and the following several years, publicly listed corporate chains built approximately 100,000 beds, at a cost of roughly $750 million. It is hard to tell just how much public investment that represented. Nursing home stocks frequently sold at substantial multiples of book value, but whether individual entrepreneurs unloaded their own holdings before the market collapsed, capturing enormous windfall profits, or experienced the feeling of being paper millionaires for a limited time without cashing in, cannot be determined. It is clear that, at the peak of the market in mid-1969, nursing home equities had an aggregate value of several billions of dollars.[23]

Market value reflected neither the inherent value of nursing home properties nor their earnings histories, since the chains always had relatively low reported earnings and paid low dividends. It reflected, instead, the speculative optimism of the time and significant misconceptions as to what nursing homes were all about. Investors, and some chain operators, most of whom had no experience in nursing homes or health care, were generally under the illusion that Medicare would pay indefinitely for a substantial fraction of nursing home care, that the increasing elderly population would automatically generate a demand for nursing home beds, and that managing nursing homes posed no insuperable problems for capable businessmen.

The prototype firm, in the public's eye, was Medicenters of America, formed by the president and board chairman of Holiday Inn, who borrowed from motel experience the principles of franchising, standardized construction plans, and uniform management policies. By February 1969, Medicenters stock was selling for two hundred times earnings, with ninety Medicenters built, planned, or in construction. But Medicenters' management strategy was grounded in a basic error. A description of its flagship facility, in downtown Memphis, which appeared in Barron's in the spring of 1969 tells the story. The "sleek and sumptuous" 270-bed extended-care facility had opened to great fanfare in June 1967, but had consistently lost money.

> ... the ECF, equipped and staffed for post-hospital extended-care, convalescent (i.e. fast-turnover) patients, somehow had filled up instead ... with the long-staying, low-paying, aged and infirm, mainly on welfare.[24]

The *Barron's* reporter attributed the problem to "inexplicable management error," on the part of the facility's administrator—who was removed. But both the reporter and higher management failed to recognize that the extended-care facility market that Medicenters was seeking to serve simply didn't exist, and that welfare patients had always been the bread and butter of the nursing home business. Throughout the industry, occupancy rates and operating margins were low, and the expansion of capacity was grounded in extravagant expectations.

By the end of 1969, the bubble had burst. The top officials of Four Seasons, one of the more publicized of the chains and the first to be listed on a major stock exchange, had been indicted for fraudulent financial reporting; Medicare cutbacks in the form of retroactive claims denials had begun on a large scale; and the stock market boom had ended with a resounding crash. The value of nursing home issues fell precipitously, and to this day, there is hardly any trading in them. Some of the chains managed to hold on, eventually completing most of the construction that was on the drawing boards in the halcyon days of the 1960s and subsisting on real estate trafficking and the trading of facilities back and forth. There were some bankruptcies, and insurance companies that extended mortgages to the chains at the height of the boom were in several instances forced to write off extensive losses.

The market share of the chains remained roughly constant from 1969 through the mid-1970s, when it began slowly to grow again. Rather than new construction, growth has taken the form of leasing or entering into management contracts to operate facilities owned by first-generation speculators eager to escape an increasingly tumultuous and stringent regulatory environment, and continued consolidation among the chains themselves. As in many other markets, the six largest firms account for roughly half of total revenue in the chain subsector, and the two largest (ARA Services, a Philadelphia-based, food-service conglomerate, and Hillhaven, Inc.) have about a quarter.[25]

The chains *look* fishy. They are always buying and selling pieces of one another. First, Hillhaven bought Merit (the renamed shell of what was left of Medicenters), then fought off an acquisition attempt by Beverly Enterprises,[26] in part by selling a package of its securities to National Medical Enterprises (NME), a proprietary hospital chain with ten nursing homes. Part of the package sold by Hillhaven to NME was in debentures secured by Hillhaven's interest in First Healthcare Corporation, a totally owned subsidiary controlling twenty New England nursing homes, which Hillhaven had acquired from CNA, the financial conglomerate which had acquired them by mortgage foreclosure.[27] Now Hillhaven is fighting off an unfriendly take-over attempt by Manor Care Inc. ARA's nursing home holdings themselves consist of three separate chains, purchased at various times.[28] If all this smacks of more financial wheeling and dealing than with the delivery of services, that is probably an accurate impression.

More than a third of all facilities managed by the chains are not owned by them, but leased or operated under contract, and some chains lease facilities to others. How much of this leasing back and forth represents legitimate "arm's length" transactions and how much is disguised self-dealing is something no one has been able to determine.

Most nursing home chains contain other kinds of businesses within the same structure, suggesting possibilities of vertical integration. Several chains own pharmaceutical suppliers; several others own respiratory therapy companies or suppliers of other highly specialized medical services. Perhaps most intriguing is Unicare Services, Inc., a Milwaukee-based firm that owns eighty-four nursing homes; operates thirty-six others; also owns Elaine Powers Figure Salons, a drugstore chain, a car wash, a franchise restaurant chain; and is a wholesaler of toys.[29]

But the impact of the chains is probably exaggerated. There is considerable qualitative variation among them, and perhaps even more variation from one facility to another within a given chain. The most notable difference between chain-operated and nonchain nursing homes is the chains' reliance on sophisticated management and accounting techniques, such as computerized billing and inventory control. If such techniques improve efficiency and if a more efficient nursing home is a better nursing home, then chain facilities may be better. But on the other hand, the problem of absentee ownership is particularly acute.

In comparison to other industries, nursing home chains make a very low profit on revenues but do rather well on return on net worth. The key is the extent of leveraging. After taxes, nursing home chains make about four cents on every dollar of revenues, but the return on net worth is closer to 7 or 8 percent; the key is the ratio of debt to total assets, which in a sample of chains used for this study was on the order of 70 percent, higher than that for any other industry examined and almost twice as high, for instance, as it is among defense contractors.[30] With a few exceptions, publicly owned nursing home corporations look strikingly like the holdings of individual speculators writ large.

The bulk of nursing home ownership remains where it has been all along, in the hands of individual entrepreneurs, although an increasing number of individual firms own more than one facility. The nursing home industry is dominated by "chains" that characteristically include two to six or seven facilities under single private ownership. Patterns of control are exceedingly complex. It is not uncommon for a single individual to own two or three facilities that he manages himself, to have a substantial financial interest in two or three others that he does not manage, and to manage yet another on a percentage-of-revenues basis. Many accountants and lawyers own substantial pieces of a number of facilities to which they provide professional services— pieces that they may have received as a supplement to, or in lieu of, their fees. Needless to say, there is substantial interlocking of ownership.[31] Individual ownership of multiple facilities is increasing as more of the first generation of owners leaves the business. The orginal "moms and pops" are now largely gone (except when they have managed to convert into operators of minichains of newer facilities), and the first generation of entrepreneurial investors is also beginning to leave the industry. Many are nearing retirement, others are just tired of managing in an increasingly complex environment and are eager to get out with their capital gains if they can; a few are being driven out by regulatory agencies or prosecutors. The supply of proprietary nursing homes for sale (at high prices) in many parts of the country now substantially exceeds demand, and most of those who are buying already have an ownership interest in the industry.[32]

The real owners of the industry are the banks. Apart from unrealised gains (created by inflation of facilities' market value over time), most owners have little equity in their facilities. The banks hold the mortgages. It is not difficult to imagine a situation in which—as a result, say, of crackdowns in reimbursement—many owners, facing operating losses, walk away from their facilities, defaulting on their mortgages and leaving the banks to worry about it. That is a classic pattern in speculative real estate. The political and policy problems such a situation would present to state governments are frightening—which is why operators threaten to do it—and the possibility is not entirely remote.

The more likely future pattern of nursing home ownership is continued consolidation, with the industry increasingly dominated by firms controlling five to ten facilities. These operations are able to attain some of the economies of managerial scale (especially in purchasing, inventory, and managerial overhead) while remaining within the bounds of the capital that a single individual or partnership can raise. There is also likely to be continued growth in corporate chain operations, through leases and management contracts rather than ownership. In some states, there may be some buying out of proprietaries by voluntaries. But the big money has already been made and is now largely gone. Profits will have to come from operations, not real estate wizardry—or, as the nonprofit market share continues to grow, not come at all.

Profits Without Honor

Expansion of nonprofit ownership is seen by some observers as the only way to improve the nursing home industry. They see for-profit ownership as the original sin at the root of many of the industry's problems because of the inherent conflict between the provision of high quality services to the dependent elderly and profit maximization. As most other kinds of health care institutions are operated on a not-for-profit basis with apparently happy results, public health professionals tend to be made uneasy by profit-seeking firms. So it is not surprising that a number of studies of the nursing home industry have concluded with calls for eliminating proprietary interests,[33] and, though formal limitations on proprietary ownership have not been adopted in any state, the trend toward slowly increasing market share for the voluntaries continues. Policymakers have sought to limit the spread of proprietary interests to other areas of health care, most notably to the provision of home health services, presumably to avoid repeating the errors of nursing home history. And many proprietary interests are convinced that states discriminate against them.

The motivations, or actual behavior, of profit-seeking firms may run counter to the well-being of nursing home residents. Proprietary facilities tend to be physically smaller than voluntary ones, especially in the provision of public space. They have incentives to discriminate against Medicaid recipients and against admission of sicker patients. They are more likely to cut corners on supplies and staffing. And there can be no denying that most of the really scandalous conditions found in nursing home investigations have been in proprietary facilities.

However, the few studies that have attempted to compare performance of proprietary and nonprofit facilities have found no statistically significant differences in the quality of care.[34] It would be a mistake to conclude too much from any of those studies; the measurement of quality is still much too primitive, and controls were inadequate for differences in preadmission patient status. But it can be said that there was no evidence so marked as to permit a *prima facie* proof of the qualitative superiority of nonprofit facilities. A more impressionistic finding, based on my own observations and interviews, would be that, on the average, voluntary facilities are somewhat better than proprietary ones. The best voluntary facilities are the best there are. The worst nursing homes are almost exclusively proprietary. But in the middle ranges, there is substantial overlap. The best way to visualize the difference might be to conceive of the range of quality in each of the two types of nursing homes as a quasi-normal distribution, as in figure 2. The two distributions overlap markedly, with the mean for the voluntaries slightly higher than the mean for proprietaries, and with voluntaries having a shorter low-quality tail. However, the great majority of facilities of both kinds fall into the middle range, and there are many more proprietary facilities than voluntary ones. The distribution for publicly operated nursing homes is much less regular; there are both very superior and very awful public nursing homes.

Although there are many economic disincentives to high-quality care in proprietary nursing homes, voluntary homes labor under incentives and disincentives of their own. They tend to have substantially larger administrative complements, which may lead to improved services but may also just be self-indulgently wasteful. They tend to drive much less hard bargains with suppliers and to have the same labor relations problems—or worse. The voluntaries may not be profit-maximizers, but they invariably operate under the constraint of trying at least to break even, and they may be less competent at meeting that objective than the proprietaries are at meeting theirs.

In low-reimbursement states, voluntaries may discriminate more

FIGURE 2

Hypothetical Quality Distributions—Proprietary and Nonprofit Nursing Homes

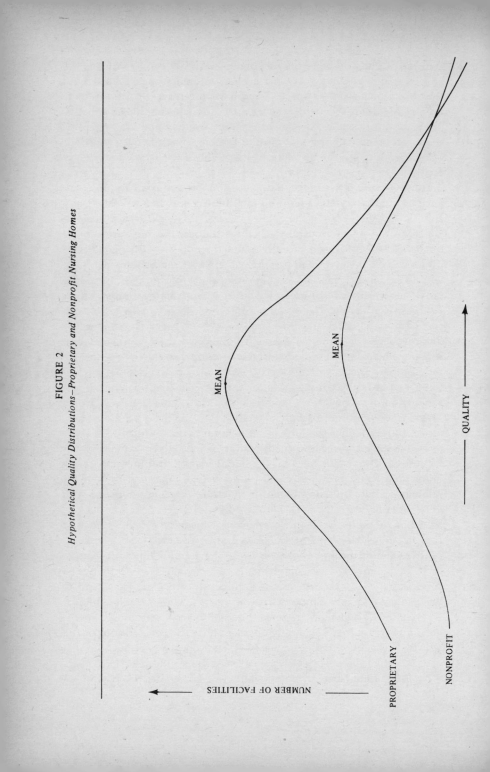

MEAN

MEAN

PROPRIETARY

NONPROFIT

NUMBER OF FACILITIES

QUALITY

heavily against Medicaid recipients than proprietaries do and be even more reluctant to accept sicker residents. In California, for example, the proportion of Medicaid residents is higher in for-profit than not-for-profit homes. Many voluntary homes elsewhere simply refuse to admit patients who need intensive services, insisting that priority for those services must go to those already in residence whose disability increases. And the record of nonprofit homes in many parts of the nation on racial discrimination is not distinguished.

Nursing homes, for-profit or not-for-profit, are complicated institutions, responding to a wide range of motives and incentives, both economic and noneconomic. Even the most rapacious proprietary nursing home operator must be concerned to some degree with the image of his facility, the safety of his investment, and his personal legal liability; even the most purely motivated administrator of a voluntary facility has a board of trustees, some of whom worry about the bottom line. All other things being equal, voluntary organizations should operate substantially better nursing homes than profit-seeking firms, but all other things are hardly ever equal.

If the existing size of the industry is to remain constant, let alone increase, there is no way of getting rid of proprietaries. The voluntaries have been concerned with taking care of their own, but not sufficiently concerned with the needs of the larger population. As recently as 1978, the New York State Health Department was desperately eager to find a voluntary sponsor to assume control of the Park Crescent, Bernard Bergman's most important property, a 500-bed nursing home on the west side of Manhattan. While a number of nonprofit organizations expressed interest, none was willing to assume control at the reimbursement levels the state was offering to provide. (As of this writing, the home is still in receivership.)

Encouraging voluntary ownership of nursing homes, at the expense of proprietaries, raises other issues of public policy.

The first arises from the fact that "voluntary" and "not-for-profit" tend to be synonymous in the health industry but mean two different things. The tax code's definition of not-for-profit, which is probably the only one usable for purposes of government relations with the nursing home industry, potentially incorporates many institutions that would not qualify as "voluntary" in common parlance. A group of physicians, for example, could convert their proprietary hospital into a "nonprofit" firm by building around it a closely held corporate shell that turned all surplus revenues over to a charitable foundation that they controlled. There is already some evidence of nursing home pro-

125

prietors transforming for-profit nursing homes into nonprofit corporations and finding other ways to benefit from the corporation, such as high salaries or the employment of relatives. Policing potential abuses of nonprofit status is a formidable task; barring for-profit firms from the nursing home sector might just create a whole new set of problems to replace those it was attempting to solve.[35]

The second issue is more fundamental. Many of the best nursing homes are operated by religious and ethnic groups, which got into the business to provide needed charitable services to their members. Religious responsibility or fraternal solidarity may be important incentives for high-quality services and should be encouraged in nursing home services, where caring and support are probably far more important to the well-being of residents than the technical skills of service providers or the efficiency with which services are delivered.

But encouraging such groups is not easy for governments to do. To begin with, there is the First Amendment, which appears to bar reimbursement for clergy employed in clerical activities in nursing homes. There is also a civil rights problem, insofar as an institution receiving public funds discriminates against nonmembers of the religious or ethnic group running the facility.

It may be constitutionally permissible for governments to subsidize individuals, through a vendor-payment system, who wish to receive services in religiously-operated institutions, so long as those institutions comply with antidiscrimination requirements. It is also possible for governments to make the distinction between nonprofit agencies, as a class, and for-profit firms; but the former may include any number of organizations that don't have the characteristics governments are trying to encourage. These indirect strategies have been partially successful at encouraging religious and ethnic organizations to take an active role in the nursing home industry, but they suffer from certain limitations.

Some ethnic or fraternal groups have more internal resources than others. Lutherans, Jews, and, to a lesser extent, Methodists have long supported nursing homes with their own community resources and were able to use the funding of Medicare and Medicaid to expand their services. But black Protestants have gotten the short end of indirect government support for ethnic groups since their limited internal resources have not, in most parts of the country, been great enough to attract unearmarked public capital.

While it may be politically acceptable but legally difficult for governments to favor religiously based nursing homes, it is legally acceptable (with some limitations) but politically difficult for governments to favor publicly operated facilities. In most of the country, the role of public nursing homes is highly circumscribed. They exist to serve those with exceptionally great political influence (veterans) or extremely great need (those too sick to be accepted by private facilities). Newly constituted public authorities are competing effectively with private nursing homes in Tucson, Arizona, and Holyoke, Massachusetts, and the rural upper Midwest has long supported community-based county facilities, but these are rare exceptions to the rule.

When government agencies seek to remove certain proprietary operators from the business, they prefer nonprofit agencies to assume control of the facilities, shying away from doing it themselves, partly in reflection of the traditional weakness of public enterprise in this country. The commissioner of health in New York, for instance, has the power to seek imposition of a civil receivership on substandard nursing homes and to recommend the receiver to be appointed. That power has been used sparingly, at least partly because the Health Department has been reluctant to assume those receiverships if voluntary agencies prove unwilling to take them on.

Entry and Exit

Government now controls the entry of new nursing home capacity through the "health planning" process. There is currently an elaborate three- and sometimes four-tiered system of federally-funded, health planning agencies. Among them, they determine the permissibility of constructing every new health facility. In the past, this power has been only sparingly utilized. In the future, the situation is likely to be different.

Beginning in 1965, a number of states, with New York in the lead, enacted "certificate-of-need" laws, which required a prior determination that a new or expanded facility was needed before it could be granted a license to operate. The initial logic of "certificate of need" drew heavily on certification of "public necessity and convenience" in the franchising of public utilities. It was accelerated by the adoption, as part of the 1972 Social Security amendments, of Section 1122 of the Social Security Act, which provided for the denial of Medicare and

Medicaid reimbursement of capital costs to any facility without appropriate certification. The National Health Planning and Resources Development Act of 1974, enacted in 1975, made it mandatory that all states adopt "certificate-of-need" procedures.

In other words, if Joe Blow decides to go into the nursing home business, he must now go beyond demonstrating that he is of sound moral character and competent to operate such a facility; he also must convince both a local "Health Systems Agency" and a state "Health Planning and Resources Development Agency" of the "need" for a new nursing home in his community.

Evaluations of "certificate-of-need" processes in those states that first got into the business have concluded that they have been largely unsuccessful at their primary objective of slowing the rate of growth in the supply of facilities.[36] The major reason is the absence of powerful political incentives to deny certificates to individual applicants. A secondary cause is the difficulty of defining just what the "need" for any number of health facilities might be. This difficulty is even more severe in the case of nursing homes than in that of hospitals, which have been the principal focus of attention in the "certificate-of-need" process, and about which there is a great deal of data and a reasonable measure of agreement. It is widely accepted that there are too many hospitals in the nation as a whole and in almost every geographical subdivision, but opinions on the appropriate number of nursing home beds vary substantially.

When HEW, as mandated by the 1974 Health Planning Law, issued its first set of "guidelines" for planning agencies, hospital bed supply and occupancy rates were the first items considered. In contrast, no guidelines whatsoever were provided for nursing homes. Officials within HEW were unable to come to agreement even among themselves on the appropriate "need" criteria.

Yet in an apparent paradox, the very fragmentary evidence available suggests that the "certificate-of-need" process has had a much more substantial impact on nursing homes than hospitals. Growing political hostility toward nursing homes since the scandals of the early 1970s is partly responsible. Nursing home operators also face greater difficulty in mustering the necessary financial, legal, and consulting resources to prepare adequate applications and shepherd them through the complex certification process. And it is not unlikely, since "certificate-of-need" proceedings include financial feasibility determinations, that many applications have run into problems on those grounds.

Whatever the reasons, the growth of the nursing home industry has slowed considerably in the past few years, especially in those states with the most advanced regulatory mechanisms. Total industry capacity in California, Connecticut, Massachusetts, and Minnesota has remained static.[37] New "certificate-of-need" approvals were frozen in New York for several years, but due to a backlog of projects in process, total capacity has continued to increase slightly. Overall, growth in the supply of nursing homes has leveled off, at least in part because of "certificate-of-need" laws. Governments have finally begun to put on the brakes, even while their feet remain on the reimbursement accelerator.

Capacity and Incapacity

To the extent that they thought about it at all, public officials in the 1950s and 1960s were eager for a substantial expansion of the supply of modern, fireproof, well-equipped nursing homes. They got it. They were hardly eager to supply windfall profits to speculators or to encourage entrepreneurs with no background or real interest in long-term care of the elderly to get into the business, and they had no desire to see the industry dominated by thinly capitalized, financially marginal facilities. But they got these too. Critics of programs for the elderly contend that the nursing home industry is so large and consumes so much money that noninstitutional services delivered to the elderly in their homes or in the community have atrophied. That, too, is an unforeseen and unwanted consequence of the way in which the industry has grown.

It is too late to undo the past, or even to substantially limit some of its consequences, but there are important lessons to be learned. Governments in the United States appear to be increasingly loath to do things for themselves, preferring to buy goods and services from private firms. It is often noted that the growth in federal budgetary expenditures over the last two decades has not coincided with a significant expansion in federal civilian employment; a large part of the reason may be that more and more of those who work "for" the federal government receive paychecks from private firms.

In nursing homes, part of the problem may well have arisen from the tendency to confuse buildings with services. Admittedly, most governmental units lacked the capacity, and perhaps the will, to provide nursing home services, so there is much to be said for letting private firms provide them. But there was no reason why those private firms had to supply the physical plants in which the services were provided. The process of generating physical capacity through real estate speculation has been inimical to the service objectives of public programs. It has also been extremely expensive.

There was ample precedent for doing things differently. By the end of World War II, almost all the physical plants in which private airplane manufacturers assembled their products were owned by the federal government. The exigences of war had demanded an extremely rapid increase in the industry's capacity; with capital allocation a pressing problem, the government had simply gone ahead and built the factories and then leased them to manufacturers. Wars are extraordinary situations, in which standard operating procedures are more easily discarded. But there is no reason why a similar process could not have been adopted once it was decided that a several-fold increase in nursing home capacity was needed.

Such a process would have had several advantages.[38] It would have broken the linkage between ownership of physical plant and operations, easing the problems of regulating the industry. Under existing practice, the operator of a nursing home is both a state licensee for the provision of services and the owner of a physical asset. It is one thing to remove the license, another to transfer the asset to a more desirable or efficient operator since the ownership of property is constitutionally protected, and not easy to take away without substantial compensation. When a physical plant is publicly owned, the potential reassignment of responsibility for operating it can be used as a policy tool in all sorts of creative ways, as when the federal government, after World War II, used the "conversion" to private ownership of wartime aluminum plants as a means of weakening the power of the aluminum monopoly.[39]

In the case of nursing homes, the separation of building and operations might also have prevented entry into the industry of some of its least desirable entrepreneurs, the real estate speculators. A system of leasing or contracting out operating rights would probably have attracted miscreants and low-lifes of its own, but it would have been easier to get rid of them.

It would also have been cheaper. Even when it costs more for the government to build a given facility than it would private concerns, the government can borrow money at lower cost. More to the point, it only makes economic sense to let private firms do the work—with the implicit promise that they will profit if the work is successfully completed—if they share the risk of that activity. Yet, there was no real risk for the builders of nursing homes. A flow of Medicaid patients was all but guaranteed, and the failure to enforce service standards meant that it would always be possible to divert enough revenue to meet the mortgage payment.

Adopting a different method of capacity-building would have required policymakers to face the problem much more squarely than they ever did. The growth of the nursing home industry was widely anticipated and generally desired but hardly *planned*. Given the high degree of uncertainty surrounding the critical questions of how much nursing home capacity would be "needed" or how services would be paid for, there is something to be said for simply letting the private sector run its own course, pushed from behind by public dollars. Doing so permitted governments *not* to make decisions about how many nursing homes there should be, or where they should be located. It also disguised budgetary impacts since construction appropriations have to be explicitly made, while Medicaid obligations appeared to arise spontaneously from the growth in "demand"—and, necessarily, after the construction had been completed, and thus in later fiscal years.

Those "nondecisions" produced unhappy results, partly because the private sector was somewhat different from what the policymakers visualized. Again, they were trapped by the overriding image of the hospital. The growth of the hospital industry was similarly unplanned, and we now have too many hospitals that have cost, and continue to cost, far too much. Nevertheless, windfall profits have been relatively rare, and service standards have remained high. The people who built nursing homes were very different from those who built hospitals and responded very differently to equivalent incentives. Hospitals took the generosity of reimbursement formulas to construct opulent workshops in which physicians could employ the most esoteric scientific technologies; nursing homes took the money and ran.

Investment in physical facilities is much less flexible than social policy. Hospitals and nursing homes last a long time, often far longer than the need for the services they provide when they are built. If the government is successful in closing some of the excess hospital capacity it has fostered, the landscape will be littered with empty hospitals (not very useful for any other purpose) just as it already is with empty state mental institutions and hundreds of elementary schools.

The problem is especially acute for nursing homes because public policy does not deal very well with the phenomenon of sunk costs, and because the existence of a physical plant creates an irresistible temptation to use it. People will be unable to think of other uses for the buildings and will feel obliged to continue throwing good money after bad. The question should be how many of them we need, not how many there are. But the process of policy-making approaches the problem in the opposite direction: if we have them, we must need them.

It is often said that government has a tendency to throw money at problems, but it would be far more accurate to say that it throws bricks and mortar—and then gets stuck with the consequences. It might be far wiser to spend the marginal dollar on people or programs. If an expansion of "community mental health services" is needed, spend the money for social workers and psychologists, not "community mental health center" structures. Pay teachers, not contractors; nurses, not engineers; nurses' aides, not real estate speculators.[40] But Americans tend to think no institution is worth its salt unless it has its own edifice, with its name over the door and carpeting in the hallways.

Construction activity involves a different constellation of political forces than service provision. Banks, contractors, insurance companies, and the building trades get into the act, and the fact that their campaign contributions are the lifeblood of state and local politics is neither accidental nor unrelated. Construction means "growth," that Holy Grail for every chamber of commerce. Programs can be discontinued, employees laid off when the fads in social policy change course, as they always do. Buildings have mortgages of twenty-five years, or longer.

The final lesson to be learned from the history of capacity building in the nursing home industry is that incremental policymaking leads governments to attempt to reach public ends through indirection, in ways that frustrate achievement of those ends and create other social costs. The political system resists government involvement in capital allocation, but it seeks to encourage investment in commercial real estate. So it writes the accelerated depreciation tax shelter into that most incrementally created of all statutes, the Internal Revenue Code. That loophole encourages such investment, but at the cost of substantial foregone revenues for the public fisc and increased inequity in tax burden among the citizenry. It is also an extraordinarily blunt tool. Its benefits fall on the nursing home speculator and the well-motivated "mom and pop" alike. They fall equally on the developer of shopping centers and the builder of nursing homes, which may give the former the idea of becoming the latter; while many of the people who might run nursing homes have never even itemized their deductions, let alone heard of depreciation.

One reason the system of property reimbursement under Medicare and Medicaid broke down so completely in the case of nursing homes was that policymakers tried to hang too many objectives onto the frail reed of reimbursement systems. Incrementalism leads to a tendency to try to load multiple, sometimes competing, objectives onto a single policy tool, rather than inventing new ones. The notion of "reasonable cost" makes relatively good sense for a labor-intensive service, but not for real property, where it becomes hopelessly entangled with the complex problem of value. Just what is a 100-bed nursing home worth? Market prices are no help because so many transactions are artificial and because the market wouldn't exist at all if it weren't for the dominant buying role of governments. Construction costs are somewhat more useful, but in an inflationary period, the level of reimbursement becomes a function of when the facility was built. And income-generating potential is no help at all because that is also entirely contingent on what the states are willing to pay at any given time. But the reimbursement tool was readily available, and because it was less controversial politically than the alternatives, it was used.

The Game of Levels

JUST AS policymakers attempted to use reimbursement mechanisms to finance and direct the growth of nursing home capacity, they attempted, with even less success, to control costs and enhance quality through the notion of "levels of care." The federal government now reimburses two types of nursing homes under public medical programs: skilled nursing facilities (SNFs), covered under both Medicare and Medicaid; and intermediate care facilities (ICFs), covered under Medicaid alone.

An extensive and growing body of law, regulation, and procedure surrounds this classification, most of it concerned with matching residents and facilities to ensure "appropriate" levels of care. But implementation of levels of care runs afoul of cost and reimbursement pressures on the states, and ownership patterns in the industry has become entangled in a web of federal-state conflict, and assigns to physicians a technically impossible administrative task.

The Logic of Levels

The concern with levels of care and appropriateness of placement arises from a number of sources. One has been the desire to ensure that public medical programs will pay only for medical services. Since the time of Kerr-Mills, policymakers have been unwilling to use health care dollars to pay for "merely custodial" services. Policymakers feared that if medical need were not a precondition for the receipt of benefits, demand for subsidized room and board would be uncontrollable. At the same time, policymakers sought to avoid tainting health care programs with the stigma of income maintenance. Defining eligibility for services in terms of medical "need" establishes physicians as gatekeepers for the receipt of benefits and provides political legitimacy, even if the preponderance of public dollars are going for custodial care.

The concept of "levels of care" assumes that a physician's diagnosis defines a level of "need" for a bundle of medical services. According to federal regulations, the services defined as "skilled care" consist of:

> ... those services furnished pursuant to physician order which
> 1) require the skills of technical or professional personnel, e.g., registered nurse, licensed practical (vocational) nurse, physical therapist, occupational therapist, speech pathologist, audiologist. ...
> 2) are provided either directly by or under the supervision ... of such personnel.[1]

Intermediate care services entail:

> ... health-related care and services to individuals who do not require the degree of care and treatment which a hospital or skilled nursing facility is designed to provide, but who because of their mental or physical condition require care and services (above the level of room and board) which can be made available to them only through institutional facilities.[2]

The notion then follows that differing bundles of service can be provided in distinct institutions, each meeting a different set of "needs." It is then argued that institutions reserved for those with the least severe needs can be operated with fewer professional personnel (and hence, more cheaply) than those caring for sicker residents. This argument is bolstered by evidence that, since the early days of Medicare and Medicaid, anywhere between 10 and 40 percent of all nursing home residents have been at the "wrong" level of care—generally too "high" a level.[3] Those findings have embodied the worst of policymakers' nightmares: expending public funds to provide social welfare recipients more than the bare minimum required to meet basic needs.

The logic of "levels of care" has serious flaws. It assigns to physicians, whose skills lie in determining services for the maintenance or rehabilitation of their patients, the task of assigning the chronically ill elderly to one of two ambiguously defined bureaucratic categories. Further, the condition of frail, older people changes constantly (especially under inadequate institutional care). An assessment of the "needed" level of care will be accurate for only a limited time.[4] Finally, the logic of levels of care confuses institutional capability with institutional performance and ignores the fact that most institutions function more effectively and economically when they serve clients with varying needs.

For the levels of care idea to work usefully in practice, the mix of institutions would have to conform to the distribution of "needs" in the population, and policymakers would need to have effective control over the processes through which individuals and institutions were matched, both at initial placement and throughout the lifetime of the client. Neither of these conditions has ever held, nor are they likely to in the near future. In their absence, "levels of care" policy has largely collapsed and may soon be scrapped altogether.

Trickling Down

The desire to recognize and separately pay for different levels of institutional care for the nursing home population reflected reasonable and humane motives. Nothing is more widely agreed upon among experts in gerontology than that "overmedicalization" of long-term care services is damaging to recipients and that the "medical model" as embodied in a narrow construction of SNF regulations fosters excessive dependency, destroys individual competence and self-esteem, and accelerates deterioration of body, mind, and spirit. Since "medical model" institutions appeared to be more expensive, many policymakers were eager to foster the development of institutions modeled on traditional homes for the aged, few of which provided their residents with more than rudimentary medical services. Many believed that delegating "level of care" determinations to physicians was preferable to bureaucratic regulation.

But these legitimate objectives were subverted by powerful political and economic pressures. The ICF category became the repository of those facilities that could not meet Life Safety Code Standards. A rationally based distinction between the two levels of care would instead revolve around staffing standards. SNF residents should require more total nursing, more skilled (RN or LPN) nursing, and much more occupational and physical therapy. But the federal SNF standards, and those in most states, are so minimal that it is nearly impossible to construct ICF standards that are less demanding but still satisfy congressional insistence on "health-related" care. With a few minor exceptions, the federal SNF and ICF standards are now effectively identical, and the definitions of "skilled" and "intermediate" care entirely circular. Skilled care is that provided by skilled nursing facilities, intermediate care that provided by intermediate care facilities.[5]

Those states that have taken the idea of "levels of care" seriously have established substantial differences in facility qualifications, generally requiring far more nursing hours per patient day in SNFs. But those states are a small minority. The proportion of SNF and ICF beds varies enormously from state to state, making a mockery of the underlying logic of "levels of care" (see table 4).[6] There is no reason to believe that Medicaid recipients in Georgia or Pennsylvania are ten times as likely to need skilled care as those in Oklahoma or Oregon, but they are ten times as likely to get it, or at least to get something called "skilled care."

There is very little difference between the services provided by SNFs in, say, California (which essentially has no ICFs) or Pennsylvania, and those provided by ICFs in Oklahoma or Tennessee. The difference lies in how they are licensed by the states and, to a lesser extent, what they call themselves. Oklahoma and Oregon were two of the states that reclassified most of their SNFs as ICFs as soon as the Miller amendment became effective, partially to save money, partially to avoid having to close many facilities that would not meet SNF standards. Georgia and California had reimbursement systems that were more lucrative for SNFs than ICFs, and operators had only to make marginally greater investments to qualify for SNF status.

If the federal regulations are given the narrowest possible interpretation, only 10 to 25 percent of all nursing home residents need "skilled care." The 47 percent figure in table 4 (which excludes many states with a high proportion of Medicaid patients in SNFs) suggests a serious mismatch between bed availability and the "needs" of the clientele. A far *higher* proportion of private patients (and all Medicare patients) are in SNFs. In seven out of eight states on which data were available, the proportion of private-pay patients in SNFs exceeded that of Medicaid patients by an average of three to one.[7]

In most states, operating a SNF is more profitable than operating an

TABLE 4

*Proportion of Medicaid Patients in
SNFs and ICFs, 32 States, 1973*

State	Percentage in SNFs	Percentage in ICFs
Alabama	65.3	34.7
Colorado	52.0	48.0
Delaware	16.3	83.7
Florida	89.3	10.7
Georgia	86.3	13.7
Illinois	18.9	81.1
Kentucky	64.8	35.2
Louisiana	1.8	98.2
Maine	6.0	94.0
Maryland	50.0	50.0
Michigan	46.4	53.6
Minnesota	33.0	67.0
Mississippi	81.1	18.9
Missouri	22.4	77.6
Montana	57.6	42.4
Nebraska	10.8	89.2
New Mexico	26.7	73.3
New York	78.9	21.1
North Dakota	54.4	45.6
Oklahoma	2.0	98.0
Oregon	5.6	94.4
Pennsylvania	77.4	22.6
Rhode Island	31.1	68.9
South Dakota	43.5	56.5
Tennessee	2.2	97.8
Texas	12.3	87.7
Utah	33.1	66.9
Vermont	23.4	76.6
Virginia	9.1	90.9
Washington	80.0	20.0
West Virginia	5.8	94.2
Wyoming	25.9	74.1
TOTAL	47.9	52.1

SOURCE: Community Research Applications, Inc., *Excerpt Summary of A National Study of Levels of Care in Intermediate Care Facilities (ICFs).* Prepared for Health Services Administration under Contract Number HSA-105-74-176, April 1976. (Issued by Bureau of Quality Assurance, Health Services Administration, Public Health Service, U.S. Department of Health, Education, and Welfare.) Appendix A, p. 3.

ICF. The more lucrative private market tends to be attracted by the trappings of the "medical model," and SNF status makes the facility potentially eligible for Medicare, the most generous of all third-party payers. It invariably ensures a higher reimbursement rate under Medicaid, and thus, even when costs are proportionately higher, higher revenues, which increase property value and property-related profits. ICFs are those facilities that cannot compete, cannot pass muster for SNF certification, or are located in states that award SNF status only grudgingly. In general, ICF facilities are solely creatures of Medicaid.[8] The major exception to that pattern is the growing number of voluntary ICFs specifically constructed to serve clients primarily needing custodial services. Too many people are in SNF beds because there are too many SNF beds. Since the federal government has not been willing to control that process through its standards-writing activity, the elaborate mechanisms designed to ensure "appropriate" placements provide no protection.

The continued, though diminishing, preponderance of SNF beds also says something about the working of economic "incentives" and their relationship to the placement system. Before 1972, all federally certified nursing homes were "skilled." The growth of the ICF category has come largely from the trickling down of inferior facilities. Because running an SNF is more profitable, proprietary operators have retained SNF status as long as they could. They have had considerable success except in those states that, for budgetary reasons, eliminated SNFs altogether. But for all states, ICF care is cheaper, so their incentive is to move *residents*, if the beds are available.

The Placement Maze

The figures in table 4 are statewide aggregates, and there is substantial variation within the states. In many communities, there may be no SNFs or no ICFs; even where there are both, under conditions of tight supply, there may be beds available only in one category. The availability of beds is an all but overwhelming constraint on efforts to operate a rational placement system.

According to federal law, states must establish, under their plans for Medicaid administration, a system of "utilization control" that "safeguards against unnecessary or inappropriate utilization of care and services." The system is based on utilization review committees in each SNF and ICF, audited periodically by the state on a sample basis. Those committees, consisting of physicians and other professionals not otherwise employed by the nursing home, are supposed to review the status of each patient on admission, and then every ninety days (for SNFs) or six months (for ICFs) thereafter, to assure that they are in need of the level of care they are presumably receiving. Only if residents are certified as being in institutions of the correct level of care are state Medicaid agencies supposed to reimburse for services rendered them.[9]

Under existing law, this utilization review system will be superseded by the activities of Professional Standards Review Organizations (PSROs), federally funded and governed by locally elected physicians charged with monitoring the quality and appropriateness of care rendered under all government payment programs. As opposed to the current system, in which utilization review committees are operated by individual providers, PSROs will be dominated by professionals outside the individual nursing home.[10]

Most "level-of-care determinations" enforced by utilization review ratify the status quo for individual residents. Those that do not usually determine that the resident should be discharged to a "lower" level of care. When practiced aggressively, utilization review gives the appearance of saving the state money by ensuring that residents are not receiving more expensive care than they "need."

Utilization review entails transferring residents from one facility to another. Thirteen percent of all live nursing home discharges are transfers to other nursing homes, although not all transfers result from utilization review.[11] These transfers eject helpless, disoriented old people from the places they have lived for months or even years to facilities, not of their own choosing, that they have never seen before. The evidence is overwhelming that, without extraordinary preparatory efforts that are hardly ever made, *any* move is harmful for the preponderance of the frail elderly; the technical term is "transfer trauma."[12] Gains that accrue from ensuring that, at any given time, the individual is in a facility capable of providing the appropriate level of care are bound to be far outweighed by the costs of moving people around to those appropriate levels. For Medicaid agencies, the greatest savings do not arise from the difference in rates between SNFs and ICFs, but from the fact that recipients moved from one level of care to another tend to die much more quickly than they would otherwise.

Many states have refused to comply with utilization review. In many nursing homes that practice utilization review, it is done mostly on paper, to satisfy record-keeping requirements. State regulators generally wink at such noncompliance, unless they are out to get individual facilities for other reasons. But HEW officials, citing congressional demands for a relatively painless way to save money, have kept the heat on, even when they have recognized that they were pursuing a chimera.

The whole charade of utilization review and other appropriateness mechanisms, with its disastrous consequences for many nursing home residents, can be seen as a continuing skirmish in the war between federal and state agencies. The ICF category and utilization review came about because the federal agencies did not trust the states to limit expenditures of federal matching funds to recipients truly in need, to refuse to subsidize medical services for those in need of custodial care, or to certify facilities only to render care of which they are capable. Sometimes, federal distrust of state officials was so great that they were by-passed altogether. States are required to see that utilization review systems are in effect, but those systems are staffed by nongovernmental physicians.

Most physicians engaged in utilization review recognize that transfers are traumatic. Since "skilled" and "intermediate" are statutory rather than medical terms, it is easy for physicians to give the benefit of the doubt to whatever level the resident is already in. The physician's continued employment in the utilization review process may depend on his not making too many waves. Utilization-review physicians cannot help but be aware that a facility's certification as "skilled" has little to do with whether its residents are receiving "skilled" care. It is therefore not surprising that so many participants in the process consider utilization review to be a meaningless exercise in bureaucratic hoop-jumping. But in most nursing homes, utilization review is the major thing physicians do.

While utilization review causes great damage to public charges by forcibly moving them from one facility to another, it is presumably tied to "need" for services and partly motivated by concern that those in need of custodial care not be "overmedicalized." But thousands of nursing home residents are forcibly transferred from one facility to another each year solely for reasons of profit. In many areas of the country, where there is a substantial divergence between private and Medicaid rates and where bed supply is tight, individuals who enter facilities as private patients, but exhaust their assets and qualify for

Medicaid, will be summarily discharged as soon as placement in a facility accepting Medicaid can be effected. No one knows just how many such economic discharges there are (the practice is relatively localized, in a number of areas including northern New Jersey, Ohio, and parts of Massachusetts) but they comprise a sizable fraction of the 100,000 or so annual discharges from one nursing home to another.

Since 1976, some state governments and private consumer advocates have moved against this practice, generally by strengthening residents' protections against discharge, or by amending licensure laws to require service to some proportion of Medicaid recipients in facilities that have Medicaid certification. But where private demand is sufficiently great, facilities can afford to forgo Medicaid certification altogether, and there appears to be little the states can do to prevent it. Because private patients are likely to be in SNFs, many of those transferred move from SNF to ICF for reasons that have nothing to do with a change in their medical or psychiatric condition.

Keeping the Gates

The point at which the logic of "appropriate" placement and utilization review makes the most sense is exactly where it has the least impact—initial admission into a nursing home. It is one thing to forcibly eject a sick, old person from the facility in which she has been living, quite another to prevent her from entering it in the first place—especially if she does not "need" it. But governments have been incapable of taking control of initial admissions because utilization review and "levels of care" are tied to the payment process and because nursing homes have *been there* when no other solutions appeared to be available.

More than half of all admissions to nursing homes are from general hospitals.[13] The impetus for many of them is utilization review or some similar process in the institutions making the placement. They are under pressures of their own to get the client out of their facility and are eager to certify their "need" for whatever beds are available in the community. Welfare agencies are greedy for the apparent, but illusory, savings in moving their beneficiaries to lower levels of care. Admitting facilities with vacant beds are unlikely to determine that a newly admitted resident does not need the service. Each institution has an incentive to find "need."

The worst nursing home facilities, run by the most unscrupulous operators, could never have existed or persisted so long without the passive complicity of placement agencies. By and large, Medicaid beneficiaries do not admit themselves to the worst nursing homes; they are placed there by others. There have been rumors of bribes and kickbacks by nursing home operators to social workers in hospitals or welfare departments,[14] but that has probably been relatively rare. Operators have not had to bribe placement agencies to get admissions.

For any placement agency, the pressures and incentives are to make as many placements as quickly as possible, regardless of quality. Social workers in hospitals and welfare departments have been highly constrained in their ability to exercise professional discretion. Speed has important financial consequences; except for specialized agencies dedicated primarily to nursing home placements (of which there are very few, all of them young), those institutions that have provided much of the flow of nursing home admissions have had no concern with the quality of different nursing homes. It is not their job. Control of quality has been the responsibility of state health departments (hospitals in particular have tended to look down on nursing homes and to treat them all with equal indifference). Among those making nursing home placements, there is often total and sometimes willful ignorance of the quality of different facilities.[15]

Beds are often tight. Something must be done with the elderly individual not qualified for, or no longer in "need" of, hospital care, and nursing home placement, regardless of its quality, is something. The tighter the bed supply at the time of placement, the greater the likelihood of ignoring the quality of an available bed.

For the other nursing home admissions, those from the "community," placed by families, friends, or social agencies, the limitations of utilization review or other appropriateness controls stem from the fact that only a small proportion *enter* nursing homes under the auspices of public programs. While, at any given time, more than two-thirds of nursing home residents are Medicaid beneficiaries, because of Medicaid "spend down," the proportion on admission is far smaller. Nursing home operators are under no legal obligation to restrict admission for "self-pay" patients on the basis of need, and they have incentives to admit those with low needs, who will be cheaper to care for. Nothing, however, is so likely to create an elderly person's need for institutional services as several months' residence in a nursing home; by the time the resident spends down to Medicaid eligibility, it is probable that she will be worn down to "needing" the nursing home according to Medicaid criteria.

Searching for a Technological Fix

The apparent failure of utilization review to substantially reduce the proportion of Medicaid recipients in too "high" a level of care has led policymakers off on a complex wild-goose chase. The problem has been identified as the inadequacy of the forms people are required to fill out. The solution has been sought in a sophisticated assessment "instrument" on which it is impossible to cheat. If the form is fancy enough, it was thought, it will automatically produce an answer as to where the client belongs.

Thus, the ONHA and its bureaucratic descendants over the past five years developed the Patient Assessment and Care Evaluation system (PACE)—a form calculated to generate both a "level of care" determination and a technique for assuring that care is of high quality.[16] New York State implemented its own controversial DMS-I form, a two-page, eleven-item questionnaire, with a numerical coding system attached. Each answer is assigned a score. Incontinence of urine is worth 20 points; of stool, 40. Difficulty in walking scores 35 points, feeding 40. Occasional abusiveness is worth 25 points, constant abusiveness 50. If the score exceeds 180, the patient is entitled to reimbursement in an SNF; if it falls between 60 and 179, in an ICF.[17] At last report, the PACE form was at least ten times as long as the DMS-I.

Use of the DMS-I form has engendered considerable controversy in New York. The form is too medically oriented, it is claimed, and ignores the importance of psychological and social characteristics. It leaves too little room for professional judgment. It counts some things too heavily and others too little. It is arbitrary and artificial to use as the basis for important decisions about people's lives; the difference in needs between someone with a score of 179 and someone with a score of 180 can't be that great.

These complaints notwithstanding, assessment is not that difficult.

There are those who would argue that the DMS-I form is too long. The problem is that the logic of assessment is out of kilter with a system that requires physical transfer of a resident whose assessment has changed, yet cannot guarantee that a more "appropriate" bed will be available. Nor can the system require effective assessment of all residents at admission, the only time such determinations can be acted on without serious harm.

Assessment and Alternatives

One of the justifications provided by advocates of sophisticated assessment procedures is that they could be used to determine whether an individual belongs in a nursing home and to define the services needed to maintain an elderly individual in the community. Assessment procedures would constrict the gateway to nursing homes while offering some hope that those kept out will not be left without care.

It is far easier to determine that an individual needs a service than to provide it. For the past fifteen years, policymakers have agreed that an expansion of services outside of institutions is desperately needed, but those services have not always been forthcoming. The original Medicare statute listed home health benefits as a covered service immediately after "post-hospital extended care"; since the outset, states have had the option of covering a more generous package of home health services under Medicaid. In the past several years, home health services have begun to grow more rapidly, as policymakers have promoted them more aggressively. But the availability of "alternatives" to nursing homes is still extremely limited.

For those doing the placing, nursing homes are once-and-for-all solutions. After the social worker or family member arranges a nursing home placement, the problem is solved. The nursing home will be of assistance in obtaining the appropriate reimbursement and will assume day-to-day supervision of the resident. But an individual remaining at home requires services that must be bought from a variety of agencies, the supervisor or caretaker must fight with Medicare and Medicaid directly, and, when institutional placements are involved, the hospital or welfare staff worker will have to continue to carry the case. Even if assessment procedures were refined, more "alternative" services available, and reimbursement policies simpler, it is still unlikely, without more administrative and financial incentives, that a large number of people would be deflected from nursing home care.

The Inappropriateness of Appropriateness

The SNF/ICF distinction is probably doomed. Several states are moving in the direction of granting facilities a single SNF/ICF license and then assessing individual residents as a basis for reimbursement and staffing decisions. HEW is talking about consolidation of SNF and ICF standards. Lawyers representing nursing home residents are increasingly successful at delaying or deterring transfers based on utilization review or payment-status considerations. Still, there is strong political support for "levels of care," and it may linger on. If it does, it will continue to inflict pain on thousands of dependent citizens without producing benefits for anyone.

"Levels of care" has become the most unmitigated failure of public policy toward nursing homes. The motives behind it were, in large part, honorable, and the underlying logic sound, but the notion ran contrary to the economic and political realities of the nursing home industry—and the needs of nursing home residents.

146

7

The Quality of Mercy

DIRECT REGULATION of the quality of nursing homes and the services they deliver has been an important government activity for at least a generation. The principal components of the regulatory process are the formulation and promulgation of standards, the inspection of facilities to determine the extent to which standards are being complied with, and the imposition of sanctions when standards are not met.

Quality of care standards in nursing homes are set simultaneously and overlappingly by state and federal governments. Federal law establishes "conditions of participation" and "standards" for facilities seeking reimbursement under Medicare or Medicaid. Those standards defer to prevailing state law on such matters as sanitary codes and personnel licensing. State standards are embodied in licensure laws. (One of the federal conditions of participation is that the facility be licensed in the state in which it is located.) The federal standards are minimums that the states must meet but are permitted to exceed. But by and large, the state standards closely parallel those of the federal government.

Inspections are conducted primarily by the states. Those inspections are buttressed (or duplicated) by federal inspections of a sample of facilities participating in federal programs—a process that is supposed to "validate" and ensure the adequacy of state inspections.

The only available sanction against a nursing home that has consistently failed to meet standards has been denial of its ability to do business, through termination of its "provider agreement" under Medicare or Medicaid or removal of its state license. These sanctions have rarely been invoked, even for severely substandard nursing homes. Partly as a result, states have begun to experiment with other sanctions, such as pecuniary fines and the imposition of civil receivership.

The conduct of standards setting, inspection, and sanctioning by both state and federal governments has been widely and justifiably criticized for its inadequacy and ineffectiveness. Yet the general level of quality in precisely those areas to which regulation has been addressed appears to have risen, although rather slowly.

It is the prevailing wisdom among public policy theorists that direct regulation is one of the ways in which governments can respond to "market failure," such as the inability of consumers or their surrogates to assess effectively the quality of care rendered by nursing homes and to act as rational buyers. The others include the provision of economic incentives or disincentives, most commonly through taxes or tax subsidies; the provision of better information to consumers; and the provision of services directly by government.[1] Policy theorists have ignored delegation of responsibility for correcting market failures to a private group or profession and the potential impact of the government's use of its market power, apart from economic "incentives" contained in any pricing mechanism. These different approaches are all employed in nursing home policy, to varying degrees, by different units of government. An assessment of nursing home regulation is thus partially an assessment of those alternatives, in keeping with the contemporary debate over "regulation" and "deregulation."

The Quality of Quality

The problem to be regulated should be crucial to the choice of regulatory instrument; what works for Sunday closing hours may not make much sense for the level of coliform bacteria in a municipal water system or the consumption of marijuana on a college campus. What works for the reduction of fire hazards in nursing homes will not work for the quality of nursing services or for seeing to it that hot foods and served hot and cold foods cold.

High quality nursing home care consists of the maintenance of a clean and pleasant environment, in which the food is good, that there is plenty to do, assistance is readily given with dressing and bathing, people are nice to each other and respect each other's privacy and personal dignity, and good medical and nursing services are provided to those who need them. This may seem like a simple set of requirements, but in practice, it is not.

Few nursing homes are of high quality by these standards. It is inherently difficult to provide intimate personal services to severely disabled, often hostile or disoriented, physically and emotionally frail people, especially when most of those providing the services are untrained and poorly paid and when the facility's operator is trying to make a profit on $25 a day, at least 10 percent of which goes to mortgage payments. Only the most exceptional institutions provide really good food. The customary practice of medical care is potentially inimical to personal privacy and dignity. And ensuring that everyone is kept busy too easily shades into regimentation and manipulation.

If it is difficult to provide high quality care, it is more difficult still to measure or control it. Moreover, both the medical and psychological makeup of nursing home residents and nursing homes are highly unstable. What is appropriate care for a resident one week may be scandalously inadequate and inhumane the next, if her condition deteriorates, or demeaning and patronizing, if it improves. A first-rate nursing home can become a terrible one in the course of weeks if it loses a good nursing director and a good cook.

Finally, most nursing homes are small, informal, nonhierarchical, and nonbureaucratic—characteristics that are otherwise desirable but that make regulation substantially more difficult. The large number of separate facilities further exacerbates this problem, since the greater the number of sites to be inspected, the greater the workload of the inspection system.

Standards

The basic sources of nursing home standards are the "Conditions of Participation" for SNFs and "Standards" for ICFs contained in the Social Security Act.[2] These have been translated into more detailed regulations, which have the force of law, and then into still more specific instructions and guidelines, which are the effective operational standards for inspectors and nursing homes, although the legal status of the guidelines is somewhat vague.

The "Conditions of Participation" occupies twenty double-column pages of the Code of Federal Regulations.[3] After three-and-a-half pages of definitions and a brief statement of the requirement that SNFs must conform to all applicable state laws including licensure, they are broken into seventeen major "conditions," which are subdivided into eighty-five "standards." The seventeen "Conditions of Participation" are:

1. Requirements related to the governing body and management, including standards for disclosure of ownership, qualifications and duties of governing boards and administrators, a number of managerial duties, record keeping, and the "patients' bill of rights."
2. A requirement that there be a medical director and a statement of his duties and responsibilities.
3. Requirements related to physician services to residents.
4. Requirements related to nursing services, including the roles of director of nursing, charge nurses, staffing, and description of nursing responsibilities.
5. Requirements related to dietary services, including staffing, nutritional, and sanitary standards.
6. Requirements related to specialized rehabilitative services (physical therapy, speech pathology and audiology, and occupational therapy), essentially stating that if such services are ordered for residents by a physician, the nursing home must be able to provide them.
7. Requirements related to pharmaceutical services, including standards of supervision, control, and accountability.
8. Requirements related to laboratory and radiological services, essentially saying that the SNF knows where to get them when its residents need them.
9. Requirements related to dental services, standards for which are much the same.
10. Requirements related to social services, with a specific statement that facilities do not need to provide them (but how they should be provided if the facility wants to do so).
11. Requirements related to patient activities, which say there must be some and that a staff member must be assigned responsibility for running them.
12. Requirements related to medical records, which detail at some length how such records are to be maintained and managed.
13. Requirements related to transfer agreements.
14. Requirements related to physical environment; these incorporate hundreds of pages of the Life Safety Code of the National Fire Protection Association relative to fire, electrical, and structural safety and provide for

waiver of some of those requirements. They also include standards for patient rooms, dining and activity rooms, nursing stations, kitchens, and so forth.

15. Requirements related to infection control, which subsumes housekeeping and linen supply.
16. Requirements related to disaster preparedness, which essentially call for staff training.
17. Requirements related to utilization review.

The ICF standards, which appear in an entirely separate volume of the Federal Regulations (under public welfare, rather than social security), occupy only seven-and-a-half pages. They are much less well organized than the SNF standards and somewhat less detailed, but they are substantially identical.[4] The differences include weaker requirements for charge nurse, nurse staffing, and physician service, and the absence of the requirement for medical direction.

The federal standards are extremely detailed in some areas but extraordinarily vague in others. It is required that no patient room contain more than four beds and that "single patient rooms measure at least 100 square feet, and multipatient rooms provide a minimum of 80 square feet per bed."[5] Yet the standards for public areas require only that "the facility provides one or more clean, orderly, and appropriately furnished rooms of adequate size designated for patient dining and for patient activities. These areas are well lighted and well ventilated."[6] Three meals a day are required, at regular hours, with no more than fourteen hours between supper and breakfast (a provision made necessary by the practice of corner-cutting facilities to employ only one shift of dietary staff and to serve all three meals in an eight-hour period), and nighttime snacks, which is pretty specific;[7] but the standards require only that "foods are prepared by methods that conserve nutritive value, flavor, and appearance, and are attractively served at the proper temperatures and in a form to meet individual needs."[8]

The SNF/ICF standards rely heavily on record keeping. Each resident must have a formal "plan of care," a medical record, a nursing record, a pharmaceutical record, a dietary record, and, if provided, plans of care and supporting records for rehabilitative, dental, and social services. The facility must maintain payroll and staffing records and minutes of its utilization review, pharmacy, and budget and planning committees.

State and federal standards are essentially the same, with some exceptions. Many states require a specific quantitative ratio of total nursing hours to patient days—generally in the range of two to three hours per twenty-four-hour day—and some have slightly more stringent sanitary codes. New York traditionally required that nursing homes provide social services, although it recently relaxed the standard that had necessitated a master's degree-level social worker in each facility to one that accepts a bachelor's degree-level social worker. Many states have adopted patients' bills of rights much stronger than the federal version. Overall, though, state standards are patterned after federal standards.

In many critical areas, the prevailing nursing home standards are terribly weak. The requirement that there be at least one LPN (for SNFs) or aide (for ICFs) awake and on duty at night hardly provides adequate coverage in a three-story, 150-bed facility. Except in a few states, there is no requirement that a nursing home ever serve fresh fruits or vegetables, get residents dressed or out of bed, or provide adequate space for residents to store their personal possessions. Nursing homes must have nurse-call systems, but the standards do not require that they respond to those calls;[9] they must maintain an adequate supply of linen but are not required to change dirty sheets.

Nursing home standards are weak primarily because the industry has been able to exert pressure on the budget, the most vulnerable part of governmental anatomy. State governments, and the federal government as well, have been reluctant to expend lots of money on nursing home care but have been eager to ensure abundant availability of nursing home beds because of the illusion that they were cheaper places for public charges than hospitals. Regulators have always been told by regulatees that stronger standards would entail substantial costs in the form either of higher reimbursement or the inability of many facilities to participate in public programs. To some extent, the industry has been bluffing, since most nursing homes could not survive without public subsidy. But it has almost always won. When told that specific standards should be strengthened, regulators often reply, not that doing so would be inherently unreasonable, but that many facilities would have great difficulty meeting them.

Apart from their laxity, nursing home standards have also been criticized for distorting priorities, deferring to professional status, ignoring the client, and emphasizing "inputs" and "process" rather than "outcomes."

An example of distorted priorities is the fire-safety issue. Nursing home fires are visible, scandalous disasters, embarrassing to regulatory agencies and quick to attract the attention of otherwise indifferent legislators. Because they have difficulty getting around and are frequently disoriented, the frail elderly are especially vulnerable to fire, and the prevalence of converted frame structures in the earlier years of the nursing home industry made this concern logical and proper. But the degree to which prevention of fire hazards has been a preeminent regulatory focus may well have exceeded its importance to the overall welfare of nursing home residents. Many excellent, homelike facilities were closed because of their structural deficiencies, and investors have been forced to sink their money into fire doors rather than pleasant places for people to sit and talk with one another. It is now almost impossible to die in a multiple-fatality nursing home fire, but the slow deaths from indifference, callousness, or inadequate nursing services are still not only possible but largely untouched by the regulatory process.

The emphasis on fire safety does not arise solely from political concern. Its source is at least partially technological.

When policymakers went looking for ways to deal with the problem of nursing home fires, the highly detailed, technically sophisticated Life-Safety Code was readily at hand. A great deal is known about minimizing fire hazards in building construction, and all of it is tangible, quantifiable, and stamped with a professional seal of approval. Superior nursing care, dietary services, or activities programs are harder to specify and much harder to measure. The more variable, personal, and intimate the service, the more difficult it is to write a detailed standard for it.

In American law, regulated firms are entitled to administrative and judicial oversight ensuring that regulatory agencies are neither "arbitrary" nor "capricious"—if standards are to be usable, they must describe activities or tangible objects that are observable, measurable, and capable of uniform definition and interpretation. But it is almost impossible to "prove" that aides are harsh with patients, that food is unnecessarily bland, or that the director of activities is condescending or indifferent. Technologically "hard" phenomena, however secondary in importance, tend to be regulated better than technologically "soft" phenomena, however critical they may be.

The distorted regulatory emphasis on paperwork and reporting requirements derives from similar concerns. No complaint is more frequently voiced by nursing home staff, nor more worthy of sympathy, than that the backbreaking load of regulation-induced paperwork can only detract from the quality of care. But patients' charts and other records are tangible and observable; they give an inspector something to look at. It would take an omniscient regulator to appreciate whether a nursing home regularly provides a diet that is both nutritious and pleasantly varied, but anyone can read a menu plan.

The volume of paperwork is also closely tied to the role of professionals in nursing homes. Regulation-writing tends to be parceled out to professional groups that lobby for inclusion of their services while seeking to maintain their autonomy. Nursing home standards identify half a dozen independent services (nursing, dietary, pharmacy, rehabilitation, activities, social services) for each of which the professional in charge must maintain quality. Since most nursing homes are too small to usefully and efficiently employ full-time professionals in any service other than nursing, the regulations permit (except for nursing in SNFs) use of part-time "consultants." Because consultants are hardly ever there, the only way for an inspector to have any sense at all of their activity is to examine the paperwork.

The system of professional consultants is the source of many of the most serious abuses, pecuniary and qualitative, in the nursing home industry. Consultants receive exorbitant fees at public expense, essentially for filling out forms. Nursing homes are really run by their administrators and nursing directors, who must implement the orders written by consultants. But standards-writers have been reluctant to assign too much responsibility to administrators. Although administrators must be licensed by the states, qualifications for administrators' licenses have been minimal, partly because smaller nursing homes have been unable to afford full-time administrators outside the owners' family, and partly from the need to grandfather-in administrators already in practice when licensure laws were adopted. Many states still do not require that an administrator have a college degree. Happily, the quality of nursing home administrators is improving considerably as a result of substantial investment in education and of turnover from one generation to the next.

Current law lodges excessive nursing home responsibility in physicians. According to the regulations, the receipt of almost all specific services by a nursing home resident is conditioned on their having been ordered by a physician (or in some instances in ICFs, by a nurse). In addition to prescribing drugs or laboratory tests and X-rays, nursing home physicians are supposed to superintend patient diet, rehabilitative services, and personal care. Existing federal standards also assign to physicians the power to constrain the exercise of residents' rights to free association, religious observance, mail communication, conjugal relations, and control of personal property.[10]

The power assigned to physicians reflects the policymakers' emphasis on medical need as a criterion of eligibility for public subsidy, as well as an almost blind adherence to patterns of hospital organization. It has been widely criticized as ignoring the fact that the problems of the dependent elderly are predominantly psychological and social, rather than medical.

The "medical model" in nursing homes is less inappropriate than irrelevant. There is precious little medicine practiced in most nursing homes. Physicians are given extensive authority by the standards, but they are hardly ever around to exercise it. The control they are supposed to have is delegated de facto to administrators and nursing directors.

The flip side of the emphasis on professional responsibility is the limited role given residents, their relatives and representatives, and other external, nongovernmental groups. It is almost literally true that a nursing home can be inspected for standards compliance without the inspector ever seeing a resident and certainly without talking to one. However confused or blindly approving their responses, residents could be asked their opinions of the food, the quality of nursing services, or the attractiveness of activities. But the regulations give no weight to their views or their feelings.

The need for government regulation arises from the weakness of consumers of nursing home services. But it would seem plausible to expect that there is something to be gained from strengthening that role rather than giving up on it. The patients' bill of rights is extremely limited, and it is not reinforced by specific remedies. Under the federal rules, and in most states, the only recourse for a resident whose rights have been violated is to seek to have that fact recorded in the inspection/enforcement process. The federal version of the patients' bill of rights provides no guarantee of access for visitors or representatives (most states do better) and provides no enforcement or monitoring mechanisms for its requirement that patients who complain about the facility be free from discrimination or reprisal. In contrast, the state of Minnesota requires nursing homes to assist in the formation of resident councils, and seeks, with limited vigor, to provide them with a direct communications link to regulatory authorities. It is difficult to demonstrate any direct effect of this practice on the quality of nursing home care in Minnesota, which by national standards is relatively high, but it does no harm.

Another criticism of existing standards is that they are concerned almost exclusively with "inputs" (such as staffing and physical facilities) and "process" (such as paperwork) rather than with "outcomes." For example, a former state official told me that "there is nothing in our regulations that says a nursing home may not permit a patient to starve to death"; they only require three meals a day meeting minimal nutritional standards. The regulations appear to be founded in the rather heroic assumption that requiring nursing homes to have certain characteristics and to do certain things will ensure that residents are getting good "care," whatever that may be.

There has been considerable discussion over the past few years about developing more "outcome"-oriented standards for nursing homes. This approach would give individual facilities freedom to hire whomever they choose and provide as many nursing hours as they feel like so long as their residents do not deteriorate any faster than they are supposed to. Presumably, regulators should be able to predict, at least on an aggregate, statistical basis, how well newly admitted residents will do over six months or a year if they receive superior care; their status at the end of any given time period could be thought of as an "outcome." The PACE system is supposed to eventually provide the mechanism through which such judgments could be made.[11]

Apart from the fact that neither PACE nor any of its competitors have yet been shown workable in terms of setting "outcome" standards, there are other reasons to be skeptical. The "outcome" for most nursing home residents, after all, is death. The multiple degenerative problems of nursing home residents do not lend themselves to easily measurable "outcomes." And the linkage between the care delivered and the "outcome" is problematic for the kinds of difficulties experienced by nursing home residents.

If the rationale for "outcome" standards lies in the notion that regulation is seeking some level of performance, then the "outcome" desired from nursing homes is good *care;* and care is a *process.* It should make all the difference in the world whether an eighty-year-old woman slowly dying of coronary disease spends her last year in a human warehouse or in a place where people are nice to her and where she has more to do than watch television.

"Inputs" also matter, and where they do, the verdict on prevailing regulatory standards must be relatively favorable. The death rate in nursing home fires is now very low. So is the rate of poisoning from inadequately refrigerated foods and the rate of electrocution from inadequate wiring. There are literally dozens of instances in day-to-day nursing home life where regulatory standards have led to marginal improvements. The fourteen-hour rule on meals, the requirement that there be some activities program, even the transfer agreement requirements have all had some effect. The specification of quantitative nursing-hours standards (however minimal) in some states has had an impact, although nursing-hours standards can accomplish only so much.

The basic form and content of regulatory standards are largely unavoidable, given the exigencies of the standards-inspection-enforcement system and especially the insistence of policymakers that nursing homes be medical facilities without much medicine. The primary problem with the standards is that, in a political environment of industry pressures and budgetary concern, they can establish only a minimum common denominator that may be very minimal indeed. The federal Conditions of Participation and ICF Standards, as well as all the state codes, are filled with compromises between what was desirable and what was feasible. The standards are minimal, but for an industry where the preregulatory performance fell below mediocrity, the attainment of mediocrity by most facilities amounts to a significant accomplishment.

Inspection

The inspection, or "survey" process, as it is generally known in health-care regulation, has long been a weak link in the regulatory process, although it has improved substantially over the last several years.

The structure of the survey process is irrational. It has grown up piecemeal and been "reformed" any number of times in a reflexive, partial, and usually shortsighted way.

In the beginning, state health departments were charged with enforcement of state licensure laws. Medicare delegated to those departments, under the vague supervision of HEW, responsibility for certifying extended-care facilities. Medicaid, as always, took a different path, giving the states total responsibility for arranging inspections and, until 1969, total discretion over standards. Many states turned this role over to health departments, often to different units from those charged with Medicare and state code inspections. In some states, it was possible for a facility participating in both Medicare and Medicaid to be inspected by Medicare inspectors, Medicaid inspectors (sometimes from the health department, sometimes from the welfare department), and still a third time by the state's own facility code inspectors.

Since 1974, Medicare, Medicaid, and state surveys have largely been consolidated, but other developments have led to a further proliferation of inspectors. The Nixon nursing home reforms of 1971–72 created a cadre of federal inspectors, based in HEW's ten regional offices, who "validate" state surveys by resurveying roughly 10 percent of homes visited by the states. Concern with Life-Safety Code enforcement led to the creation of special "structural" surveys by both federal and state governments. Fleshing out of utilization review regulations required the states to employ special "Medical Review" teams (for SNFs) or "Independent Professional Review" teams (for ICFs) to inspect patients. And as public attention to nursing homes has increased, municipal and county health and building departments have begun to take more seriously their responsibility to enforce local sanitation, health, and building codes.

Consequently, a single nursing home may be inspected several dozen times a year by a dozen different agencies, each concerned with a different feature of its operations. This does not even include the armies of auditors and accountants enforcing—separately, of course—the cost-reporting requirements of Medicare and Medicaid. Nursing home operators have a perfectly legitimate complaint when they say inspection process is duplicative, wasteful, and time consuming. That complaint would be still more valid if those inspections had more content or force to them.

There are more than fifteen thousand nursing homes in the country. A decent general inspection requires at least a couple of days just to fill out all the forms. Form SSA–1569, the "Medicare/Medicaid Skilled Nursing Facility Survey Report," is sixty-eight pages; its ICF counterpart is only twenty-four but is frequently supplemented by additional state forms. (The size of these documents reflects the failure to decide what is important and what is not in the standards themselves, but a complete top-to-bottom inspection of a good-sized nursing home should require the collection of a lot of information.)

Many states use two- to four-person teams (a nurse, a "sanitarian," an "administrative generalist," and perhaps a nutritionist) for their surveys, so a single inspection can easily take eight man-days. There are perhaps 3,000 people in the nation who devote at least part of their time to nursing home inspections. But the number of available full-time equivalents is such that many states have difficulty meeting the federal minimum of one complete survey per facility per year, especially because, when serious deficiencies are found, resurveys are invariably required. And nursing homes are so unstable that a facility that corrects a deficiency in one area is likely to have another spring up somewhere else in the interim. Since nursing home inspections are conducted by different people looking for different things, none of whom talk to one another, no general view is ever recorded. More frequent inspection by agencies with broad, general jurisdiction would be more valuable.

The variability of nursing home argues for unpredictability in the scheduling of inspections. It is relatively easy for nursing homes with serious nonstructural deficiencies to erect Potemkin villages on short notice. It has long been common practice for nursing homes to schedule annual cleanups, to purchase additional linen and supplies, and even to rent equipment or add staff in anticipation of inspection, only to revert to less-satisfactory practices once the inspection is past. Yet until recently, it was routine practice to give facilities considerable advance notice of when the surveyors were coming. In many cases, this practice was rationalized on the grounds that it made the surveyors' work easier if the facilities had their records in order and staff members were accessible. This practice was tied to a concept of surveyors as "consultants," not police. And sometimes it was the result of political pressure.

In 1973, Minnesota enacted a law requiring unannounced health department inspections of nursing homes. Somehow, though, the facilities always seemed to know when the inspectors were coming. Rumors of intrigue and corruption filled the air. A special committee of the state legislature investigated. It found that federal regulations required the states to inspect nursing homes certified for Medicaid at least once a year, thirty to ninety days prior to expiration of their Medicaid provider agreement (presumably to give the facilities time to correct deficiencies before the provider agreement was renewed). Nursing homes knew that surveys would have to be conducted within the two-month span. But the state health department was short of staff and always behind on inspections. It rarely met the federal requirements with more than a day or two to spare. It was very simple for nursing home operators to look at the expiration date on their provider agreement and subtract thirty-two or thirty-three days.[12]

The obvious solution in the Minnesota case, and everywhere else, is to increase survey staffing or to train "generalists" who can do the work of more than one surveyor. Since the nursing home scandals of the mid-1970s, many states have increased the size of their inspection operations. But even though the federal government picks up a large share of the cost, elected officials would rather spend scarce budget dollars on increased benefits to constituents than on inspection, despite the fact that inspection can improve the delivery of those benefits.

Given the enormous variation in quality among nursing homes, it would make sense to devote most of the inspection effort to the most inadequate homes and to check the better ones more sporadically. Yet the existing regulations are interpreted by HEW to require that each nursing home receive the full top-to-bottom survey at least once a year and to hold that partial or spot checks are impermissible. With the exceptions of New Jersey and South Carolina, which have received special waivers from HEW, the states make no special effort to establish priorities in inspection or to concentrate their efforts on the worst problems. The appearance of evenhandedness in policing facilities is important to the legal enforceability of standards. It is also compelling in the political arena, where bureaucrats are generally eager to cover their legislative flanks. The director of a facilities branch of a state health department has no desire to receive a memo from the commissioner attached to a letter from a member of a powerful legislative committee inquiring about the apparent harassment of his constituent whose nursing home has been inspected half a dozen times in the past year while his competitor down the street has only been visited once. No matter how much sense that situation may make, it may be difficult to explain to the legislator. Finally, there is considerable bureaucratic inertia in the failure to schedule surveys in a manner responsive to variations in facility quality. It is easier to run through the list from alpha to omega and then start all over again.

Special terms of state surveyors whose function is to respond to complaints have become increasingly popular. Most often, these teams have been established as a result of failure to respond to an inquiry that the press revealed to have been well founded. In some states, these teams have been required by the legislature in response to pressures from consumer groups. The availability of complaint teams provides health departments with a kind of special, flying squad to concentrate on special problems. But most of those involved in the survey process believe that the correlation between complaints and serious deficiencies is tenuous and that, when manpower is scarce, responding to spontaneous complaints may not be the best way to employ it.

Rules designed to curb the worst facilities must be imposed identically on the best. Standards must be highly explicit and detailed in order to prevent the worst operators from finding additional corners to cut and even to anticipate inadequacies in the quality of care they may not yet have dreamed up. These details, when enforced in the cases of the better facilities, may appear to be the worst kind of nit-picking and red tape. But equal justice requires that surveyors cite a first-rate nursing director for being behind on keeping patient charts the same as they cite incompetent nursing directors who could not maintain a decent chart if they tried.

At one time, nursing home surveyors had substantial discretion. From the time state health departments became active in the survey and inspection of health facilities, they defined their role as "consultants" rather than "cops," reflecting the deference of public health agencies to private professionals—especially the fraternity of physicians.[13] Government agencies sought to make allies, not opponents, of such powerful groups. Most surveyors, and their supervisors, liked to think of themselves as professionals too, and thus colleagues and peers of those whose facilities they were surveying.

In the early years of nursing home surveys, the quality of most institutions was so low that the only alternative to playing a consultative role was to insist on the closing of an overwhelming proportion of all facilities—a politically unacceptable approach.

There is no gainsaying that nursing home regulators and those they regulated developed, as in many areas of government regulation, a mutually interdependent relationship. The nursing home owner or administrator is in a position to make the surveyor's job much easier and more pleasant. Americans tend to be uncomfortable with authoritarian face-to-face relations. As sociologist Jerome H. Skolnick has pointed out, relations between adversaries, like those between nursing home administrator and surveyor, tend to "regress" into cooperative ones.[14] Although there is very little overt evidence of corruption in the survey process, there is also little evidence that, until recently, surveys were rigorous or effective. The overall pattern was one of insufficiently frequent, scheduled inspections, inadequately performed by overworked and undertrained surveyors.

The scandals of the early and mid–1970s changed all that. Above all, they changed the political balance, from one in which rigorous inspection was more trouble than it was worth to one where the greatest fear was of revelations by a newspaper or legislative investigator of shocking conditions in a nursing home that had been found adequate by the survey process. Consultants became policemen overnight. Minor problems could no longer be overlooked. Even in the best facilities, every nit had to be picked. This swing of the pendulum was undoubtedly a good thing, on the whole, but at the expense of possible pettiness and overrigidity. Greater discretion is the cure for rigidity, but discretion can become laxity. A delicate balance must be found.

Sanctions

If inspections have been the weak link in the regulatory process, sanctions have been the missing link. One of the cardinal failures of government policy has been the failure to close substandard nursing homes. While governments have become much more aggressive since 1975 in imposing penalties on nursing homes, the process is still extremely limited by few and inadequate enforcement tools.

The impact of standards and inspections has been seriously limited by the weakness of sanctions, but it has not been entirely destroyed. A high proportion of the population obeys the law more or less spontaneously, because it is the law, and public censure or criticism, unaccompanied by stronger punishment, will serve to deter most of the rest.

Unfortunately, though, the nursing home industry has a large number of recalcitrants. Investors concerned with short-term profit maximization generally found it cheaper to ignore standards than to comply with them; welfare agencies continued to ensure a flow of paying customers; and peer pressure has been weak. The failure of enforcement has been a real problem.

In order to do business, a nursing home must have a license in the state in which it operates and often a local license or a certificate of occupancy. In order to be reimbursed by Medicare or Medicaid, the nursing home must have a "provider agreement" in force. Federal law provides that a nursing home found to have deficiencies be granted a period of time to correct them. If, on reinspection, those deficiencies are not corrected or in the process of being corrected, the provider agreement is canceled or not renewed. Similarly, until recently, state licensure laws generally required initiation of license-revocation proceedings when a facility was found to have serious deficiencies.

As the only available penalty for noncompliance with standards, termination of provider agreements or licenses is too severe. It is analogous to a criminal code in which execution is the only penalty; little room is left for rehabilitation. And the innocent are penalized along with the guilty. Lifting a facility's license or provider certificate imposes serious burdens on nursing home residents as well as on those nursing home operators at whom the sanction is directed.

The reluctance of states to use so blunt-edged a tool has long been reinforced by the perceived shortage of nursing home beds.[15] No theme is more persistent in the annals of nursing home investigations than the rationale provided by state officials for the failure to remove licenses: the beds were "needed."

Legal constraints have also contributed to the reluctance to close facilities. A facility license creates a property right. Under the Fifth and Fourteenth Amendments, it can be removed only under due process of law, which includes a formal evidentiary hearing, a decision based on the facts adduced at the hearing, and the opportunity for judicial review. Some courts have found that a provider agreement constitutes the same kind of property right, although it is unmistakably a fixed-duration contract.[16] Removal of a license or a provider agreement is no easy task for a state agency.

While the evidentiary hearing is readily waived in instances of imminent life-threatening hazard to residents, and while states generally have little trouble convincing their own hearing officers of the justice of their cases, it is an expensive and time-consuming process. For example, it took the state of New York almost two years to remove Bernard Bergman's license to operate the Park Crescent Nursing Home in Manhattan, even though the commissioner's discretion over facility licenses is greater in New York than in any other state.[17] Even a year is a significant fraction of the expected lifetime of nursing home residents living in a bad facility.

The prospect of judicial review has a chilling effect on the states' enforcement activity. While the number of license revocations or provider agreement terminations that have been overturned by the courts is not great, the states have often been enjoined from enforcing those determinations until the judicial process has been completed. Given the backlogs in court calendars and the ability of skillful legal counsel to stall for time, state agencies often wonder whether decertification is worth all the trouble.

Bureaucrats tend to be afraid of litigation and to overreact to the threat of being overruled in court. The revision of standards is now colored by fears of judicial judgments about unconstitutional vagueness or arbitrariness, and surveyors are now routinely taught that their records must be of a quality that would pass muster in a formal trial setting. The potential of judicial review engenders considerable bureaucratic caution and rigidity—as indeed it is supposed to—but also considerable timidity. The ultimate effect is to discourage aggressive regulation.

There are situations in which the courts are reluctant to intervene, notably when the Life-Safety Code is involved. Most regulatory closings of nursing homes have involved structural deficiencies or safety hazards. The Life-Safety Code can certainly not be described as unconstitutionally vague, nor are judges immune to the image of elderly people dying in a nursing home fire.

In the area of quality of care (nursing services and the like) the penalty of delicensure appears to some courts to be too harsh, especially when those deficiencies can be easily remedied (assuming good faith on the part of the operator). States therefore generally attempt to close only those facilities with the most flagrant and self-evident abuses. Even then, the courts often grant the operator thirty, sixty, or ninety days (on top of the numerous extensions the state has already granted) to remedy the violation.

Judges also tend to be receptive to arguments by nursing home lawyers that closing facilities would cause "transfer trauma" for their residents. The evidence on transfer trauma suggests that moving the elderly from a bad environment to a good one is substantially less damaging than other kinds of moves. But while the facilities' argument may be willfully disingenuous, they often succeed.

In the wake of the 1975 scandals, a number of states searched for more usable penalties. Six states now have adopted systems for issuing fines for standards violations. When an inspector finds a deficiency, he issues a citation. The facility then has thirty days, give or take, to make corrections. If the deficiency has not been remedied by the time of reinspection, a fine is incurred. Generally, violations have been graded into three categories, with the most serious incurring fines of $250 to $1,000—in Minnesota, $250 *a day*, until the violation is corrected.[18]

There are substantial problems with fines, which is why the states have been so slow to adopt them. To begin with, fines are subject to the same due process considerations and to the same need for hearings and formal proceedings as delicensure actions, even though the penalties are much less severe. They also require increased record keeping, more follow-up inspections, and probably more staff. It is also feared that, to pay them off, nursing homes that incur fines will divert revenues from patient care. This last argument is dubious because paying fines out of patient care revenues is likely to lead to still more fines.

The increasingly popular sanction for nursing home noncompliance is imposition of a civil receivership. Half a dozen states have now granted their health departments statutory authority to go into district court and seek a temporary receivership for inadequate facilities; in a number of other states, attorneys general have succeeded at obtaining such receiverships under their general common law powers.

Receivership has several advantages. It involves the least disruption for residents, since moving them is not required, and the only changes made are those the receiver thinks will improve the quality of services. Standards of proof for imposition of a receivership are less stringent than they are for removing a license. And a receiver, once installed, has freedom of action that the state cannot otherwise obtain— through a receiver, the state can correct deficiencies. A receivership can be active rather than reactive. Receiverships directly address the ends for which regulation exists—improving services—rather than the means of enforcement through punishment.[19]

The major problem is finding receivers. State health departments have been reluctant to take on the job. So have administrators of other nursing homes, not eager to improve the operation of what, in essence, is the competition. Voluntary organizations have been somewhat more forthcoming but are often reluctant to get their hands dirty or to devote their scarce resources to putting out other people's brush fires.

Another problem with receivership is that the receiver is responsible for protecting the assets of owners of seriously deficient nursing homes. The public desire for retribution is hardly satisfied by a receivership that puts operating profits into an escrow account that will ultimately be returned to the malfeasor. These obstacles to successful implementation of receivership will perhaps be worked out as experience accumulates. For the time being, receivership remains a very limited enforcement tool.

Delicensure, fines, and receiverships essentially exhaust the list of currently available sanctions for noncompliance with nursing home standards. One sanction that has not been widely employed, but that might be effective if used in conjunction with those already in place, is the fiscal sanction available through Medicaid. While it is probably unacceptable, politically and legally, to cut off Medicaid funds for those already residing in substandard nursing homes, it is quite another to cut off the flow of Medicaid admissions, the major source of revenue for most facilities. Yet only two or three states have employed the "Medicaid hold" on a regular basis.

This reluctance arises from conflicts between federal law and state fiscal and managerial concerns. Medicaid recipients are guaranteed "freedom of choice" among providers, which can be interpreted to mean that the states cannot channel beneficiaries away from nursing homes holding valid provider agreements. Yet if the state challenges the provider agreement, it runs the risk of losing the federal share of Medicaid payments for residents already in the home. Those states that have used the Medicaid hold have prevailed on federal regional officials to look the other way. In most states, however, fiscal responsibility for Medicaid is lodged in welfare agencies much more concerned with maximizing federal financial participation than with helping the survey agency enforce its quality-of-care determinations. Those states have been unwilling even to run the risk of negotiating the issue with federal officials.

Another underused enforcement tool has been publicity. Inspecting agencies have not only been reluctant to publicize their findings; they have even sought to deny public access to them. Mal Schecter, an editor of the magazine *Hospital Practice*, had to take HEW to court under the Freedom of Information Act before it agreed to make survey reports available to the public. New York and California now require nursing homes to post their latest deficiency notices and make them available to prospective residents and their families, but most other states have not followed suit.

One cause for such secrecy is that health professionals assume the ignorance and incapacity of the general public. Another is that even very good facilities are bound to have some deficiencies that sound serious, while the worst facilities might not sound so bad—again, neither starving patients to death nor drowning them is a specific violation. There may have been fear that publicity about deficiencies would seriously affect the morale of residents and their families. Mostly, the survey agencies have simply been afraid of the scandals. They knew that they were countenancing the existence of many seriously deficient facilities. As the number of substandard homes has declined, the reluctance to make survey findings available to the public has diminished.

So long as beds are limited and half of all placements are made by bureaucratic agencies, it is unlikely that survey findings will have much of an effect. But prospective residents, their families, and the general public should be entitled to that information.

A third enforcement tool that has not been widely used is tort liability—suits for malpractice. But malpractice is extremely difficult to prove, even in instances of the most flagrant abuses. Even when it can be proved, there is little in the way of "damages" that can be recovered. Nursing home residents are not earning very much money and are not about to; punitive damages cannot be relied on, given public ignorance about nursing homes and their residents. Thus, few families bring suits, and negligence lawyers do not seek them out; the costs of litigation will almost inevitably exceed the potential recovery.[20]

A final enforcement tool is being experimented with in New York State. New York has adopted regulations requiring those holding professional licenses who work in nursing homes to inform on colleagues engaging in verbal or physical assaults or other abusive behavior, and has backed that up with extensive investigation of such complaints and the threat of aggressive action to remove professional licenses.[21]

Apart from the somewhat unsavory reliance on informers, the general proposition is sound, to the extent it is directed at those licensed professionals who exercise control: administrators, medical directors, attending physicians, and nursing directors. But the brunt of the new enforcement effort in New York is being borne by lower level, subordinate employees. No physician has yet lost his license for being medical director of a terrible nursing home, but some LPNs have lost theirs. There is also a problem that fear of punishment might discourage professionals from working in nursing homes at all, when there is already a serious problem of attracting enough good ones. For that reason, states are likely to be slow in following New York's example.

Outcomes

No one has bothered to keep count, but since 1972 at least several hundred, and probably on the order of a thousand, substandard nursing homes have been closed. Those that remain are relatively fire-resistant, keep some records, do not store soiled linen in the kitchen, generally keep controlled drugs in a safe place, and worry at least a little when the inspector comes to town. Each succeeding wave of increased regulation has been accompanied by gradual improvement.

But while the regulatory process has been reasonably effective at generating improvements in building standards and record keeping, it has imposed costs that may have detracted from the more important aspects of quality: kindness, consideration, and care in the nontechnical sense.

The costs of complying with regulations have directly contributed to driving smaller operators and facilities out of the nursing home industry. They have been replaced by impersonal corporate managements operating more modern but often less homelike facilities. Smaller firms are less able to afford the administrative overhead regulation requires and are less able to attract the capital regulation frequently demands, such as that needed for sprinklers or smoke alarms to meet the Life-Safety Code. As regulatory activity increases, smaller firms tend to consolidate, sell out, or drop out, and that has clearly been the case with nursing homes.[22]

One shortcoming of the regulatory process, the duplication of inspections, is soon likely to be corrected. Many states are now moving to a consolidation of general surveys, Life-Safety Code surveys, and medical review/independent professional review. There is substantial talk in the federal government of consolidating Medicare and Medicaid surveys and of encouraging the states to further rationalize their efforts. If these reforms permit more frequent inspection of the worst facilities, the benefits will be significant.

But the major shortcomings of the standards-inspection-enforcement process are not likely to be remedied in the foreseeable future. In part, this is because of the unwillingness of standards-writers to promulgate stringent requirements, for fear that many nursing homes will be unable to meet them, and that those that do meet them will do so only at great, eventually public expense. It is also because the problem of formulating legally defensible standards for the important aspects of care is truly formidable and possibly irresolvable.

Alternatives

The real trick is to control the components of quality care that regulation cannot reach. One approach is to rely on outsiders, neither professionals nor public officials, to keep an active eye on what is going on in nursing homes. There is empirical evidence that the mere presence of outsiders—be they relatives, volunteers, or representatives of religious groups—in nursing homes is associated with high quality care.[23] To the extent that outsiders share familial, religious, ethnic, or social ties with residents, they can bring a sensitivity to the least tangible aspects of nursing home life, toward which regulation is inherently incompetent. If they are provided channels through which they can communicate with administrators, staff, and regulators, they can perhaps goad them into action in these areas.

Regulation can help strengthen the ties of nursing homes to the community outside or at least remove some of the obstacles to development of those ties. Visiting hours can be made mandatory; volunteer programs can be required; facilities can be asked to appoint community members to a board of visitors. The Central Arizona Health Systems Agency, a federally funded planning body, is training volunteers to assess nursing homes under a statutory mandate from the state that will guarantee those volunteers access to facilities. The Community Services Department of the AFL-CIO has undertaken similar volunteer training efforts.

While lay groups have an important role to play in assuring nursing home quality, the central role must be played by professionals. Regulators, industry officials, and other professionals *know* which are the good nursing homes and which are the crummy ones. An experienced nursing home administrator, nurse, or surveyor can tell within half an hour whether a facility is very poor, very good, or somewhere in between. In a day and a half, they can tell with some precision and some detail how good it is. But those are "subjective" judgments that do not meet legal standards of evidence and thus are unusable for regulatory purposes.

The way to use that sort of "subjective" determination in regulating the performance of institutions is through "peer review." "Peer review" has acquired a bad name because of the unwillingness of professional groups to impose punitive sanctions on their own members and because of the way governments have bureaucratized, and thus vitiated, the process in organizations like the PSRO. But nursing home care would appear to be exactly the kind of activity to which it could be best applied.

In health policy, peer review is assumed to mean review by physicians. But physicians are willing and able to exercise control over only a small fraction of the activities that go on in a nursing home. Others who could profitably become involved in peer review, in descending order of importance, are administrators, nursing directors, nutritionists, pharmacists, and social workers. If each state identified its five or ten best facilities and asked two or three professionals from each to visit five or ten other facilities a year, the states could, at an absolute minimum, use their findings to determine which nursing homes merited the most frequent surveys. Another way to provide peer review would be for the states to reinstitute their consultative role. But in order for that process to work, it would have to be insulated from the survey process and would require a substantial increase in manpower with no immediate political payoffs.

It might seem attractive to tie peer review to licensure or reimbursement—as PSROs are supposed to do—but the essence of peer review is contradictory to the legal requirements for either system. Peer review is highly subjective, judgmatic and unquantifiable, and it works best when it is relatively informal; regulation and reimbursement require formal, objective, measurable standards.

The choice of a specific mechanism for peer review is less important than ensuring that the principle is promoted. The blatant failure of the organized professions to protect the public interest in many areas, of which nursing homes are a striking but hardly exceptional example, has generated increasing reluctance by policymakers to countenance their continued autonomy. (The unwillingness of governments to blindly accept decisions of individual physicians on nursing home admissions illustrates this point.) The tendency of the public-policy pendulum to swing from one extreme to the other creates the danger of discarding valuable professional judgment. The question is how that judgment can best be employed, controlled, and held accountable.

One answer is to combine peer review with elements of the existing regulatory process. In areas like charge nurse requirements, residents' rights, control of prescription drugs, and many aspects of the Life-Safety Code, there is no acceptable alternative to stringent standards, stringently enforced. The trick is to regulate through standards-inspection-enforcement those things that standards-inspection-enforcement can effectively control, while not trying to get indirectly, through paperwork proxies, at those things it cannot, for which peer review or public scrutiny is a preferable substitute.

A strategy for improving the quality of care in nursing homes should consist of the following:

1. Substantial strengthening of standards in those areas where they can be sensibly formulated (patients' rights, staffing, sanitation, the frequency and content of meals, and the control of drugs) combined with stringent enforcement. Most record-keeping requirements could be abandoned.

2. Mandatory peer review of all administrators, nursing directors, and medical directors, with continued licensing predicated on satisfactory performance. To provide reciprocal checks and reinforcement, peer reviewers and regulatory surveyors should have to take each other's findings into account. (Reviewers would have to demonstrate extraordinary extenuating circumstances, for example, to justify continued licensing for an administrator whose facility had repeated sanitary deficiencies, while finding such deficiencies would cast serious doubt, and should generate sanctions, on peer reviewers.)
3. Creation of formal mechanisms, such as visiting committees or governing board representation, to engage outsiders in monitoring nursing homes. These outsiders should formally report both to the facilities and the regulators, and both should be required to respond.

The Limits of Regulation

In the promotion of quality of care in nursing homes, regulation is both indispensable and inadequate. For regulation to work effectively, administrators must be able to ignore the peccadilloes of the good guys while coming down hard on the slightest transgressions by the bad guys. They must be able to distinguish legitimate good faith from ritualistic adherence to requirements and to consider intentions as well as performance. And they must be able to draw on a flexible range of standards that can be applied with some degree of arbitrariness.

The American legal system will not stand for that. Every administrative act is, potentially, subject to judicial review as well as to legislative oversight. The precise extent to which courts restrict administrators fluctuates with the cycles of history, but we seem to be in a period of relatively strong judicial antipathy to administrators. The granting of an injunction against the closing of a nursing home, the overruling of a determination that a provider agreement should be cancelled, the denial of a state's cutoff of Medicaid funds to a noncomplying nursing home, the requirement of a formal hearing before a fine can be imposed for a life-threatening safety or pharmacy violation—all make it difficult to administer a regulatory regime in an industry where qualitative concerns bulk so large.

Governments stand before the bar with the inherent powers of sovereignty limited and suspect. Since regulated industries have a considerable economic stake in the process and seek out the best legal counsel, while state governments rely heavily on patronage appointees and recent graduates of the state university's law school, the administrator comes to court with two strikes against him—and knows it before he ever gets served with papers. Much of the red tape, inflexibility, pickiness, and caution in the regulatory process are the result.

Closely related to this primary legal problem is a problem that might be described as technological. It has been suggested that one of the reasons "health and safety" regulations have come under increasing political attack is that governments have attempted, in recent years, to extend regulatory authority into more complex and sophisticated areas, where it is difficult to establish standards. Perhaps even more difficult to regulate are human services, such as those provided by health-care or social welfare institutions, where the basic "technology" consists of a professional sitting down and working with a client. As the nursing home experience suggests, the more engineering content there is to an activity, the easier it is to draw regulatory standards; the more the activity resembles social work or individual counseling, the harder it is.

The combination of this technological problem with legal constraints is a major source of the regulatory emphasis on "input" or "process" as opposed to "outcome" standards. Since the service being delivered is so hard to define, let alone to measure, regulators rely on professional licensure (inputs) or peer review (process).

The regulation of inputs or processes, rather than outcomes, also permits society to avoid directly confronting problems of overwhelming moral and political complexity. The "outcome" of air pollution is so many respiratory deaths per year; of automobile accidents so many deaths, so many spinal cord injuries, so much permanent disability. The short-range outcome of optimal nursing home care is retarded deterioration of residents. From the viewpoint of classical welfare economics, the optimal social choice is an outcome standard that precisely equates the cost of preventing the marginal death with the value society places on preventing that death. Any other standard is technically inefficient. But the political system, reflecting, one suspects, more widely shared attitudes, refuses to address problems in these terms. It chooses, instead, to mandate what seems to be reasonable from the viewpoint of common sense and professional judgment and to deliberately refuse to attempt to find the technically "correct" solution.

Regulation is a profoundly political process. In the United States, politics is the art of displeasing the smallest number of potential voters by attempting to do a little something for everybody, even if those "everythings" become contradictory. Government policies often work at cross purposes because interests in society are often at cross purposes. There is no law that requires any legislative body to be consistent. The courts do often require administrators to be consistent. As a result, regulation is frequently a mess.

The implicit message to nursing home regulators from the Congress and state legislatures, from whom their authority derives, has been: Maintain the highest possible standards of nursing home care without requiring more than incremental increases in Medicaid expenditures and don't stir up a political fuss. Avoid visible disasters like nursing home fires at all costs, but keep the industry off our backs. Don't appear officious, arbitrary, or capricious. The people in nursing homes must be protected, but remember that nursing home operators are constituents too.

In response to such conflicting signals, the classic bureaucratic response may well be to do nothing, and that is often what nursing home regulators have done. Those dedicated to doing something more have tried to do the best they could within those difficult constraints. There are many instances of inefficiency, stupidity, and irrationality in the regulatory process. But on the whole, governments have gotten just what they have asked for.

8

Robbers and Cops

"Trust everybody, but cut the cards."
—Mr. Dooley

THERE HAS long been a considerable element of cops and robbers—sometimes of keystone cops—in government–nursing home relations. The nursing home industry has exhibited an extremely high level of criminal activity, and that activity has been a continuing object of government concern. The extensive inquiries of New York State's Moreland Act Commission were triggered by revelations of financial manipulation. Congressional committees and investigative bodies in other states have also been preoccupied with the problems of theft. The major congressional initiative in nursing home legislation since 1972 was the Medicare and Medicaid Antifraud and Abuse Amendments of 1977.

There is good political capital in crime. Everybody loves a parade of nervous witnesses. Pecuniary scandals make great public relations for the politicians who "uncover" them. And focusing attention on criminal behavior permits policymakers to avoid the more complex and controversial issues. Crime, like cancer, is something to which everyone can safely appear opposed.

But the preoccupation with stealing in the nursing home industry is not misplaced. If only 2 percent of every dollar expended for nursing home services winds up in the wrong pockets, that comes to a quarter of a billion dollars a year. At least half that money is public—dollars toward which citizens feel a certain proprietary protectiveness. Moreover, these dollars were intended for the provision of care to needy and helpless individuals, so that deprivations resulting from their diversion are particularly reprehensible. It has been widely argued that there is a direct, causal connection between the degree of stealing and the extent of inadequate care in the nursing home industry. If that argument holds, then "program fraud and abuse" deserves special attention.

Theft from government programs has a number of important consequences. While it is logically distinct, and sometimes actually separated, from the corruption of public officials—defined as the shaping of policy in exchange for illegitimate inducements—the two often go hand in hand. Political corruption raises serious questions in any society with democratic ideals. Moreover, theft from government programs imposes an inequitable and often burdensome tax on both the general public and, especially, intended program beneficiaries. And in the long run, awareness of the diversion of public funds into the wrong hands discredits government action in general, further reinforces the innate suspicion of many Americans toward the public sector, and thus weakens legitimate public activity. In the sphere of public opinion, bad policy tends to drive out good, and one scandal of six-figure magnitude can cripple an effective and worthwhile multibillion dollar program.

Varieties of Crime

The criminal activity frequently associated with the nursing home industry (presented in table 5) includes embezzlement of patients' assets, extortion from the families of residents, vendor kickbacks, reimbursement fraud, capital finance fraud, fraudulent attempts to appear in compliance with regulatory standards, criminal abuse of patients, thefts from nursing homes by owners and employees, and tax fraud. The big money is in the first five. The most pervasive, until recently, was embezzlement of residents' assets. In a sizable minority of the nation's nursing homes, a large proportion of Medicaid residents' $25 "personal needs" funds were routinely embezzled by nursing home operators for their personal use.[1]

Many nursing home residents are not competent to manage funds on their own behalf, nor do many have families capable of playing an active role in their care. It is not uncommon for the nursing home or its administrator to be assigned the status of legal guardian of the resi-

TABLE 5
Major Forms of Nursing Home Crime

Type	Order of Magnitude (in dollars)	Comments
Embezzlement of residents' assets	Tens of millions per year	Small sums but widespread practice
Extortion from residents' families	Tens of millions per year	"Consumer fraud"
Vendor kickbacks	Tens of millions per year	Especially pharmacy
Reimbursement fraud	Tens of millions per year	Different forms in cost-related and flat rate states
Capital finance fraud	Hundreds of millions in 1965-75 period	Now largely passé
Fraudulent regulatory compliance	?	Thin line between civil and criminal abuses
Patient abuse	—	Thin line between civil and criminal abuses
Employee theft	Tens of millions per year	High similarity to hospitals and other industries
Tax fraud	?	Largely as byproduct of other forms

dent and his or her assets. Even when such formal guardianship is not established, the resident generally receives only a single social security check that he or she signs over to the nursing home, which then has the responsibility for segregating the personal needs amount. Since personal needs allowances are spent almost entirely within the facility, it has appeared to make sense for the nursing home to assume responsibility for managing residents' accounts. That is not a simple administrative task. When it is performed correctly, separate ledgers must be kept for every resident, and hundreds of nickel-and-dime transactions must be recorded every month. The temptation to take short cuts has been overwhelming. So, apparently, has been the temptation to steal.

Until recently, many states did not even require nursing home operators to maintain separate accounts for residents' personal funds. Most nursing homes routinely skimmed off whatever interest residents' funds earned; many appropriated the entire amount. It was easier than keeping track of separate accounts; most of those from whom the money was taken never knew it was missing, and a complete accounting was never demanded.

In those states that did regulate resident funds, somewhat more sophisticated devices were employed to steal them. In Ohio, where facilities were required to segregate residents' funds from their own, one nursing home was afflicted by a series of armed robberies, always at night, when only one staff person was on duty. Through an amazing coincidence, the robbers were unable to penetrate the safe containing the nursing home's petty cash but cleaned out the safe containing residents' funds every time, to the owner's expressed amazement and chagrin.[2] Less creative methods have included phony charges for services or items to which the resident is entitled under Medicaid but never received, or exorbitant charges at the "company store" for routine items like Kleenex or toothpaste.

Assuming that, at any given time, there are 750,000 nursing home residents receiving Medicaid, then the flow of personal needs funds approaches $225 million a year. Illegal diversion of any substantial proportion of that total comes to a lot of money. Since the inception of Medicaid, it is likely that the total amount stolen, from residents' accounts alone, amounts to hundreds of millions of dollars. The Medicare-Medicaid Anti-fraud and Abuse Amendments (H.R.3) now require that nursing homes maintain separate accounts for residents' funds, with complete, audited, bookkeeping.[3] If enforced, as they may be for at least a few years, those requirements may largely eliminate the problem. The cost of doing so will be considerable in bookkeeping alone, but there appears to be no other way of handling the problem aside from establishing an entirely separate instrumentality, which would itself have to be policed, to handle those funds.

While big money, in the aggregate, may come from the millions of nickels and dimes in residents' accounts, larger individual sums have come from residents' families. The less-scrupulous nursing home operators have adeptly played on the guilt, naiveté, and fear of thousands of families for millions of dollars in unreported income. Despite the fact that Medicaid, by statute, relieves all relatives but a resident's spouse of any financial responsibility for a beneficiary's nursing home care, the flow of funds from families of residents to nursing home operators must be on the order of a billion dollars a year, much of it illegal.

Those residents not receiving public assistance have lacked the most elementary kinds of consumer protection in purchasing nursing home services. Many contracts between nursing homes and families turn over all of the residents' assets to the facility, as well as all pension and other income, and then add additional charges, with the most minimal accounting for services rendered. Goods and services such as special diets or nonprescription medication, which by law or practice should have been included in the monthly rate, have been billed separately, whether actually provided or not. More direct extortion has taken the form of threats, explicit or implied, that the family member will not receive the best of care or will be discharged altogether, unless supplementary payments are made. The extent of consumer fraud practiced against self-pay nursing home residents and their relatives and the fact that they are almost entirely defenseless has received the recognition of the Federal Trade Commission, which is now conducting a formal industry-wide investigation.[4]

Voluntary nursing homes have often relied on an entirely legal form of extortion from families and fraud against the tax laws: requirement of a "charitable contribution" to the facility as a kind of admission charge. Given long waiting lists, the voluntaries have been able to exercise considerable selectivity about admissions and have, in many instances, exacted contributions of thousands of dollars from anxious families in a hurry to make a placement. Such contributions in exchange for a specific favor have been outlawed by H.R.3; while families can still be required to pay an admissions fee, they can no longer take it as a tax-deductible "contribution."[5]

The "life-care" contract, long employed by voluntary nursing homes, has also led to serious problems and is increasingly being abandoned. Under the life-care concept, employed primarily by religious groups, a resident would pay a substantial fixed fee on admission (in recent years, as much as $50,000) supplemented, in some cases, by a nominal monthly fee. In exchange, the nursing home would guarantee to care for the resident for the rest of the resident's life. Life-care contracts were employed by many organizations with limited financial resources as the means of raising capital to get facilities off the ground, literally and figuratively. Many older individuals, who had accumulated some assets but feared they would outlive them and have no one to take care of them, were reassured by the security life-care arrangements appeared to provide.

Many institutions financed by life-care arrangements found their residents outliving actuarial assumptions, while inflation and changing regulatory standards drove costs up beyond projections. In many instances, bankruptcies have been averted by exacting additional fees from residents or their families; in some cases, sponsoring bodies have had to chip in from other resources. And some institutions have gone bankrupt, leaving their residents substantially worse off than they were to begin with. In order for a life-care institution to be financially successful, its residents must live no longer than predicted; the better the care, and therefore the longer the residents live, the greater the risk of bankruptcy. The fact that there have been so many near-bankruptcies suggests that ineptitude rather than cupidity has been the principal characteristic of the operators of life-care facilities.

To return to illegal practices, extortion from residents' families quickly shades into fraud against Medicaid. Supplementation of Medicaid payments is in violation of the law. It is widespread, although often on a small scale, taking the form of "bribes" or "tips" to employees of the nursing home. Double billing of families and Medicaid for "ancillary" services not included in the basic rate, notably for prescription drugs and medical supplies, has also been common, as has billing of families, Medicaid, or both for ancillary services never supplied. Nursing homes have also been known to bill Medicaid for several months after residents have died or been discharged.

Abuses in Medicaid billing often involve professionals other than nursing home administrators, either in cooperation with the operators or as free agents. Physicians, podiatrists, and physical therapists have billed Medicaid for "gang visits" to nursing homes in which, in paper compliance with the regulations, they have "visited" dozens of patients in an hour or so without actually laying eyes on most of them— sometimes without even appearing at the facility but conducting their "examinations" by phone.[6] There is substantial phony billing or inflated charging for prescription drugs as well. In pharmaceutical service, these practices are often related to kickback arrangements.[7]

All these practices are now illegal. In some states, until recently, many were not. (Ohio, for example, had no statutory ban on provider fraud.)[8] The response of Congress and state legislators to revelations about these practices has been to substantially increase penalties and sometimes to appropriate additional funds for enforcement activities. Nursing home interests have complained that the complexity of the administration of Medicaid has led to many honest billing errors, now prosecuted as felonies. But it is apparent that many "errors" have not been entirely inadvertent and that prosecutors have been too reluctant, rather than too eager, to prosecute.

The most elaborate Medicaid and Medicare frauds involved falsification of cost reports in cost-related reimbursement systems. The most dramatic cases have been in New York, where Rembrandts, Cadillacs, and private yachts were billed to the Medicaid program under one phony category or another.[9] In total, the special prosecutor has identified $70 million in Medicaid overpayments alone.[10] While it is true that "allowable costs" is a complicated bureaucratic matter, subject to differing interpretations, it is clear that the bulk of the $70 million involved egregious violations, and that the special prosecutor has only brought criminal indictments in cases of transparent fraud.

Most of the special prosecutor's indictments have involved vendor kickbacks. For example, a nursing home operator conspires with a supplier, say, of meat or cleaning services, who bills at an inflated rate or delivers fewer or lower-quality goods than those specified on an invoice and then kicks back a large part of the difference to the operator. The illegally inflated cost is then passed along to the reimbursement system. Most of the vendor kickback cases in New York have followed that model.[11] In other states, especially those with flat-rate reimbursement, kickbacks have been most common in ancillary services, notably pharmacy. The franchise to supply drugs to a nursing home is a valuable concession for a pharmacist. Individual nursing home operators have sold those opportunities to local pharmacists, who recoup the costs, in some instances, by stealing the difference from Medicaid, often in collusion with the nursing home operator.[12] In states with flat-rate reimbursement systems, kickbacks from vendors have been less common, except for those services (laundry is a frequently cited example) where they are a standard business practice not limited to nursing homes.

Large sums have also been stolen through capital finance fraud. The devices employed entail inflating the price of a facility, generally through phony transactions in which operators essentially sell to themselves, in order to increase paper depreciation and both the reimbursement of depreciation and tax shelter it provides. Medicare put its foot down on this practice as early as 1969, but states often continued to pay the inflated amounts for some time thereafter.

There is not way to estimate how much money has been involved in these "big five" forms of stealing in the nursing home industry. Nor is there any other way to determine what proportion of facilities have participated in these shenanigans. On the basis of what little hard evidence is available, a reasoned guess would be that over the last few years prior to the enactment of H.R.3, the total volume must have been in excess of $100 million a year and may have run to several hundreds of millions. The number of facilities engaging in such activity has probably fallen continuously since the early days of Medicaid, and there has probably always been substantial variation from one area to another. It seems safe to say that in some parts of the country, some of the practices described here have been engaged in, to some degree, by the overwhelming majority of facilities, while only the most avaricious operators have engaged in all of them all of the time. As public exposure has increased and as regulatory efforts have been expanded, it is likely that only a distinct, but still sizable, minority of operators (somewhere between 10 and 20 percent) have been stealing on all but the most modest scale.

One hundred million dollars comes to only 1 percent of total industry revenues; $500 million, probably an extremely high estimate, would still only be 5 percent. That volume of stealing is not inordinately high compared to stealing in other enterprises. The estimate of 10 to 20 percent of dishonest operators is not out of line with dishonesty in other industries. On the other hand, $500 million would roughly equal reported after-tax income for the industry as a whole, and illegally obtained income is untaxed. And all of it is other people's money.

Causes

The opportunities for crime in the nursing home industry have been vast, because of the way in which money was dispensed and the weakness of those on whose behalf it was purportedly being spent.

There has been an enormous volume of money flowing into the nursing home industry. Individuals seeking to make a fast buck tend to gravitate to sectors of rapid economic growth, especially those sectors that are not already dominated by a few large firms. The involvement of real estate speculators in the nursing home industry reflects this pattern, as does their gradual outmigration as the nursing home industry has begun to consolidate. The tenfold growth in nursing home revenues since 1965 created a boom-town atmosphere and morality in which controls were something that could be worried about tomorrow.

Nor was much of that money dispensed with great care. For its size, Medicaid was, and in some parts of the country still is, one of the most poorly administered public programs in recent memory. Part of the problem arose from the division of responsibility between federal and state governments, and between the states and the counties. Part of the problem arose from the decision to be deferential toward the providers of medical services in order to elicit as much cooperation from them as possible. But the core of the problem was the inability of welfare agencies to cope with a vendor payment operation.

Medicaid administration involves certification of beneficiary eligibility and the processing of reimbursement claims from providers. The agencies administering Medicaid at the state level were very conscious, if not conscientious, about problems with certification but totally lacked controls on reimbursement. Claims processing was often subcontracted to Blue Cross or other insurance companies that were efficient at writing checks but had no mandate to root out fraud. Administrative controls that would have at least required those bent on stealing to exert some effort, let alone controls that might have actually made stealing difficult, were very slow to develop. Auditing of claims was almost nonexistent, and unanalyzed records were stored in shoeboxes despite the fact that technologies to do a moderately effective job were already being employed or developed by the Social Security Administration in another branch of HEW.

While middle-class service providers were stealing millions, public officials concentrated on beneficiary fraud—"welfare cheats"—and such administrative controls as were instituted focused almost entirely on eligibility determination. Knowing that benefit recipients, and thus their programs, were vulnerable to charges of fraud and theft, welfare administrators sought to downplay the issue of stealing and to concentrate on getting the dollars out. They defined their job as dispensing benefits, not law enforcement or "interference" in the private lives of their clients. Nor, until recently did the federal government, despite its considerable financial stake, push the states to improve Medicaid administration.

Medicaid beneficiaries were in no position to defend their own interests. The very causes of institutionalization render nursing home residents especially vulnerable to exploitation of all kinds. Relatives, whose emotional and practical position is analogous to that of people buying funeral services, are not in a much stronger position. Moreover, poor people, almost by definition, are less able to fend for themselves in the marketplace.[13] If welfare recipients are more likely to be cheated in their purchases of food or housing, they are also likely to be cheated in their "purchase" of nursing home care.

Another source of consumer incapacity is embarrassment. So strong is the stigmatization attached to the receipt of welfare benefits of any kind and so often humiliating are the procedures imposed on prospective beneficiaries that relatives of nursing home residents are too ashamed to make complaints against the system. Medicaid-financed nursing home care is the one "welfare" benefit received by large numbers of middle-class families to whom the very idea of welfare is anathema, and shenanigans they would not put up with for a minute if attempted by those who sell them cars or houses—or by their own physicians—are unopposed when engaged in by those providing nursing home care to their relatives.

The incentives to steal from Medicaid were very great, and the likelihood of resistance from residents and their relatives very low. The chances of being caught perpetrating most of the forms of stealing were also very low, the chances of being prosecuted and convicted if caught only somewhat higher, and the odds of being punished in some proportion to the size of the crime almost infinitesimal.

It has been widely observed that prosecuting agencies at all levels have been reluctant to vigorously pursue "white-collar" crime. While that is largely accurate as an historic generalization, it was perhaps never more true than in the late 1960s and early 1970s, when the public appeared terrified by violent street crime and law-enforcement agencies were preoccupied with the phantom specters of political protest and counterculture radicalism. In the United States, most prosecuting agencies in most jurisdictions are headed by elected officials who, when they are not concerned with reelection, are generally running for higher offices. When newspaper headlines are filled with reports of murders, assaults, rapes, political demonstrations, and drug abuse, crimes such as Medicaid fraud are unlikely to be allocated a large share of scarce law-enforcement resources—unless those frauds are committed by minority-group beneficiaries. Nor do most nursing home criminals fit the public stereotypes of dangerous criminals. They are neither young, black, nor, in most instances, Italian. Instead, they are typically moderately affluent small businessmen, a sociological type generally viewed favorably by the public. This is not just a matter of public appearance; one of the reasons judges are so often reluctant to impose stiff sentences on white-collar criminals, it has been argued, is that those criminals are so much like them in social and economic background.[14]

Until recently, the penalties for Medicaid fraud have been disproportionately light compared to the amounts of money that have been stolen. When convictions were obtained, fines were only a fraction of the money taken (restitution of the amount illegally obtained customarily would have involved a payment many times larger) and prison terms were rarely meted out. From the viewpoint of a narrowly calculating individual not much affected by compassion for his clients or concern for his public reputation, *not* stealing from Medicaid was an economically irrational thing to do, even if the likelihood of being caught was calculated as much greater than it really was.

Much of the illegal activity committed in the nursing home industry is also very hard to prove in court. Residents do not make good witnesses, which is a primary reason prosecutors have brought so few cases involving physical abuse. Families are easily intimidated. Difficulties in measuring, or even defining, the quality of care rendered provide a great obstacle to criminal prosecutions. In cases of overbilling or duplicate billing, the provider's criminal intent must be proved in court.

Edwin Sutherland, the sociologist who literally wrote the book on white-collar crime, coined the term "differential association" to describe the theory that white-collar crime is a learned behavior that flourishes in certain institutions and not in others.[15] To borrow a term from other criminologists, certain kinds of stealing may be characterized by a "contagion" phenomenon.[16] Somebody starts doing it and gets away with it; others observe and follow suit.

The rapid expansion of nursing home revenues attracted a number of shady characters into the industry, anticipating a Medicare boom. When that boom fizzled, they found themselves holding expensive bags. In some places at some times, the only way to make a comfortable profit was to cheat. Those who didn't were driven out of the industry, often selling out to those who did. Nursing home operators soon caught on to the fact that stealing was going on successfully. When it was not resisted by public agencies, stealing, in certain forms and in certain areas, became contagious. Differential association began to take over, as relatively honest operators were driven out and new operators quickly became educated into customary ways of doing business. That such sociological phenomena were occurring seems to be demonstrated by the fact that the proprietary industry in metropolitan New York City, as well as a number of other metropolitan areas, was pretty thoroughly corrupt, while there was less stealing in some upstate cities. The nursing home industry in Texas has long had a particularly unsavory reputation, while neighboring Oklahoma has had less of a problem; the levels of stealing in Massachusetts have been high, while in Connecticut they have been low.

Reducing the level of corruption in an industry in which it is widespread is a very different, and much more difficult, problem from minimizing its development in the first place. Someone in the New York Special Prosecutor's Office said that if you put a million dollars on a table, 10 percent of the population won't steal it no matter what, 10 percent will try to steal it even if it is guarded by policemen with machine guns, and the other 80 percent will steal it only if they think they have a good chance of getting away with it. But, after a decade of widespread stealing in the state, experience suggests that the last category has shrunk considerably, and the middle group has grown to far exceed the first.

The pattern of nursing home corruption differs substantially from the more traditional forms of stealing from government, in which firms in industries dependent on government contracts seek to ensure their prosperity by bribing politicians. Political corruption has not been absent from the nursing home arena, but it has been less closely tied to stealing. In the nursing home industry, the pattern is that governments seek to provide benefits to dependent groups through intermediary contractors, who then defraud the beneficiaries by overcharging, delivering less than promised, or extorting additional income. Stealing has arisen in areas where administrative controls have been weak and where a contagion process appears to have occurred (see table 6).

Stealing and Quality

Since any dollars stolen are in some sense being subtracted from those available for the care of nursing home residents, the tie between poor care and degree of corruption would appear logical. It might also be expected that the most rapacious and greedy operators would be the most indifferent to the well-being of their residents.

But officials in the office of the New York Special Prosecutor insist that they have found no systematic relationship between the extent of stealing and poor care. In fact, they found that many of the biggest

TABLE 6

Patterns of Stealing from Government Programs

Type	Characteristic Pattern	Contagion Effect	Relationship to Political Corruption	Program Growth	Administrative Controls	Intended Program Beneficiaries
"Traditional"	Firms highly dependent on government obtain favors through political corruption or patronage. Examples: construction; land-use planning and regulation.	High	Contingent on such corruption	Low	Varying	Diffuse general public
"Welfare Fraud"	Individuals obtain benefits to which they are not entitled, or, if entitled to benefits, more than they are entitled to obtain. Examples: Unreported income by welfare recipients; phony disability claims.	Low to Moderate	At lower administrative levels only, and not frequently	Low	Stringent, often counterproductive	The ones doing the stealing
"New Welfare Fraud"	Government provides benefits through contractors, who overcharge or deliver less than promised or extort additional income from beneficiaries. Examples: nursing homes; school lunch programs.	Moderate to high	Not uncommon, but not necessary	Rapid	Weak	Residents Students

crooks ran moderate to very good nursing homes, while some of those who ran poor nursing homes were more incompetent than dishonest.[17] Officials in other states have reported similar observations. The most intelligent and far-sighted crooks might endeavor to run especially good facilities in order to maintain good relations with regulatory authorities, stay out of the public eye, and develop a positive professional reputation.

To give some sense of the complexity of the problem, a nursing home operator could make a legal deal with a beauty parlor to provide services to his residents at $20 a shot, receive a 50 percent "concession" fee, and maintain the integrity of his residents' personal needs accounts in order to ensure the flow of those fees. Or, he could arrange to have the beauty shop charge only $5 and steal the rest directly from the residents' accounts. Residents may be worse off in a nursing home run by an honest incompetent from whom the staff steals most of the linen and cleaning supplies than in one run by an efficient crook who—in part because he has a kickback arrangement with a supplier—sees to it that there is plenty of both. On balance, however, entrepreneurs more concerned with extracting quick windfalls than establishing stable businesses with assets in "good will" can hardly have been beneficial for nursing home residents.

It could be contended that some states have unconsciously accepted a situation in which nursing homes, like medieval armies, have been paid bare subsistence plus all they could steal. For the nursing home operator, taking his residents' $25-a-month personal needs allowance is almost equal to an additional dollar a day per resident in reimbursement rates, and public officials may have winked at the diversion of the former in order to avoid having to pay the latter. There is reason to believe that some legislators have not looked askance at the supplementing of the personal needs allowance by the families of Medicaid recipients—so long as it was done covertly—since it deflects political pressures to do something about the quality of care by raising reimbursement rates. Some members of the nursing home industry will argue that in order to get by under low reimbursement rates it has been necessary to steal. Such attitudes have probably not played a central part, but they have contributed to the general pattern of stealing in the nursing home industry.

Policing

The scandals of the mid-1970s dramatically increased the political attractiveness of crackdowns on nursing home fraud and abuse. A major impetus for those crackdowns was the belief that, over time, they would produce substantial dollar savings for public programs.

The intensified effort to prevent or prosecute stealing in the nursing home industry was embodied in H.R.3, which increases the incentives for public officials to prosecute stealing. It expands and tightens the definition of vendor kickbacks; mandates new procedures for management of residents' funds, violation of which is subject to strengthened penalties; and outlaws extorted "charitable contributions" as a condition for admission to, or special consideration by, a nursing home. It upgrades most forms of provider fraud from misdemeanors to felonies to which are attached penalties of up to $25,000 in fines and up to five years' imprisonment. Reflecting a major shift in emphasis, it kept beneficiary fraud a misdemeanor. Perhaps more important, it required that those convicted of crimes against Medicare or Medicaid be suspended from participation in those programs, and that their cases be referred to state licensing authorities. In the past, such suspension was not automatic.[18]

A year prior to the enactment of H.R.3, in the only new health legislation Congress was able to pass in 1976, an office of inspector general had been created in HEW. H.R.3 expands the inspector general's access to information and grants him additional powers of prosecution. H.R. 3 also encourages the states to establish special Medicaid investigation and prosecution agencies by providing 100 percent federal matching funds the first year, 90 percent the second, and 75 percent the third.[19] This provision was specifically modeled on the office of New York's special prosecutor for nursing homes, as is demonstrated by the requirement that the prosecuting function be separated from the state agency directing Medicaid. Charles J. Hynes, the deputy attorney general who created New York's office and ran it for its first three years, argued strenuously that administrative agencies charged with disbursing benefits were inherently incapable of policing their own programs, and that the complexities of Medicaid and other public programs supporting health services required special prosecutors with their own staffs and technical expertise.[20]

H.R.3's primary emphasis is on expanding and completing the system of administrative controls that should have been present from the beginning. It mandates, *for the first time,* the development of a system of uniform cost accounting and reporting for Medicare and Medicaid providers; establishes performance standards for the payment of Medicaid claims; establishes recordkeeping and reporting requirements for residents' personal funds; and further expands requirements on the reporting of ownership, possible conflicts-of-interest of employees, and relationships with vendors.[21]

Had all these requirements, as well as those contained in the 1972 Social Security amendments, been incorporated into the original Medicaid statute, it is very likely that the volume of stealing would have been substantially less. H.R.3, and related developments in the states, will probably have a significant dampening effect on the volume of nursing home crime, at least in the short run, particularly in those states that create special prosecutors' offices. But that effect will be achieved at much greater cost than it would have been if such controls had been instituted earlier. The problem is the contagion effect. The nursing home industry now requires a lot more policing than it would have if stealing had been more actively discouraged before it became so common a practice. A considerable hard core of shady operators was permitted to grow up in the industry, and it will take a sizable administrative effort to keep them in line.

Unfortunately, periods of rapid programmatic expansion are precisely the times when willingness to worry about program controls is hardest to come by. Because the initiation of innovative, expansive social programs is so irregular and infrequent, and because it tends to result from ephemeral political circumstances that everyone recognizes as transitory (thus creating a sense of urgency), all the emphasis is on getting things under way and starting the flow of benefits. Program controls can be worried about tomorrow.

James Sundquist has likened the creative burst of the Great Society Congress to the breaking of an ice-jam behind which unmet demands and unredressed grievances had collected for a generation.[22] The flood of legislation that burst forth carried many things with it and temporarily swept aside patterns of legislative and administrative caution and thoroughness. In the prevailing ethos of incremental policymaking, administrative controls were something that could be worried about later, tacked onto programs once they had rooted themselves in an incremental world that precluded their abandonment or abolition.

In other words, incremental policymaking practices contribute in two ways to the development and perpetuation of "new welfare" fraud. First, they create the illusion that stealing from government programs can be limited by the addition of standards and administrative requirements once the program is under way. Second, and a bit more subtly, a system predominately characterized by incrementalism may be particularly ill equipped to cope with nonincremental innovation. Such nonincremental change is, and is widely recognized as, atypical, and those who support it seek to get as much as they can as quickly as they can, knowing the opportunity may not soon come again. Once the period of creativity is passed, stealing from new programs does reach the political agenda—not least because it is one of the few avenues that those who have opposed the benefit all along can employ to attack a program already in place. Benefits once conferred are not, again, easily withdrawn, and one of the few strategies available to those who would limit them, if not eliminate them altogether, is to attack program administration, especially where it is most vulnerable. The pressure for controls against stealing increases as impetus for program expansion decreases, in an almost perfectly inverse relationship. Controls do eventually get imposed, but only after a lot of money has disappeared into thin air.

The cycle of program expansion and consolidation is preeminently political, and therein lies a central distinction between all forms of stealing from government and other forms of white-collar crime. Unless they seek to publicize it as part of an overall control strategy, the institutional *victims* of shoplifting, embezzlement, computer fraud, or industrial espionage generally try to suppress information about being victimized. This curious conspiracy of silence is, indeed, a principal reason why so little is known about white-collar crime, and why so few cases reach the criminal justice system. But there are often political advantages to exposing crimes against government, reaped by those who oppose specific programs or the people administering them. Macy's does not hold press conferences to decry the amount of shoplifting at Gimbels, but members of the minority party are always eager to ferret out scandals in the majority's administration.

In so doing, they find willing allies in the press, which in this area generally conforms to its stereotypical image of total unconcern with either causes or the recording of good news. Imagine the following lead: "Despite inordinate administrative complexity, as reflected in a 14-page application form and a 200-page instruction manual for minimally trained clerical workers, the State Welfare Department correctly processed, on the first try, 87 percent of all applications for Medicaid coverage, it was learned today from reliable sources."

The problem of stealing from governments is complicated, in other words, by the ways in which it impinges on, and is impinged upon by, the political dynamics of the press, the party system, and the separation of powers between administrators and legislators. Policy and politics are inextricably interconnected. Changing the former requires moving the latter; battles must be fought on two fronts simultaneously.

The Art of the Possible

POLICY CHOICES do not emerge from thin air. Analysis of public policy may be conducted in the abstract, but policy change always requires concrete decisions. Policy and politics are inseparable. Proposals for reform, no matter how soundly conceived or well formulated, are just proposals—until the political process has done its work.

In some respects, the politics of nursing home policy closely resemble those of other arenas, such as liquor regulation or milk pricing, in which individual industries are highly dependent on government largesse. A comparatively small group, concerned with the details of relatively technical issues, exerts pressure and influence on busy legislators who have no particular interest or expertise in the area. There is low public visibility and limited public interest, except at those times when scandals spur spasms of media attention. But the relationships between executive agencies and their constituencies, both in the nursing home industry and among nursing home consumers, are atypically weak, at least in part because of the status of nursing homes as a bastard stepchild of both welfare and health policies.

Lobbies

There are two commonly held misconceptions about nursing home politics. The first is that the nursing home industry constitutes one of the most powerful lobbies in Washington and in many state capitals.

The second is that the weakness of "consumer" representation on nursing home issues is due to the fact that older Americans are inadequately represented or protected in the political process in general.

The nursing home industry, while it does a relatively good job of presenting its views to public officials, is no more effective or skillful than many other such industries. The success that it has had is due as much to the weakness of the opposition and historical accident, as to its own strength. The weakness of the opposition derives not from the political impotence of the elderly (the elderly are among the most powerful and well-served interest groups in society) but from the relative indifference of general-purpose organizations of the elderly toward nursing home issues. Those "consumers" who do care about nursing homes tend to be the immediate families of nursing home residents, a group that is, indeed, small, unmobilized, and politically impotent.

Nursing home interests are represented at the national level by three trade associations. The American Health Care Association (AHCA; formerly called the American Nursing Home Association, ANHA) is the largest and most influential. Claiming to represent roughly half the nation's nursing homes, it is the trade association of the proprietary sector of the industry, although its membership is open to nonprofit facilities as well. Housed, inevitably, two blocks from the White House, AHCA maintains a professional "government services" staff of seven and draws heavily on outside legal counsel. The American Association of Homes for the Aging (AAHA), a much smaller organization, represents about 1,500 voluntary institutions. The National Council for Health Care Services (NCHCS) represents eighteen major nursing home chains that broke away from the then-ANHA in the early 1970s out of dissatisfaction with what was perceived as that organization's embarrassingly defensive posture. AAHA and NCHCS each have one full-time lobbyist. The function of all three organizations is primarily to deal with government, so the number of employees directly engaged in "lobbying" is misleadingly small. Moreover, all rely heavily on part-time leadership from the industry itself to carry a large share of the public representation burden.

The most obvious political weakness of the nursing home industry is its internal division. AAHA and AHCA rarely cooperate on anything, at least in public. While AAHA is much smaller and less generously endowed, it has special legitimacy as a representative of voluntary organizations, many of them church-sponsored. Thus, the industry often speaks with two conflicting voices—or three when

NCHCS takes a still different position. Some 25 to 30 percent of the nation's nursing homes do not belong to any of the three national organizations. More constraining still are the political tensions within each of the three associations—especially within AHCA, which is essentially a federation of state affiliates, each of which has its own concerns and priorities.

In many respects, the states are where the action is for nursing home policy (where reimbursement rates are set and regulatory activities controlled) and so it is at the state level where the most active and important lobbying is conducted. The variation is striking. The California affiliate of AHCA, for instance, under skillful leadership, presents a relatively united front for the proprietary industry in dealing with state government. The industry in Ohio, on the other hand, has long been split into factions. There, the "flat raters" largely by-pass the state nursing home association and seek influence through the governor's office, while the more "progressive" in the industry work through the weakened state association. In New York State, New York City's proprietary nursing homes have their own association, which has often been fragmented into as many as four competing factions. Oklahoma is *sui generis*. Officials of the Department of Institutions, Social and Rehabilitative Services (its welfare and Medicaid agency) have bargained directly with the state association, while legislators and everyone else have been pretty much excluded. Often, the nursing home association finds itself allied with the department in budgetary and jurisdictional fights with other political groups. So unusual is the Oklahoma situation, and so atypical the political perspective of its association, that the state affiliate has dropped out of AHCA.

There is disunity among AAHA affiliates as well. Many member facilities do their primary political lobbying through church affiliations and look to church sponsors for the leadership, technical assistance, and information provided in other instances by trade associations. Thus, there is a separate national organization of Jewish homes for the aged, and the orientation of many Catholic and Lutheran facilities is to a regional denominational organization rather than to a statewide association.

Another constraint on the national associations is that the reasonableness and willingness to see the broader perspective that is so necessary for effective representation of industry interests in Washington may conflict with members' perceptions of what they are paying their lobbyists for. Still more serious is the need for the national associations to maintain an appropriate public relations front in an industry in which individual facilities are always being caught doing something embarrassing. Nursing home lobbyists, as do lobbyists of all kinds, speak with great feeling of the overriding need to "educate" their constituencies, not only to "educate" them in the political process, but also to teach them to mind their manners. The political damage of scandals is so great that cleaning up the industry's appearance is a major preoccupation of all three associations, and of AHCA in particular. As AHCA's name change suggests, one approach to improving the industry's appearance has been to change its name.

Despite these constraints, the national associations and many of their state affiliates have a considerable impact on policy decisions. Part of the reason is that, over the past several years, their full-time lobbyists have been particularly skillful. The most important reason is simply that they are there. No one else able to command sizable resources of money, manpower, and legal talent has, until recently, kept track of the hundreds of policy decisions made by legislatures and administrators each year, submitted public comments on those decisions, threatened or actually brought litigation when they felt adversely affected, or even spoken out when comments from the "public" were sought.

Like most lobbyists for most industries, those who represent nursing homes spend most of their time collecting and dispensing information and arguing their constituents' cases. The national associations finance major studies of reimbursement and other issues; employ experts who can explain the most detailed arcana of accounting or regulatory practice to a congressman—or, more likely, a congressional aide—better than anyone HEW is likely to send over; appear at all the congressional hearings; and meet periodically with HEW officials. Information, which can be a scarce and valuable commodity in Washington and most state capitals, is the primary stock in trade for nursing home associations and their state affiliates.

More storied and hallowed tools of political persuasion are also employed. The proprietary industry maintains good ties with a number of legislators, primarily in the states but in Washington as well. Some of these ties are fraternal: in many communities, the nursing home proprietor is one of a number of local businessmen who belong to the same clubs as the local legislator, contribute to his campaigns, and give to the same charities. Legislators are only too happy to help out their friends and constituents by arranging an appointment with the health commissioner, writing a letter of inquiry, or otherwise attesting to the proprietor's "bona fides." The legislator is not, after all, necessarily endorsing the nursing home owner's arguments, just ensuring that they get the "fair hearing" to which any citizen's grievances are entitled.

Some of the ties are ideological. Proprietary nursing home owners are not averse to reminding legislators that they are independent, tax-paying entrepreneurs with payrolls to meet and bottom lines to be looked at. When businessmen complain about administrators, legislators generally sympathize. Voluntary nursing homes are not without their own ideological claims, the strongest of which is not community charity but denominational affiliation.

The importance of ideological legitimacy should not be underemphasized, for public imagery plays a crucial role in nursing home politics. While their for-profit status marks proprietary nursing homes as suspect in some public-health, academic, and left wing political circles, it has quite the opposite effect among many conservative, rural, and/or Republican legislators. The God-given right of every American citizen to make a buck occupies a hallowed place in much of the American political system.

Still stronger ties are cemented by what the great Boss Plunkitt termed "honest graft." As with other businesses heavily reliant on government favor, nursing homes buy a disproportionate share of legal services, insurance, and other commodities from firms in which legislators have an interest. Two of the three state legislators whose names were prominently mentioned in the New York scandals had ties with insurance firms. A surprisingly large number of legislators (apparently including the speaker of the House of Representatives,[1] several particularly influential members of the Senate, and countless state legislators) also own shares of nursing homes, sometimes conferred in lieu of legal or other professional fees, or "given" in "friendship."

There is also a fair amount of cash exchanged, both over and under the table. Most of it goes to legislators; there is very little plausible evidence of pecuniary corruption of administrative officials. AHCA's state affiliates contribute thousands of dollars to legislative campaigns, generally to members of key committees concerned with reimbursement and regulation. The national association similarly targets its contributions to its friends in high places. Just how much impact campaign contributions have on legislative behavior is one of those unanswerable questions. It would seem safe to conclude that it can't hurt. Money remains the mother's milk of politics, and its buying power undoubtedly increases at lower levels of government.

The Art of the Possible

In these post-Watergate days of public disclosure, under-the-table money is probably much more valuable than legitimate contributions. No one knows how much money flows under the table, but it probably exceeds legitimate contributions by several fold. In at least a handful of states, the state nursing home association maintains a slush fund based on contributions from its members of a dollar per bed per month. Rumors of an unreported contribution of several hundred thousand dollars in an Ohio gubernational election are widely believed. In local elections, where campaigning is less expensive and corruption more widespread, even relatively small investments in politicians can go a long way.[2]

These traditional avenues of influence are increasingly being supplanted by what AHCA's former chief lobbyist called his most important tool, litigation. Nursing homes and their associations spend a lot of money on legal fees, employ highly skilled counsel, and are well represented in court. Their hired guns are generally better paid, better educated, more experienced, and more numerous than the government's, and they win more than their share of court contests.

When HEW promulgated rules for "reasonable cost-related" Medicaid reimbursement, under Section 249 of the 1972 Social Security Act Amendments, it did so under threat of litigation from AHCA. It postponed implementation of those new rules for eighteen months and was promptly dragged into court by AHCA affiliates in at least three states, in each of which judges ruled that cost-related reimbursement must be retroactive to the date on which the regulations were issued, not the date HEW preferred.[3] The definition of allowable profit in those regulations was changed at least three times by HEW in the course of AHCA-initiated litigation in the District of Columbia Federal Court.[4] Litigation, or the fear of litigation, poses obstacles to closing substandard nursing homes. There is hardly a single administrative reform that has not been challenged in some court by industry representatives.

Given this impressive array of tools, it is surprising that nursing home interests have not done substantially better than they have. Reimbursement rates have increased substantially over the past decade, but nowhere nearly as dramatically as rates for hospitals or other health services. Regulatory initiatives have been stalled or by-passed but not negated. And while profits in the industry as a whole have been good—especially if real estate profits and illegally gotten gains are included—they have been somewhat unreliable and increasingly hard to come by. Rather than the fat plutocrat (labeled "Nursing

Home Trust"?) of turn-of-the-century political cartoons, holding a politician in every pocket, the nursing home industry might better be depicted as a King Canute trying to turn back the tide of increased regulation and tightened controls.

The industry's failure to do better is particularly striking in light of the weakness of the opposition. Nursing home "consumers" have few voices in policy debates, despite the fact that the elderly hold considerable political power. After the American Legion, the American Association of Retired Persons/National Retired Teachers Association (AARP/NRTA) is the largest mass-membership lobbying group in the country. The National Council of Senior Citizens, closely allied with the AFL-CIO and considerably to the left of AARP, claims over a million members and makes itself well heard in Congress. Elected officials are acutely aware of the fact that those over fifty-five constitute a third of all voters (they comprise just under 30 percent of those over eighteen and vote more consistently than younger people), as was reflected in the speed with which legislation to ban mandatory retirement moved through Congress over the combined opposition of major business and labor groups, or the current popularity of property-tax relief for the elderly.

But nursing homes have never been high on the political agenda of the elderly, either as individual voters or as association members. Those in institutions, or at greatest risk for institutionalization, are a small minority in the increasingly heterogeneous elderly population, the majority of whom are most concerned with social security benefits, property taxes, inflation, and crime. The principal health-related issue for associations of the elderly and their political spokesmen in the past several years has been the extension of Medicare coverage to prescription drugs.

The National Council of Senior Citizens (NCSC), provides an instructive example. NCSC was formed in the 1950s largely as a vehicle for Medicare lobbying, with ties to both the AFL-CIO and the Democratic party.[5] Health insurance has remained NCSC's first priority, and it is a major supporter of the Committee for National Health Insurance and other proponents of a comprehensive "health security" program. But the drive for national health insurance has been stymied by fears of its budgetary implications, one element of which is projected cost increases for long-term care. While NCSC has supported the standard liberal nostrums of tighter regulation, greater reliance on nonprofit sponsorship, and increased use of "alternatives" such as home care, it has been largely paralyzed on nursing home issues for fear that any major changes might cost a lot of money and thus further delay movement toward national health insurance.

Development of effective political representation for nursing home residents and their families has also been impeded by the failure of executive branch agencies, in the federal government and in the states, to engage in customary forms of constituency-building: encouraging the development of constituent groups; providing them with information, access and other forms of support; and sometimes virtually creating them—as Herbert Hoover, when secretary of commerce, organized the National Chamber of Commerce.[6] Executive agencies responsible for nursing home policy have never defined nursing home residents as their constituents.

State and local health departments, as well as the Public Health Service in HEW, have defined their constituencies as consisting primarily of their fellow professionals in the private sector. The Bureau of Health Insurance of the Social Security Administration similarly showed more solicitude for the interests of hospitals and other service providers than for its beneficiaries. Federal welfare administrators have been most concerned with the problems of their state counterparts, who, because of the political weakness of welfare recipients, have concentrated their constituency-building on voluntary charitable organizations, which often number the social and sometimes the corporate elite among their officers. The "iron triangle" based on mutual alliances between executive officials, legislators, and constituents that characterizes so much of American politics is thus largely absent in nursing home policy. (Nor, in most jurisdictions, do nursing homes occupy the place of many regulated industries as the "constituents" in a *ménage à trois* from which consumers are excluded. The industry's status vis-à-vis administrative agencies is not at all comparable to that of railroads with the Interstate Commerce Commission, or shippers with the Maritime Administration, or aerospace contractors with the Defense Department; this is one facet of the industry's weakness. But the industry can take care of itself—nursing home residents cannot.)

Agencies engage in constituency-building to generate political support for their programs and their budgets. Given the limited political resources of nursing home residents, it is not surprising that administrators have not reached out to them. State and federal welfare agencies and the Health Care Financing Administration sit astride multibillion dollar budgets that they can barely control. Many state health and welfare departments themselves operate institutions of one kind or another, and are wary of encouraging the expression of patient or consumer interests.

The one exception is the nursing home ombudsman program of the Administration on Aging (AOA), a remnant of the Nixon nursing home initiative. AOA serves primarily as a funding conduit to state and local agencies. It is built on a structure of state and "area" agencies on aging, which dispense funds to literally thousands of senior citizens' centers and special purpose programs. The nursing home ombudsman program established an administrative office in each state to receive, investigate, and act—without formal powers—on complaints about nursing home care. It was lodged in AOA in conformance with the principle that program agencies should not police themselves and that a "consumer"-based organization was appropriate for an ombudsman program.

AOA's attitude toward its ombudsman program has run the gamut from mild support to total indifference; it has been much more concerned with programs that benefit its younger, healthier, and more politically active constituents. In most states, the ombudsman's offices are only paper tigers. The few successful programs have developed where the ombudsman has engaged in constituency-building among nursing home consumers.

Most of the "consumers" to whom they have reached out are essentially unorganized. A recent "Citizens' Action Guide" to nursing homes, compiled by the National Citizens Coalition for Nursing Home Reform, lists only twenty organized "consumer" groups scattered widely throughout the country, all primarily local in orientations. While that count is incomplete, the numbers of such organizations, many of which consist of one full-time staff member and a handful of part-time volunteers, is not very great. A few, notably Citizens for Better Care in Detroit and the Minneapolis Age and Opportunity Center, have had significant political impact at the state level, but they are the exception. They are also the only two such groups supported financially by local governments.

The existing "consumer groups," and those that ombudsmen have attempted to create or foster, all suffer from the literal and figurative weaknesses of their constituencies, and all are open to the charge of being self-appointed, middle-class (and middle-aged) "do-gooders" claiming to speak for nursing home residents. A single exception is the Nursing Home Residents Advisory Council in Minnesota, which (with the help of a less-than-middle-aged staff) has lobbied effectively in the legislature.

The most effective "consumer" voice in nursing home politics is that of "public interest" lawyers. Most are young and work for federally funded legal services organizations for the poor or for local legal aid societies. As litigation has become more important as a political tool, these lawyers increasingly have represented nursing home residents in court and have helped to fight back against the highly paid, experienced legal counsel employed by the proprietor. The transfer cases and the requirement that homes accept Medicaid recipients, discussed previously, constitute their most noteworthy victories. The National Health Law Project and National Senior Citizens Law Center, both "back-up centers" in the federal Legal Service Corporation system, have served as indispensable clearinghouses and information resources for advocates for nursing home residents.

Legislators

This consumer activity is small potatoes when compared to the resources the nursing home industry can command. Nonetheless, the industry has not done better politically for several reasons: imagery, agendas, and budgets.

The nursing home industry has a lousy public image. Although politicians, bought or otherwise, may be sympathetic to the industry's interests, they are reluctant to appear sympathetic in public. Nursing homes may have limited organized enemies, but they also have few public friends. Nursing home residents, on the other hand, are ideal objects of public concern: deserving, dependent, entirely unthreatening.

The manipulation of political imagery is central to much of nursing home politics. Industry spokesmen seek to establish themselves as representatives of their helpless residents, who deserve a slightly larger pittance from penurious state officials. Those officials, in turn, pose as vigilant guardians of the public purse against raids by avaricious and unprincipled nursing home owners. Consumer groups portray owners as vicious abusers of resident welfare and state officials as cowardly bureaucrats secretly in league with the enemy.

All three groups are assisted in their image-making by the mass media. There are fewer than a handful of reporters in the United States with more than a rudimentary understanding of nursing home issues. If industry associations, in reimbursement battles with state officials, threaten to close their facilities and dump their residents into the streets if rates are not raised to "minimally adequate" levels, those hollow claims are straightforwardly passed on in the daily press. (In one such battle in Michigan, the proprietary association printed thousands of bumper stickers bearing the message, "Governor Milliken is mean to old people," as part of such a campaign.) Consumer groups seeking to recruit volunteers or solicit support invite TV cameras on "inspection" tours of carefully selected nursing homes and are not displeased if they are denied admittance, so long as the tape is rolling. Sometimes, the press itself creates distortion. With "investigative journalism" the prevailing fad, a young reporter seeking to make his mark can always uncover a nursing home scandal. (There was a wave of such scandals after John Hess of the *New York Times* was nominated for a Pulitzer Prize for his investigative reporting on nursing homes in New York.)

Thus, nursing home policy issues tend to be defined in distorted terms, generally but not always to the industry's disadvantage. This is not to say that the industry does not deserve its poor reputation, only that the causes of problems are more complex than is usually depicted and that responses generated by enmity toward proprietors may not resolve them very well. For example, per diem reimbursement rates, which are often the focus of the most visible political conflicts, are only one part of the quality-of-care problem; the intimately related questions of staff qualifications, or standards, or regulatory enforcement are totally ignored.

Because of its poor public image, the industry's political posture is essentially defensive. It must devote most of its political energies to putting out fires. Nursing home issues only get onto the political agenda when propelled there by scandals or other untoward events. The nursing home industry lacks the support for policy innovation in its behalf that has proved so helpful to other health services or other programs for the elderly. Nursing home lobbyists devote much of their energy to preventing proposals from being acted upon. They are good field, very little hit.

Compared to nursing home consumers, providers may seem mighty, but they are puny in comparison to the banks, insurance companies, liquor dealers, retail druggists, or hospitals that tend to be the really powerful interests in state politics. (A former New York legislator described nursing home lobbying as "nickel and dime" stuff in comparison to that of the banks.) Occasionally, nursing home interests are able to ally themselves with more powerful lobbies, as when savings banks in New York State pushed for increased reimbursement rates to ensure that nursing homes could cover their mortgage payments. More typically, nursing homes fare poorly competing against such groups for scarce legislative time and attention. The difficulty of bringing nursing home issues to the forefront can actually work to the industry's advantage. For example, many legislators might be sympathetic to expansion of regulatory activities if forced to confront the issue: but it tends to get neglected for more politically pressing concerns until scandals erupt.

The greatest political constraint on the industry is budgetary. Its primary political objective is almost always increased reimbursement, but nursing home payments largely come from welfare budgets and, even more unfortunately from the industry's perspective, from Medicaid budgets, which are generally the last thing that state politicians want to increase. Since hospital costs, which the states are required to reimburse on a "reasonable cost" basis, increase inexorably, and since the supply of nursing home beds has also steadily increased, there has been little left over for increases in the per diem rate, especially in a climate of widespread mistrust of the industry.

An example of the power of budgetary restraints occurred in California in 1976. A coalition of "consumer" advocates, liberal legislators, nursing home interests, and, crucially, the state AFL-CIO, added several million dollars to the state Medicaid budget with the proviso that all of the per diem increase be passed along to aides and other nonprofessional employees in the hope of attracting and retaining better staff. That increase was removed by Governor Brown, who made control of the Medicaid budget a central political claim of his administration.

In sum, nursing homes do rather poorly in extracting funds from state governments. When public attention is focused on the industry by unfavorable publicity, it has trouble resisting punitive measures. Little affirmative legislation in the industry's interest ever sees the light of political day. But the industry is effective at limiting expansion or strengthening of state regulation. And in hundreds of individual cases involving "certificate-of-need" determinations or license revocations for noncompliance with standards, or rate appeals, it is well served by individual legislators all too happy to intervene as a "casework" service for favored constituents. These ad hoc, *ex parte* legislative interventions in the administrative process are a recurrent and pervasive phenomenon in American government, but in the nursing home arena, they have a substantial effect on the overall shape of policy. They contribute to the demoralization of administrative agencies and often make it possible for industry interests that are defeated at the broad legislative level to prevail in specific individual cases.

Federalism

This picture is substantially complicated by intergovernmental politics. Federal-state fiscal relations have been a major political issue since the early years of the Nixon administration, and a concern with the impact of federal policy decisions on state finances has significantly colored Medicaid policy. Congress delayed the effective date for reasonable cost-related reimbursement largely from a desire to postpone the expected additional costs for state governments. HEW was even more sensitive to the states' concerns, both further delaying the implementation of those requirements and then writing the regulations in a way intended to minimize their financial impact—by permitting various forms of ceilings and other quasiflat rates.

Federal officials' concern with the states' fiscal problems is not motivated entirely by beneficent altruism or a commitment to abstract principles of good government. To the contrary, one of the fastest-growing and increasingly powerful lobbies in Washington is that of state and local government. What Professor Samuel Beer has called the "public sector lobby," which first visibly coalesced around the passage of General Revenue-Sharing in 1972,[7] has been particularly vocal on matters relating to welfare and Medicaid. State and local officials are influential in Washington because congressmen know who controls local election laws and local party machinery—and every member of Congress must be reelected from a locality. The National Governors Conference, National Conference of State Legislators, and National Association of Counties have all had special Medicaid task forces, and while none has focused primarily on nursing homes, the message of state and local fiscal burden has been clearly communicated.

Since a direct connection between increased quality and increased costs is widely accepted by Washington policymakers, empathy with the fiscal plight of the states has provided a perfect excuse for failure to move aggressively to strengthen either the content of nursing home regulations or their enforcement. It might be embarrassing for congressmen or HEW officials to take the position that they are prepared to accept substandard care in order to save federal dollars, but a reluctance to require greater expenditures from the states seems more acceptable. The industry and its friends in Washington are not averse to reinforcing this lassitude. Pro-reform groups, which tend to be highly localized in membership and orientation, have little clout in state capitals and even less in Washington.

Another reason for the weakness of federal pressure on the nursing home industry is jurisdictional problems in Congress. Both the House and Senate Committees on Aging serve primarily as spokesmen for constituent interests. For more than a decade, the Senate committee has been the leading platform for antiindustry views—although with the retirement of Senator Moss and the creation and aggrandizement of the House Aging Committee, it is losing its status to that of its counterpart from the lower chamber. But neither committee has any legislative jurisdiction whatsoever. They may only recommend. Responsibility for federal nursing home legislation rests with the Finance Committee in the Senate and the Ways and Means Committee in the House; responsibility for Medicaid rests with the Health Subcommittee of the House Committee on Interstate and Foreign Commerce. As their names imply, all these bodies have an enormous number of matters to deal with, of which nursing homes are far from first in importance.

Given their jurisdictional turf, both Finance and Ways and Means see nursing homes as a part of the more general issues of Medicare and Medicaid, despite the fact that it is nowhere contained in Holy Writ that nursing home care must fall under the existing Medicaid financing formula. These essentially conservative committees, preoccupied with overall program costs, the federal budget deficit, and the soundness of the Medicare Hospital Insurance Trust Fund, are hardly eager to have the federal treasury assume any greater share of nursing home costs. Both Ways and Means and Finance have expressed a total willingness to contemplate any nursing home reforms so long as they don't cost any extra money. (H.R.3 was sold politically as a cost-saving measure.)

Congress is prepared to let the states do whatever they please so long as minimum standards are observed and the federal budget is not affected. The federal system is supposed to encourage diversity and experimentation by the states, but the states are unlikely to engage in program innovation without federal support. When dollars do flow stateward, the federal agencies always try to attach strings to them. The experience with general revenue sharing, which was supposed to redress the fiscal imbalance and encourage the states to innovate, has reconfirmed this: rather than embark on new ventures, the states used revenue-sharing funds to reduce taxes or to avert tax increases.

If federal policymakers are reluctant to increase budgetary liabilities, either for themselves or their state and local counterparts, another way in which new ventures could be financed would be by reducing the financing of old ones. Since the growth of nursing home expenditures under public programs is more a result of increased utilization than increased charges, the way to make funds available for new programs would be to stem the growth of the industry, and perhaps even reverse it. But doing so would encounter political problems of a very different order. It is hard to withdraw benefits once conferred. So the nursing home industry finds itself in a very favorable position. While little additional aid may be given to the industry, it is unlikely that very much will be taken away.

Gathering the Threads

In sum, the likelihood of continued incremental change in nursing home policy is great, while the chances for radical innovation are substantially less. That bodes poorly for the future, since better policy requires a dramatic change from current directions. Before looking ahead, though, it may be useful to take a brief look backward.

A principal reason that nursing homes have fared as poorly as they have in reimbursement is that hospitals have been first in line at the public trough and have left very little behind for the stragglers. Nursing home interests have been best served in the political process when they have managed to align themselves with hospitals, as in the provisions for reimbursement of depreciation under Medicare or, a bit more subtly, in the general passivity of inspection agencies, most of which are responsible for hospital as well as nursing home surveys. The hospitals' superior political position is in part explained by their greater economic importance. But other factors are even more important. Citizens and communities value their local hospitals but are largely indifferent to nursing homes, which suggests that "voluntary" institutions can do perfectly all right for themselves in competition with profit-making firms. Many of the nation's most prestigious and respected figures sit on the boards of voluntary hospitals. Perhaps most important, doctors care enormously about the well-being of hospitals that are so crucial to their own well-being. In the mystery of nursing home policy, the physician who wasn't there thus again turns out to be a critical clue. To the extent nursing homes resemble hospitals, they are deflected from providing a pleasant place for frail and isolated old people to live. But it is just such identification with hospitals that leads to more generous treatment from governments.

The centrality of intergovernmental relations to nursing home policy and politics has also been a factor. The recent stalemate between state and federal governments on nursing home policy illustrates the extent to which the federal system focuses on questions of money—or more precisely, around the struggle to let someone else's constituents pay the taxes—far more than on questions of programmatic content. The sharing of powers between federal and state governments permits politicians at all levels to pass the buck on difficult problems such as "levels of care" policy, the creation of reimbursement methods, or quality-cost trade-offs.

The dependence of governments on private firms supplying them with necessary services has had a significant impact on the regulatory process. These private firms, as "constituents," have called on legislators for help in dealing with government regulation. Increasingly, legislators collectively enact regulatory statutes and then individually undermine them by seeking ad hoc exemptions for the politically powerful in their own districts.

The love of the press for clear-cut, bilateral conflicts often gives complicated, ambiguous relationships between regulators and the regulated an extremely misleading appearance.

Finally, it should be emphasized that "booze, bucks, and broads"—the stereotypical lobbyist's stock in trade—are being replaced by lawyers in pinstripe suits. There are things to be said for preferring the blindness of justice to other forms of human frailty, but the increasing resort to litigation holds no guarantees of upholding the public interest any better than the old practices.

Shaping the Future

Existing public policy toward nursing homes reflects a relatively stable balance of political power that will not yield readily to significant change. But the prospects for policy innovation are not entirely bleak.

The most plausible avenue for substantial change lies in the increasing importance of the AOA as a constituency-oriented service bureaucracy. Despite its rapid and certain-to-increase growth in both budget and influence, AOA has had difficulty defining an overall mission apart from dispensing funds to its state and local counterparts. There are, however, potential reforms in the provision of long-term care in which it would be natural for AOA, or at least its local grantees, to take a leading role. In most communities, once an individual has reached a certain degree of disability and dependence, nursing homes have had the service market largely to themselves. More generic programs for the aging could begin to alter that balance of market forces. General-purpose agencies involved in such programs could establish, for the first time, a powerful organizational base competing with nursing homes for the right to serve—and income derived from serving—that clientele. The organized elderly have not shown much concern for long-term care issues, but that does not mean they cannot be inspired to do so. AOA has the resources to inspire them.

A second avenue for change would be the involvement of community hospitals in care for the frail elderly. The indifference of hospitals to the needs of the people served by nursing homes has been emphasized repeatedly, and in some sense, the nursing home industry has developed and thrived because it has provided hospitals the valued service of taking from them customers they didn't want. But the nation's hospitals, especially those in inner cities or those affiliated with medical schools, are undergoing a period of unprecedented turmoil.[8] Many of them, if they are to survive, will have to rethink their services to the frail elderly. If it can be demonstrated that they have a real stake in the care of the nursing home population, their interest could have considerable significance. No interest group is better situated to compete with the nursing home industry than the hospital industry, and if direct conflict should ensue, this observer would give odds on the hospitals. While agencies on aging are moderately interested and moderately influential, hospitals are not yet interested but are extremely influential.

Finally, there is some slim chance that the political balance could be undermined by a direct assault on its conceptual underpinnings. Public officials believe that people in nursing homes by and large need to be there. They believe that the most frequently discussed alternatives to existing nursing home policy would be frightfully and uncontrollably expensive. Mostly, they believe they have no other choice. All of those beliefs are wrong, in whole or in part. The vast majority of the nation's nursing homes can never be induced, through reimbursement or regulation, to rise above a level of shabby mediocrity. There is no money to be saved from kicking people out of hospitals to put them in nursing homes. Many nursing home residents would be better off almost anywhere else. There are potential allies for those who would attempt to alter the status quo. What remains to be demonstrated is that there is something else that can be done—something that is reasonably manageable both in terms of administration and budget, and that will provide better services than existing policies, which, in any event, are likely to collapse under their own weight.

Doing Better

ACCORDING TO the Congressional Budget Office (CBO), if there are no major changes in public policy, government expenditures for nursing home care can be expected to *triple* between 1975 and 1985, approaching $22 billion a year by the end of that period.[1] The study on which that estimate is based abounds with dubious assumptions and questionable assertions, but there is no doubt that expenditures for nursing home care will increase substantially.

The most reliable figures in the CBO study are demographic. The number of Americans over seventy-five, those most at risk for institutionalization, will increase steadily. By the end of the century, the over seventy-five population will have increased by 60 percent—by 5 million people. While the elderly population as a whole is actually growing less rapidly, relatively, than it has at any time in this century, the old are getting older, and those projections are conservative: everyone who will be sixty-five or older by the year 2000 has already been born, and estimates of the future elderly population are based on an assumption that there will not be significant changes in death rates.[2] Should major breakthroughs be made in treating cardiovascular disease or cancer, the number of the very old will increase even more. There is also some reason to expect that as mortality from those diseases declines, survivors will be afflicted with a high incidence of senility and other completely disabling intractable conditions, and thus be especially in need of intensive services.[3]

While these demographic changes appear inevitable and while no one is very happy with existing nursing home services, policymakers in both state and federal governments and those who advise them in the academic and professional communities seem to be largely at a loss as to what to do. While everyone agrees that a substantial expansion of "alternative," home-based services is imperative, policymakers are appalled at the budgetary implications of any expansion that would even begin to approach the extent of "need" they believe exists. (The CBO study just cited estimates that comprehensive insurance for noninstitutional long-term care services would cost between $7.4 billion and $28.9 billion by 1985.[4]) Since the political impetus for change is extremely limited while reducing the overall federal budget deficit is a major priority, the likelihood of continued drift and small-scale incremental change is substantial. No one, except perhaps those in the nursing home industry, is very happy about that either.

The Limits of Reform

Some meliorative changes in nursing home policy should be possible within the bounds of the existing balance of political forces. In the summer of 1978, for instance, HEW announced plans for a major revision in federal regulatory standards.[5] Those revisions—part of the Carter administration's push for reexamination of all regulatory activities—constituted the first effort since the early 1950s to upgrade nursing home standards without direct legislative or interest-group prodding. The revisions process has been stalled by internal turmoil within HEW that arose, at the highest levels, from an almost obsessive concern with cost control to the exclusion of program issues. The process also has appeared, in its early stages, to be colored by the protectiveness of individual professional groups toward their occupational status. Still, it is likely that there will be some improvement in terms of stronger nursing and housekeeping standards, reduced paperwork, rationalization of the inspections process, and the development of more flexible regulatory sanctions. HEW also appears increasingly willing to move away from a rigid SNF/ICF distinction toward licensing facilities for both levels of care.

The states, in the meantime, are moving much more quickly on both the "levels-of-care" issue and the strengthening of regulatory processes. In the latter area, for instance, Michigan has just enacted a comprehensive new statute that strengthens standards, gives inspectors more discretion, and establishes both a new system of fines and procedures for imposing civil receiverships.[6] To some degree, the states are still responding to the scandals of the mid–1970s, and the cyclical return to business-as-usual has already begun in some places, but the responses to the scandals have established changes that will be hard to reverse.

Policy decisions of earlier years will also continue to have some positive effect on the operation of many nursing homes. Here, the growing number of professional administrators, divorced from direct ownership, will be most important, as the first generations of those with college degrees and special training in nursing home administration diffuse through the industry. Federally sponsored continuing education and midcareer training, especially for nursing personnel, will also have some effect. So will the regulatory changes engendered by H.R.3. The move to cost-related reimbursement systems will improve the financial management of nursing homes and state oversight of their expenditure patterns.

A thorough rethinking of the role of physicians in nursing home care could have a substantial impact on the quality of life in nursing homes. Physicians now serve the following roles in nursing homes: Every SNF must have a medical director. Every resident, in both SNFs and ICFs, must have an attending physician, who may or may not (in SNFs) be the medical director. Every admission must be certified by a physician and then reviewed under a utilization review procedure in which another physician accedes to the admission. Continuation of stay must also be periodically certified by a utilization review physician. Physicians serve on the Medical Review and Independent Professional Review Teams, which monitor facilities' utilization review processes. And physicians supervise the activities of the PSROs that are gradually assuming the utilization review function for SNFs. Often, each of these roles is filled by a different individual. Almost invariably, physicians' involvement in nursing home care is part time, cursory, and tangential to their primary activity. The confusion in physicians' roles is partly a confusion of policy: physicians are asked to serve as gatekeepers, administrators, and quality regulators as well as providers of service to individual residents, without a clear sense of who is to do what or which is more important. And partly it is a reflection of the indifference of physicians to geriatric patients, especially disabled geriatric patients.

Nursing home residents are not primarily in need of continual medical services and do not belong in medical institutions. But they do need medical care as much as other chronically ill people who are not in institutions. What is so distressing about the provision of physicians' services in nursing homes is that their residents, who are living in health-care facilities, often receive less high quality physicians' services than the average man in the street. Medical services in nursing homes must be improved, but without further "medicalizing" them as institutions.

Changes in the role of physicians in nursing homes could come about as part of the broader changes that are slowly developing in care of the elderly. But they will not follow automatically. There will need to be concerted effort to ensure that new training programs in geriatric medicine involve nursing homes and their residents, that new academic departments view nursing homes as important clinical settings, and that geriatric consultants or back-up services for general practitioners or other "primary care" physicians include an emphasis on care of patients in nursing homes. It is probably too much to hope that American physicians adopt the model of their British counterparts, who, in addition to providing medical care per se, direct nursing and social services delivered in the home. But it may not be unreasonable to expect that physicians' growing sensitivity to geriatric problems may give life to the notion of an "attending physician" for nursing home residents.

Still, given the likely shortage of physicians with adequate training or interest, reform of the physicians' role in nursing homes may have to focus elsewhere. If, for example, instead of a medical director, each nursing home (SNF and ICF alike) were to have a contractual relationship with a hospital, medical school, health maintenance organization, or even a group practice to superintend the care of all its residents, and if those organizations were reimbursed directly by Medicare for the services they rendered, and if they were held responsible for the quality of medical care in nursing homes under their supervision, and if they reported, not just to the facility administrator but to the certifying agency and the general public, then the quality of medical care in the nation's nursing homes might be substantially improved. Those are a lot of ifs, and many of them would be expensive, but they would produce real benefits.

A variant of this proposal would employ nurse practitioners—RNs with advanced, specialized training in primary care—under the supervision of independent physician groups on a full-time basis in nursing homes. The reluctance of physicians to spend time in nursing homes would be side-stepped, while the professional management of medical care would remain outside the control of the nursing home administrator. Such a system is already working, with apparent success, in the Boston area.[7]

Redefinition of the role of physicians in the care of nursing home patients would lead to a redefinition, probably beneficial, of the roles of both nursing directors and administrators. Administrators would have someone to whom they were accountable for at least a portion of the services they delivered, while nursing directors could be relieved of much of their paperwork and provided with a largely autonomous check on administrators' judgments. To the argument that a greater involvement of physicians in nursing home care would further "medicalize" what should be nonmedical institutions, the reply is that adequate physicians' services could *demedicalize* the jobs of nursing and administrative staff, who would no longer write prescriptions for drugs or have to determine when residents were sick enough to be transferred to acute-care hospitals.

The final avenue for incremental reform involves further mobilization of third parties, notably community groups, general-purpose agencies for the aging, and charitable organizations. There is much to be said for bringing outsiders into nursing homes. The employment of junior high and high school students, under federally subsidized summer-jobs programs, as visitors to nursing home residents has helped to reduce the residents' isolation. Third parties could strike directly at nursing home governance through the creation of "boards of visitors," "outside directors," or "community advisory boards." A further, crucial step would be the mobilization of third parties to fill the role of temporary or permanent receivers. The Village Nursing Home in New York City provides an example. A lay community board assumed ownership from a proprietor who walked away from the facility. With the strenuous assistance of state officials and active fund raising from the community at large, it turned a moderately decent, but bankrupt proprietary facility into a first-rate, nearly solvent, truly community-based service. A federal investment of minuscule proportions—in comparison to total nursing home expenditures—could foster this kind of activity.

The federal government, through its health planning laws and the funds it expends in support of their administration, has undertaken the recruitment, education, and mobilization of thousands of lay citizens to serve as "consumer representatives" in health planning agencies, without clear expectations of where that "consumer" participation might lead. The local instrumentalities of that process (health systems agencies) provide a potential source of third-party involvement in nursing home affairs; at present, however, there is only one such effort underway—in Arizona.

Reform of this kind, along with additional infusions of money, can make nursing homes better places. But it is unlikely to happen over the next decade. Too many proprietors, physicians, staff members, and legislators just don't care. More to the point, even if nursing homes did become as good as they could be, they still wouldn't be very good. A cage, no matter how gilded, is still a cage. Reforms can never solve the underlying problems. They will never make nursing homes places where anyone, given a real choice, would ever *want* to live. No matter how much stronger regulation, improved professionalism, or increased community involvement changes the atmosphere or quality of nursing homes, they will still be institutions in which residents will be surrounded primarily by other people as old, as infirm, and as helpless as themselves, in which life will always be regimented. Nursing homes will always serve institutional food. Nursing home residents will always be cared for by strangers. And nursing homes will never be home. The tragedy is that, even though the intrinsic inadequacy of nursing homes has long been recognized, we continue to rely on them as the principal, and often the only, vehicle for meeting the needs of the dependent elderly.

Empty Alternatives

For at least a generation, policymakers have had serious qualms about nursing homes and have recognized that providing services to people in their homes might be a better way to meet the needs of the frail elderly. But the expansion of noninstitutional services has been caught in a series of unresolved dilemmas that continue to make more than modest growth impossible.

Medicare and Medicaid will both pay for home health services (defined as those rendered by professionals, mostly RNs, under the supervision of physicians) for their beneficiaries under very limited circumstances for limited periods. Medicaid will also pay for "home-help" services (nonprofessional cleaning, cooking, and other household chores) in a handful of states. And dozens of local agencies provide home-help services with funds from the AOA or Title XX social services funds provided to the states under the Social Security Act. Expansion of home-health care has been hampered by Medicare restrictions that limit it to posthospitalization services within a given "spell of illness," by budgetary caution, and mostly by an intense if quiet political war over the participation of proprietary home-health agencies.[8] Proprietary agencies are eligible for Medicare reimbursement only in the fifteen states that license them. Expanded licensing, or dropping of the state-licensing requirement from the federal law, has been fought by those who do not want to see a repeat of proprietary dominance in the nursing home industry. It has also been fought by visiting nurses associations and other voluntary home-health agencies, which are generally limited in size but politically potent as a result of their long-standing alliances with social welfare agencies, local charities, and their board members. Those agencies, however, have nowhere near the proprietaries' capacity to provide services to the vast numbers of elderly thought to need them—and so the chicken-and-egg argument is often made that Medicare benefits should not be expanded before capacity to deliver services increases.

HEW is now promoting, in a small way, the growth of voluntary home-health agencies. It is likely that in the next several years the conditions for receipt of Medicare home-health benefits will be substantially relaxed; it is one of the few relatively uncontroversial and inexpensive gestures policymakers can make toward their disabled elderly constituents. The problem with an expansion of home-health services is that by themselves they are not what the people policymakers are worried about need. There is something to be said for the logic of the initial Medicare formulation: those who can benefit solely from home-health services are individuals in the latter stages of recovery from acute incidents who can make do in the home environment if someone comes to change the dressings or give them their shots. Anyone well enough to take care of himself or herself at home, once an acute incident has passed, is well enough to receive medical attention outside the home. Those who cannot get that outside medical attention probably can't take care of their other needs either, and it makes no sense to bring skilled nursing or rehabilitation services to people in need of cooking or cleaning or shopping.

In order to substitute for nursing homes and other forms of institutional care, home-health services must serve as an adjunct to home-help services. It is not disability that sends people to nursing homes; it is the combination of disability and isolation. But expansion of home-help services is enmired in problems of its own.

Nonhealth services lack an appropriate gatekeeper. Literally millions of elderly individuals incapable of performing some or all of the "activities of daily living" are getting by outside of institutions with the help of family, friends, neighbors, and uncoordinated, fragmented social programs operated by local welfare or aging agencies. ("Meals on wheels," which addresses shopping and cooking problems simultaneously, is probably the most important.) It is widely feared that, if help in getting by were suddenly made more generally available by governments, there would be no way to control demand. Friends and neighbors would no longer be willing to go out of their way to help; those now doing without would no longer have to, and the budgetary consequences would be staggering. As one congressional staff member told me, "I'd like somebody to come fix my roof or do my shopping for me too, but why should the taxpayers have to provide me with that?"

Expansion of nonhealth services as an alternative to institutionalization raises the prospect of "socializing" private costs. Individuals now bear, and perhaps should bear, the costs of providing those services to their relatives and friends—more in the form of time and effort than in dollars and cents. Or elderly persons themselves bear the costs of not receiving services. What are now private, voluntary, noneconomic transactions would be paid for with tax dollars and inevitably provided in a less personal, more bureaucratic fashion.

One way to justify this socialization of private costs would be to demonstrate that it actually reduced total expenditures—that it could prevent institutionalization, which is exceedingly expensive. The debate as to whether, in any individual case, it is cheaper to provide services at home or in an institution has occupied endless hours of legislative testimony and reams of published reports. The most reasonable conclusion is that it depends.[9] But such arguments are largely irrelevant. The problem with expanding home-based services has been that there are far more people who need services than are currently being provided for in institutions. For every nursing home resident there is at least one other person, and probably two, not in an institution who are just as frail and disabled. They are just getting by. Even if services delivered in the home were demonstrably less expensive, which they probably are not, there is no way of assuring that expanded in-home services will *substitute for* institutional services. It has been legitimately feared that they will simply supplement them—that every dollar spent on services in the home will be a new dollar. That fear is buttressed by the high occupancy rates for nursing homes everywhere and the apparent existence of a "supply effect" in nursing home utilization, in which available beds tend to become filled beds.

The search for an ideal gatekeeper that could limit the utilization of home-help services while ensuring that they substituted for institutional services has become something of a Holy Grail among those who make policy for long-term care. Legislation has been introduced, and a number of experimental "demonstration projects" are being conducted around the country. But the problems of design are sufficiently troubling, and the impetus for change sufficiently weak, that development of gatekeeping mechanisms will almost undoubtedly progress, for at least the next five to ten years, in an extremely ad hoc, experimental, step-by-step fashion. Because home-help services must be predicated on having an adequate gatekeeper in place, it is likely that there will be only minor expansion of those services. Nursing homes will continue to be the dominant element in public policy toward long-term care.

Crossroads

If *something* does not begin to substitute for nursing home care now, nothing ever will. There exists an opportunity that will last for five to, at most, ten years for policymakers to seize control of the future of long-term care. Thereafter it will be lost.

The crucial factor is that the growth of the nursing home industry has slowed substantially, while the over seventy-five population continues to expand. State governments are gradually catching on to the notion that controlling the bed supply may be the only way to control Medicaid expenditures for nursing home services, and the certificate-of-need provisions of the new health-planning process provide them with workable tools with which to do something about it. The incentive to act is heightened by the requirement that states move to cost-related reimbursement systems and by the likelihood that industry representatives will use the federal statutory language, in both legislatures and the courts, to compel increases in reimbursement at least parallel to the overall rate of inflation. In an inflationary economy, states and other third-party payers could "reduce" per diem reimbursement simply by failing to increase it. But it appears from preliminary reports that they will have increasing difficulty in getting away with that.

Most importantly, the regulatory and reimbursement climate has turned much chillier, and most of the speculators have departed for warmer climes. Most of the cost-related reimbursement systems adopted by the states over the past several years, while more generous on operating costs to existing facilities, substantially limit, if they do not eliminate, the prospects of exorbitant profits on initial construction and financing. The big real estate loopholes have been narrowed. And recent regulatory trends—even if they are more appearance than substance—have frightened away speculators looking to turn a fast buck. Of eight states visited in 1977 in the course of this study (California, New York, Ohio, New Jersey, Minnesota, Connecticut, Arizona, and Oklahoma), there was substantial nursing home construction in none.

But pressures to resume the construction of new nursing homes may recur very quickly. As the supply of nursing home beds remains relatively constant while the population at risk for nursing home admissions grows dramatically, a number of things are likely to happen. In the short run, an increasing paucity of beds, if combined with some kind of admission controls, will mean that the residents of nursing homes will become increasingly sicker and more disabled. That will raise the costs of providing adequate services, further heighten pressures for qualitative improvement, and reduce the proportion of "inappropriate" placements. Over time, however, the number of people who "need" some kind of institutional services will begin to approach the available supply, thus exacerbating the backup of those awaiting discharge from acute-care hospitals and further increasing pressures to expand nursing home availability.

Those pressures will be particularly acute if the nursing home industry responds to increased demand in the face of constricted supply by heightened discrimination against Medicaid recipients. Public officials are already fearful that the increasing population at risk for nursing homes will reduce the availability of Medicaid beds (recent efforts by some states to prohibit such discrimination might be interpreted as an attempt to forestall the problem). Because governments lack the means to control "inappropriate" private nursing home admissions, increasing the bed supply will be especially attractive.

Finally, constraints on supply in the face of growing "need" and the absence of other policy initiatives can only accelerate the growth of the domiciliary-care industry and the continued "trickledown" of institutional and individual residents. There are now over 100,000 elderly recipients of SSI residing in "homes for adults" or "board and care" homes, mostly under proprietary auspices. Those facilities, licensed by the states if at all, have grown up in the five years since the adoption of SSI, in a process eerily similar to that which followed creation of OAA in 1935.

Except in a handful of states, domiciliary-care facilities (DCFs) have not substituted for nursing homes on a large scale, although they have been major recipients of elderly patients "deinstitutionalized" from state mental hospitals. But without the development of other services, those who formerly would have gone to nursing homes but are unable to find beds will increasingly end up in domiciliary institutions providing only the most primitive services.[10] Pressure to improve and expand those services could well lead to redefinition of DCFs as still a third, lower level of nursing homes, so that the problem will not have been solved so much as renamed. While the funding mechanisms are different, DCF care is borne at public expense just as much as is nursing home care, and the development of regulatory standards for DCFs is strikingly parallel to that of nursing homes, just twenty-five years before. Families and social agencies experience enormous pressures to put the dependent elderly somewhere, especially when services that might permit them to remain at home are unavailable. If they are increasingly unable to make placements in nursing homes, they will turn to DCFs. But as the new DCF population starts to look more and more like the old nursing home population, DCFs will come to look more like nursing homes.

If nature and policy are allowed to take their courses, the current pause in the growth of nursing homes will someday look, in retrospect, like merely a bump on the curve, a transient disturbance in the long-term trend. If the growing preponderance of demand over supply is met with increased noninstitutional services, the temporary leveling out in the supply of institutional beds can be converted into a permanent one; if those noninstitutional services do not materialize, the pressure to start building may again prove irresistible. The CBO estimates that, if those over sixty-five continue to be institutionalized at the rates implied by current practices, we will need *2.5 million* nursing home beds by 1985, 80 percent more than we now have.[11] The economic costs would be staggering. Nor is there any guarantee that the average level of care will be substantially higher than the present minimal mediocrity. Instead of having 1.25 million citizens housed in inadequate institutions, the only major change will be the addition of another 1.25 million.

A Strategy

We can do better. A strategy for doing so can be predicated on the assumption that no one who does not absolutely have to be in an institution should be in one, so long as he or she can be maintained as well in a more homelike setting without prohibitive cost to society. It also should be predicated on the argument that if we have, even temporarily, too many people in nursing homes, then we should close nursing homes. If we don't, people will end up in them, and that will cost so much money that none will be left over for doing better things. The strategy should start with a clear understanding of who the people nursing home policy has been serving, or misserving, are.

For purposes of developing future policy, nursing home residents can be divided into three groups (see table 7). The first are those who stay only a short time. Sixty-four percent of all nursing home discharges (although a much smaller proportion of all residents) involve stays of six months or less.[12] This group can be subdivided into two smaller groups: the very few who recuperate, or at least do not deteriorate, and have homes they can return to, and those who die very soon after admission. The critical element in the provision of services to both subgroups is the acute-care general hospital, which either kicks dying patients out to spend their last days in a nursing home or sends patients who are going to recover to complete their convalescence in a nursing home in order to satisfy utilization review requirements or other internal hospital pressures. Although it is almost impossible to estimate accurately, it would be fair to guess that 10 percent of all nursing home beds are occupied, on any given day, by people who will not be there long. That proportion fits very closely to estimates, based on strict interpretation of the definitions, of those in need of "skilled" care.

TABLE 7

The Nursing Home Population

Group	Approximate Percentage of Current Nursing Home Days	Approximate Number in Nursing Homes at Any One Time	Primary Descriptive Characteristics	Primary Policy – Relevant Characteristics
I	10	100,000–150,000		Discharged from hospitals for short (under six months) nursing home stays
Ia			Recuperating from acute illnesses, with homes to return to	
Ib			Fatally ill	
II	40	500,000	Chronically ill *and* socially isolated but not entirely helpless	Can be cared for in the community at a cost comparable to institutionalization
III	50	600,000–650,000	Moderate to severe senility or other severe psychiatric or physical disability (e.g., entirely bedfast)	Need round-the-clock custodial care

Doing Better

The second group of nursing home residents includes most of those whose disabilities are primarily physical but who lack spouses or other close family members to take care of them, or other social supports. With the exception of paralysis (relatively rare in the very old) and senility (which is not rare), there is just as much disability in the elderly outside of nursing homes as inside. The second group, lodged mostly in ICFs, numbers about 40 percent of nursing home residents, or about half a million people.

Members of this second group, if they live long enough, often pass gradually into the third, those who are so disabled as to require round-the-clock custodial care. Most of those in this category are moderately to severely senile. While they do not require, and do not benefit very much from, intensive medical care (narrowly defined), their confusion, tendency to wander, and danger to themselves make taking care of the very senile an extraordinarily difficult task outside of the institutional setting. The best approximation would be that about half of nursing home residents (over 600,000 people) fall into this category.[13] It is probable that relatively few individuals with an equivalent degree of mental disability remain outside in the community, although hundreds of thousands of people with early or mild degrees of mental impairment live perfectly well either with their families or, in fewer instances, by themselves.

The core of the strategy proposed here is that *only* individuals in Group III should be in nursing homes. Group II, those less severely disabled, should be in homes—although in many instances it will not be possible for them to remain in their own homes. Group I, those who will recover or die, should be in hospitals, which are the most effective institutions our society maintains for doing either.

If this logic holds, we now have in the United States roughly twice as many nursing home beds as we need, although we will need more in the future as the elderly age. This argument, that 50 percent of nursing home beds are excessive, is built on data and assumptions that are widely accepted. The problem has been that, like the Arkansas traveler, no one has known how to get from here to there without prohibitive expense. The real sticking point has been what to do with people who are *now* in nursing homes. For the vast majority of those who are not going to recuperate from an acute physical ailment, once the Rubicon of nursing home admission has been crossed the only remaining place to go is to the Great Beyond. Yet so long as all nursing home beds are full, they consume so much money that the development of "alternatives" is foreclosed.

Closing Beds

The way to cut nursing home beds is to constrict the flow of admissions. Let me suggest the broad outlines of a plan. In each of the 213 "health services areas" into which the nation has been divided for health planning purposes, local health systems agencies, in conjunction with state certifying agencies, could identify those nursing homes with the worst qualitative performances. Once such a list has been established, with all the appropriate hearings, appeals, and opportunities for reconsideration, the states probably have the power, under existing statutes in some cases, to phase out the worst 25 to 50 percent of all beds over a two to three-year period. No one residing in a facility marked for closing would be ejected through governmental action, at least in the early stages. The legal issue of whether the states can actually remove facility licenses solely on the basis of excess supply is not entirely resolved and probably varies from state to state depending on state constitutions and attitudes of state supreme courts. But there is no question that, with appropriate minor amendment to the Social Security Act, the states could cut off the flow of Medicaid admissions to excess facilities. Regulating the flow of private admissions—because of the spend-down effect, private patients constitute a much higher proportion of *admissions* than of residents or of days—is more difficult, although publication of a list of endangered facilities might well discourage those seeking private admissions from applying to those on the list.

Under existing law, the way to get this process into motion would be publication of a "National Health Guideline," under the aegis of the National Council of Health Planning and Development, establishing the national target of a one-third bed reduction. Because there is so much variation in existing nursing home availability from one place to another, that reduction would vary across the states. In some, no reduction at all would be necessary; in others, one-third would not be nearly enough. The target should be on the order of thirty-seven beds per 1,000 people over sixty-five and should be linked to an initial target occupancy rate of 75 percent. The precise determination of how many beds should be closed, and which ones, should probably be made locally.

The median length of stay in nursing homes is approximately 580 days, or just over a year and a half.[14] That means that half the nursing home population turns over every eighteen months. With no new admissions, the average facility will be half empty at the end of that period. If admissions to excess facilities were effectively controlled, most of them would be half empty by the second year of plan implementation. At that point, it would be necessary, for humane care as well as economic reasons, to consolidate the remaining residents into a smaller number of facilities. That would impose a cost on those residents being transferred—the greatest human cost in implementation of this plan—but the long-term general benefits would probably justify the one-time disadvantages.

The objective of this phasing out of industry capacity should not be to precisely equate supply with need nor to achieve uniformly high occupancies in the remaining facilities. It would probably be advantageous if, by 1985, average occupancy rates were somewhere between 70 and 75 percent, a number heretically low to most of those engaged in health planning and policymaking. (Excess capacity is desirable for several reasons. It is absolutely crucial to effective regulation and to reimbursement strategies. When capacity is very tight, the government, as monopsonist, finds itself in a weak position, and there is no point in promoting such weakness. Also, the number of those who will need nursing home services, those in Group III, will continue to grow steadily until at least the end of the century. If it is folly to over-invest in capital facilities, it would be even greater folly to discard that investment if parts of it will be needed in the foreseeable future.)

Achieving relatively low occupancy rates will be difficult. Existing beds tend to get filled, regardless of control measures. The greatest pressures working against a bed-closing scheme (apart from the political pressure that would undoubtedly be exerted by industry interests and those to whom they owe money) would emanate from the demand for private nursing home services, which will probably grow more rapidly than total demand as the elderly become increasingly affluent relative to other groups in the population. So long as the beds are there, noninstitutional alternatives will appear risky and difficult, even though they may be preferable. One tactic that might mitigate this problem would be reimbursement practices that *reward* low occupancy rates, so that a marginal admission beyond, say, 80 percent occupancy would produce no net revenue for the operator. In order for this scheme to work, nondiscrimination against Medicaid recipients would have to be enforced.

Some operators, especially in those states where Medicaid's market share is low, would probably respond to a plan of phased capacity reduction by withdrawing from public programs altogether, seeking private patients only. There is probably no way that governments can forbid a citizen to purchase services from a licensed nursing home, although health-related police powers and general consumer powers can partially circumscribe such transactions. Beyond that, the only sound thing for governments to do with totally private nursing homes would be to ignore them.

Permitting some facilities to "drop out" of the public market altogether would deflect some of the severe political pressures that a plan for phased closings would incite. Nursing home operators, and those holding their mortgage paper, would raise the specter of governmentally induced bankruptcies and contend that governments were violating a long-standing implicit covenant to continue paying those facilities that retained their licenses.[15] Basing closing on qualitative ratings would partially blunt those arguments, but the essential reply must be that government cannot be construed to owe nursing homes, especially substandard nursing homes, a living. The provision of services to government for a profit cannot be justified unless entrepreneurs experience risk, and the entrepreneurs supplying nursing home services have been reaping comfortable risk premiums for a generation. Under the strategy proposed here, some nursing homes would go bankrupt, and they thoroughly deserve to. Banks will have to write off hundreds of mortgage loans, but that will hardly shake the foundations of the republic, although the banks will try to create the impression that it will. Those who live by the sword of for-profit enterprise should be prepared to die by it; their claim on public subsidy is hardly compelling.

Political pressure will come not only from the industry and the banks but from potential nursing home residents, their families, and advocates, who now really have no other alternatives and would rightly fear being left entirely without services.

Apart from the basic goal of shifting toward noninstitutional services, capacity reduction could introduce qualitative competition within the nursing home industry. There is now no incentive for nursing homes that rely primarily on Medicaid reimbursement to provide anything other than the minimum necessary to escape regulatory sanctions. Their performance is measured against an abstract, minimal standard, rather than against other facilities. The very process of attempting to classify facilities into even two or three broad qualitative groupings (whether or not closings actually resulted from those groupings) would probably have a salutary effect. So long as the threat of closing on the basis of low ranking remained, proprietors would have a substantial incentive to invest in qualitative improvements.

Precise measurements of quality are probably impossible, but they would not be necessary either. Rough groupings would suffice and—if the process of making those groupings were sufficiently open, participatory, and in keeping with due process requirements—should be manageable. Nor would much be lost if those facilities at the top of the lowest grouping were given the benefit of the doubt, since the precariousness of their status would, if the rating process were continuous, probably do wonders to keep them in line.

A reduction to even one million beds, which would entail the closing of less than 25 percent of existing capacity, combined with an industrywide average occupancy rate of 80 percent (as opposed to the present average of somewhere over 90 percent) would, if the ratio of Medicaid and Medicare recipients to all residents remained constant, produce a savings from 1976 expenditures of $2.3 billion. The big savings, though, would come from forestalling future growth. CBO's estimate of close to $23 billion in public nursing home expenditures for 1985 is based on their projection of total bed capacity of over two million, combined with relatively conservative estimates on inflation.[16] One million beds at 90 percent occupancy in 1985 would cost taxpayers $12.5 billion less.

If half of the more than $2 billion in possible savings were redirected to housing and home-based services, that would more than *double* the existing public expenditures for those activities. Most of the rest of the savings would go to services for Group I patients. The balance might even be returned to the taxpayer, although it is more likely to vanish into thin air; it could most productively be spent on still further expansion of housing and in-home services for those who do not end up in the nursing home system.

Hospitals

The major question about the capacity-reduction plan proposed here is what is to become of people who will "need" nursing home care but will be "backed up" in acute-care hospitals? The partial answer is that those backed up in hospitals should stay there. Those who are now discharged from hospitals to nursing homes because of utilization review requirements, insurance limitations, or the general impatience of hospital staffs with the chronically ill elderly and who can reasonably be expected to have only a short nursing home stay, because they are likely to die soon or recover soon, should remain in hospitals. Transferring them to nursing homes is inhumane, means that they will receive less competent and probably less concerned care, and doesn't really save any money.

There are now, by the most conservative estimates, in excess of 100,000 more hospital beds in the United States than are needed.[17]And the prospects for reducing excess hospital capacity are not promising. Hospitals are just as well, if not better, equipped as nursing homes to provide basic nursing, personal care, and food services. They are substantially less good at providing "psychosocial care" or a pleasant living environment, but most nursing homes don't do that well either. It is obviously insane to build new nursing home beds when hospital beds are kept empty by the constant flow of discharges to nursing homes and only slightly less irrational to close halfway decent hospitals when fourth-rate nursing homes are entirely full.

The numbers mesh almost exactly. On any given day, 10 percent of nursing home residents (about 125,000 people) fall into Group I—short-stay admissions. While 100,000 excess hospital beds is the figure most commonly cited, it is undoubtedly conservative. Moreover, advances in medical technology make shorter hospital stays or treatment on an outpatient basis possible. Given the often soundly based difference in most communities' feelings toward their hospitals and nursing homes, the motto should be: close nursing homes, not hospitals.

The only thing wrong with these figures is that elimination of discharges from hospitals to nursing homes for short-stay residents would probably have a significant impact on those patients' mortality rates. They would die less often, or less quickly. Of every one thousand frail, old people transferred from one setting to another, five to ten die in the process. The numbers involved are not large enough to undermine the estimates, although they would certainly add weight to the proposal.

Maintaining in hospitals some of those who are now discharged to nursing homes would not require very much more than a relaxation of utilization review and similar pressures. But it would probably be desirable to make some minimal capital and educational investments to create special units (floors, wings, or buildings) for those whose stays will be very long by contemporary hospital standards. Those units could be "deinstitutionalized" to some degree with painting, draperies, decoration, and the creation of common areas and dining rooms and could be provided with specially interested or trained staff. Many of the nation's older community hospitals once had such "chronic disease" or long-stay wards, which tended to be occupied primarily by those who fall into Groups II and III. The hospitals were only too glad to get rid of them when nursing homes developed. What is being described is essentially a reinvention of the extended-care facility as it appeared in Medicare legislation before the "transfer agreement" notion was added; the primary difference is that this proposal does not contemplate the creation of new p^{hy}sical plant.

The principal objection to this proposal will be that it would be frighteningly expensive. On average, hospitals charge and are reimbursed five times as much for a day of care as the most expensive nursing home. But the actual incremental costs are not that much different. Because their stays are short and the fixed costs of admissions and discharges are amortized over fewer days, old people recuperating or dying are among the most expensive residents to care for in a nursing home; they are among the least expensive patients to care for in the hospital. Hospitals should not be reimbursed at their average acute-care per diem for longer-stay geriatric patients. It is also reasonable to assert that the marginal revenue to hospitals reimbursed at, say, locally prevailing Medicare SNF rates *for beds that would otherwise be empty* would exceed their marginal costs for putting those beds back into operation as extended-care facilities.[18]

Convincing hospitals that it is in their interest to go along will be difficult. Every hospital administrator and trustee clings to the objective of increasing occupancy to effective capacity by capturing a larger market share, presumably from other hospitals. Many hospitals might close down wings rather than convert them for the use of geriatric patients. To the extent that the health planning process remains a paper tiger, threats of closure will not be very intimidating to the hospitals. But levers are available for inducing hospital cooperation. One is the health planning process itself, especially in those states that have closure powers or where funds are available to bribe hospitals to comply with planning mandates.[19] More powerful is the reimbursement process. If re-creation of extended-care facilities is seen as a desirable policy goal, then increases in hospitals' acute-care rates might be used as an inducement.

Housing

Extended hospital stays on the extended-care facility model would be appropriate for only a minority of those denied admission to nursing homes under circumstances of tighter supply. Those in Group II, while they may not have regular need of the kinds of medical supervision nursing homes are supposed to provide, do need services. Mostly, they need to be taken care of, to be assisted in bathing, dressing, food preparation, and simply getting around, to have companionship, and to have the reassurance that medical help is available when they need it. For many of these individuals, the ideal solution is what has come to be called congregate or sheltered housing. In congregate housing, which is widespread in much of northern Europe, individuals reside in their own apartments but eat communally in a central dining room and are provided housekeeping, laundry, recreational activities, transportation, and some health and social services by the organization administering the housing. Apartments in congregate housing complexes customarily contain nurse-call buttons, like those employed in hospitals, which are an important source of reassurance and security for old people fearful of being trapped, incapacitated, alone at home.

There are obvious economies of scale in providing services from a central location. Congregate housing also provides a balance, so often crucial for the well-being of the frail elderly, between independence and dependence. Most importantly, in well-run congregate housing, residents take care of one another, especially in those projects managed by ethnic or fraternal groups drawing from relatively homogenous communities. The availability of others able and willing to help with daily problems—or just to listen—is what many of those who now end up in nursing homes most lack.

Most existing congregate housing in the United States is managed by nonprofit voluntary organizations, much of it on the same "campuses" as their nursing homes. Just as the "hospital" component of this strategy involves "reinventing" the extended-care facility, so congregate housing, in a sense, is a reinvention of the older home for the aging, adjusted to contemporary standards of privacy and housing adequacy. For some voluntary organizations, construction of congregate housing means coming full circle. They began as religiously or ethnically sponsored homes for the aging, but as their clientele became older and more infirm and as funds were available for nursing home but not residential care, they converted their facilities to nursing homes or built new ones. Now many are erecting congregate housing. Where once there was a dormitory-style "home" to which a three-or five-bed infirmary was attached, there is now a 200-bed nursing home to which an apartment house is attached.

For people to be served by congregate housing, they must be prepared to move there, and the reluctance of many elderly people to leave the homes and communities of a lifetime deserves respect, not least because of the evidence that forced residential relocations can be damaging in much the way nursing home "transfer trauma" is.[20] Congregate housing also contributes to increasing "ghettoization" of the elderly, a situation desired by some older people, but far from all, and one that may be undesirable from a broader social perspective. And while congregate housing is economical, it is hardly cheap. Rents in existing congregate units range from $600 to more than $1,000 a month. (The top of that range is as much as moderately expensive SNFs and substantially more than the ICFs for which congregate housing residents would presumably be eligible.) Those amounts are not outside the means of many elderly people, especially those in a position to sell off housing assets or receive assistance from family members. But the median income for women over sixty-five is barely $3,000 ($250 a month), and those without other resources are the ones most likely to end up in nursing homes.

The major barrier to the expansion of congregate housing is not the upkeep but the initial capital investment. Construction of almost all forms of residential housing is becoming prohibitively expensive, and rentals in congregate housing are so high largely because of the burden of debt such projects carry. Luxury housing without services for the affluent younger elderly is an infinitely more attractive investment for private capital. Section 202 of the National Housing Act does provide low-interest mortgage loans to nonprofit sponsors of housing for the disabled, including the disabled elderly, and almost all congregate housing now being constructed in the United States is built with 202 funds. Even then, sponsors will not embark on projects without assurances that tenants will also be eligible for rent subsidies under Section 8 of the Housing Act, a provision that ensures that tenants who meet income guidelines will be subsidized to the extent that rents in approved low-income housing projects exceed 25 percent of their income. And Section 202 only provides about $200 million per year. At current construction costs, that will allow for barely 5,000 units— equivalent to less than a week's worth of ICF admissions.

One way to beat the high costs of congregate housing construction would be to attempt to create something like congregate housing from existing units. In many parts of the country, including inner cities as well as so-called retirement communities, there are large concentrations of old people living in conventional housing. By bringing services to these people, it might be possible to obtain the economies of scale and other advantages of congregate housing without the capital expenditures. That is the rationale behind the experiment in "enriched housing" recently undertaken by New York State, in which nonprofit sponsors will rent several contiguous apartments, make marginal capital improvements, and provide services to groups of fifteen to twenty elderly people at a time. State officials estimate that this mix of housing and services can be provided for no more than the highest rate paid for recipients of Supplemental Social Security Income living in DCFs—around $400 per month. That estimate may be grounded more in optimism than economics, but it is clear that the services component of congregate housing is, at least potentially, much cheaper than the housing component.

Assessing the costs of comprehensive long-term care programs for the elderly is very difficult. The average monthly "cost" for nursing home care could be broken down into so much for food, so much for shelter, so much for medical care, and so much for each of the other services provided. The payment for that month of nursing home care is compounded of the resident's income from social security and other retirement programs, plus a contribution from Medicaid to make up the balance. For an elderly person living in the "community," on the other hand, medical expenditures are paid for by Medicare (minus some not inconsiderable deductibles and coinsurance), and food or recreation may be provided through federally financed meals-on-wheels or senior citizens centers. The costs of housing, housekeeping, and everything else are met out-of-pocket. For most, the primary source of that income is social security. How much it will cost to provide that individual with services is thus a function not only of the costs of supplying those services but of how she is paying for the other necessities of life, and, crucially, the level of her social security benefits.

The problem of estimating costs is hopelessly complicated, since Congress keeps fiddling with social security benefits, and since those benefits are now tied to the rate of inflation in the economy as a whole. Still worse, no one has been able to make very convincing estimates of the future total income of the elderly. It will be affected by the fact that, subsequent to the 1948 Taft-Hartley Amendments, the number of those retiring with private pension benefits is increasing all the time; the further changes in pension patterns induced by the Employees Retirement Income Security Act (ERISA) of 1974; the growth in public employment since the 1950s, especially at state and local levels (with the customarily more generous pensions but also by the exclusion of roughly 25 percent of public employees from the social security system); and the increasing participation of women in the workforce—all of which should increase the relative income of the elderly. It will also be affected by the unprecedented inflation of recent years, which may reduce it.

The one assumption that can be made for purposes of budget estimation, employed by the CBO in its study, is that all new services will be provided on an entitlement basis, regardless of ability to pay. That assumption coincides comfortably with the prevailing ideology of elderly groups, which is strongly opposed to means-testing for any publicly provided benefits. But it is clear, as the CBO study demonstrates, that the provision of comprehensive services to any large part of the elderly population without taking other income into account would be prohibitively expensive. Still, tying the financing of benefits to recipients' income makes the range of possible costs literally infinite.

Old people in need of services have to live somewhere. To the extent that economies of scale in service provision amount to enough, over time, to defray the capital costs of building specialized housing, expanded congregate units should be part of any strategy for long-term care, regardless of the total funds available. As the elderly population becomes more affluent, it is also conceivable that some volume of congregate housing could become commercially feasible, perhaps with appropriate assistance and encouragement from governments (in the form of mortgage insurance or more limited subsidies, for example). No one knows exactly how many people now reside in congregate units, but if production were to double immediately, there would probably still be fewer than 200,000 units by 1985. The strategy proposed here includes the diversion of a significant fraction of the savings from closing nursing homes to the development of more congregate housing, with emphasis on those congregate dwellings than can be developed without major capital outlays. There will still be recurring costs for providing services to congregate housing residents, but those costs should be lower than the costs of providing identical services to residents of conventional housing.

Services

No matter how great an expansion in congregate housing is undertaken, there will still be many individuals scattered through the community who need services delivered at home. Estimates of how many such persons there are vary widely. If half of the 500,000 Group II nursing home residents could be accommodated in congregate housing, that would leave over 200,000 people in the community in need of intensive services, not to mention those already needing such services in the community, nor to take account of the over-seventy-five population growth.

There is enormous potential demand, and thus the problem of gatekeeping. That problem is complex, but not unsolvable. In each locality, there should be an agency, or several competing agencies, to which any elderly individual seeking services would be referred. Ideally, all such individuals would be referred there, but it is probably not legally possible to require it. The best arrangement would be one in which all those seeking public subsidy would have to be referred while those prepared to pay out-of-pocket would be encouraged to do so voluntarily.

The agency's central function would be to "assess" those seeking services and, thereby, to determine which combination of services was necessary. Debates among gerontologists about how those assessments should be performed resemble, in passionate intensity and irrelevance to practical affairs, those of Orthodox schismatics on the Stations of the Cross, but a number of different assessment procedures would probably all work equally well. The crucial element in this process would be conditioning public subsidy on the recommendations of the gatekeeping agency; if the agency determined that a homemaker was not necessary, none would be provided. Some provision for appeals from assessment determinations would also be necessary.

It would also be desirable for the gatekeeping agency to monitor the quality of services provided on its recommendation and to encourage, through grants or contractual mechanisms, development of those services inadequately available in the locality it served. Whether or not the gatekeeping agency should provide direct services itself is debatable; my own inclination is that it should not. (The gatekeeping agency could not serve as its clients' advocate vis-a-vis service providers if it provided services itself.)

The question then arises as to whether the gatekeeping agency's purview should extend to nursing homes, hospitals, physician services, and prescription drugs. Also at issue is how services should be paid for, and how the gatekeeping agency should control payment.

My own preference would be to consolidate all public funds now expended for nursing homes, home-health, and the myriad of smaller services in a given area into a single pot, with sweeteners thrown in as incentives for desired agency performance in specific areas. The agency should then be held fiscally responsible for purchasing all services received by its clients, which would furnish the incentive to bargain hard with service providers and encourage the preference of less-expensive over more expensive services. This is the optimal solution from the point of view of federal budgetary authorities. Something much like it circulated as a "long-term care block grant" during the Ford administration, as a means of controlling the growth of Medicaid expenditures. But the annual lump sum available could, in theory, be any amount. When there is more than one gatekeeping agency in a community, that sum could be divided among them in proportion to their "enrollees," or according to a formula that took both enrollment and other performance characteristics into account.

All but the most indigent clients should be required to pay some share of the costs of service they receive, on a graduated scale according to income. Here it is probably imperative that cost-sharing formulas be set at uniform, national levels, since the more "responsive" agencies are to the wishes of their more vocal clients, the less willing they are likely to be to impose progressive cost-sharing. It would also be imperative to impose stringent federal supervision of the way agencies are governed and the criteria they use to determine priorities for service, since the possibility of discrimination among classes of clients is the single greatest administrative danger the idea of a gatekeeping agency poses.

Regardless of how much client cost-sharing is imposed, there is no way to assure—short of unlimited, open-ended funding—that everyone who "needs" services will get them. When demand is effectively infinite, supply will never catch up. It makes good sense, though, to finance services in any given community from a fixed pot. How big that pot should be is a question of political and social allocations. But some determination of who will get services and who will not, and of which services they will get, must be made, and there is probably no magical computer-based formula that will make that determination automatically. That is one reason, given American mores and traditions, why those determinations should be made locally by lay-governed institutions. And that is one reason why cost estimates for a nationwide network of in-home services allocated by gatekeeping agencies are impossible to make: it will cost whatever we are willing to pay. But so long as some services like senior centers or meals on wheels are funded on an annual fixed-dollar basis, while others that may partially substitute for them are paid for open-endedly, the latter services are likely to be overconsumed.

In essence, what is being proposed here might be described as a form of long-term care Health Maintenance Organization (HMO).[21] HMOs are the currently popular device, in certain Washington circles, for controlling health-care costs. A political renaming of what used to be called prepaid group practices, HMOs undertake to provide all necessary health services for their subscribers for an annual fixed fee. Because they are at risk for expenditures in excess of that annual fee that might arise from overutilization or too-high unit prices, HMOs presumably have an incentive to economize by relying on less-expensive services and keeping their clients well. While there is no evidence that the "preventive" services provided by HMOs actually do conduce to lower costs, or even that other HMOs will be able to duplicate the enormous success of the prototypical Kaiser system on the West Coast, HMOs do have the enormous budgetary advantage of having to live within their incomes and do show evidence of using resources more efficiently.[22]

The ultimate extension of the HMO concept to long-term care services for the elderly would be to bring all health services, including those now fully covered by Medicare, within the range of covered services and within the annual single fee. A partial prototype currently exists in central Connecticut, where an organization named Triage is conducting an experimental demonstration program, under discretionary authority of the Social Security Act. Triage is basically a gatekeeping agency, but it also serves as the Medicare fiscal intermediary for its clients. For the purposes of the experiment, a range of in-home homemaker, nutrition, and chore services, as well as transportation and social services, have been extended Medicare coverage, as have prescription drugs. In its role of fiscal intermediary, Triage has been able to discourage hospital utilization—for which, in an area of tight nursing home bed supply, it appears that in-home services are more likely to substitute—to a sufficient extent to generate savings adequate to pay for the full range of in-home services. There is reason to doubt that comprehensive HMOs for the elderly could always provide such a wide range of services so economically. And the widespread extension of so much authority over medical decisions to nonphysician-dominated agencies is probably not politically possible. But the idea merits further exploration.

There is no reason why a single uniform model of any kind should be rigidly applied throughout the nation. The very core of the gatekeeping agency concept is maintenance of a high degree of flexibility, openness, and improvisation in order to serve a heterogeneous group of clients whose needs are themselves fluctuating and highly variable. This would be a particularly good place to let a hundred flowers bloom. The objective is to provide as much service to as many people as possible. It makes no sense to devote years waiting for identification of the "one best way" to do it.

There is already enough money in the system to provide adequate in-home services for those in Group II who would otherwise be channelled to nursing homes, provided that the nursing homes in which they would be placed are closed. Home care may be no less expensive than nursing home care, but for those who still have most of their wits about them and who do not need daily nursing attention, it should not be much more expensive. It is impossible to prove that those who remain in their homes will be better off. But given the quality of life in the average nursing home, it is hard to believe that most of them could be worse off.

Nursing Homes

Even if all the suggestions listed to this point were adopted, more than half a million Americans would still reside in nursing homes, and those that did would be the most helpless and most disabled. Preventing the institutions in which they resided from becoming the worst kind of human warehouses would be a formidable task. To some extent, the presence of people in nursing homes who could get by on the outside with adequate assistance provides a crucial moderating influence. It prevents the total demoralization of staff, the total insulation of staff and administration from the opinions of residents, and the total cutting off of the institution from the rest of society. Confining nursing home admissions to those in Group III would provide further justification for abolishing the SNF/ICF distinction, permit abandonment of the prevailing rhetoric of rehabilitation, and generate some minor savings. The price would be recognition of nursing homes as a place for those who are both entirely helpless and entirely beyond help.

In some form or another, this dilemma reasserts itself whenever proposals for "deinstitutionalization" of persons of any type (the retarded, the mentally ill, or even prisoners) is presented. Discharging those who might make it on the outside means leaving behind those with the most severe disabilities. By itself, that is scarcely an argument against deinstitutionalization, since it is obviously unjust to deprive those who can subsist on the outside in order to benefit those who will remain in institutions.

Those who would be left behind in nursing homes do not require an extensive range of services. They need to be kept clean, kept fed, and kept from injuring themselves or others.[23] Most societies are not particularly good at caring for such people; no one wants the job. All that can be suggested is stringent regulation, adequate funding, provision for active and aggressive third-party involvement in monitoring and oversight, and a system of rotating young people, recently graduated from high school or college, through one-year stints as nursing home aides (long enough to capture their openness and enthusiasm, short enough to get them out before total cynicism and disillusionment take over). Providing for the hopelessly disabled does not require new technologies or even vastly greater amounts of money, just a combination of caring and interorganizational checks and balances that is often hard to come by.

Making It Work

Caring for the hopelessly disabled remaining in nursing homes poses problems of administrative and political complexity of the kinds from which policymakers are often eager to flee. Limiting nursing home admissions to those in Group III; ranking nursing homes by quality; closing low-quality nursing homes; developing in-hospital, extended-care facilities; developing congregate housing in existing buildings; developing and managing gatekeeping agencies—all seem like reasonable things to do. But those are not the kinds of tasks governments are particularly eager to undertake. Public agencies are much better at writing checks or erecting buildings, and in a period of widespread skepticism about the capability of governments to accomplish anything, there is serious question as to their ability to perform the hundreds of tasks that would be necessary to implement this strategy.

Should there be government action along the lines proposed, there would be many failures, and hardly anything would work perfectly. In all probability, too few nursing homes would be closed, and some mistakes would be made—closing good ones while bad ones remained in business. Too few extended-care facility beds would be set aside, and too much provided to reimburse for them. Gatekeeping agencies would make lots of errors, and in spite of whatever control mechanisms were invented, some nursing homes populated primarily by the very senile would become hellholes. But that is just to say that those activities would be subject to the same human limitations that existing insitutions providing services to the elderly are.

The appropriate comparison for the likelihood of future imperfection is present imperfection. Perhaps the strongest argument that can be made for the proposals here is that they are unlikely to be worse than existing policies. But the difficulties of implementation have important political implications. Recognizing the complexity of more radical and innovative programs, policymakers fear that they might fail, and caution sets in. That caution is substantially reinforced by prevailing political ideologies that question the ability of governments to do anything and by a balance of political forces entirely content with the status quo.

Of course some of the proposals contained in this strategy might fail. If we extrapolate from existing programs for the dependent elderly, the odds are certainly against them. The sticking point is the criterion for success. For the timidity among policymakers these days is such that a high probability of partial success is no longer acceptable. Even Ted Williams hit safely fewer than four times out of ten. That batting average is no longer good enough, even though a 40 percent success rate in the establishment of gatekeeping agencies or the conversion of unused beds to extended-care facilities would leave thousands of citizens better off than they were before. The decision of whether to undertake a particular course of action should depend not only on the likelihood of success, but on the size of the payoff if success is attained compared to the size of the losses if it isn't. But those who make policy for long-term care are like poker players who would stand pat on a pair of threes, even when looking at a large pot.

The practical difficulties in implementing this strategy should not be underemphasized. That is why the reduction of institutional capacity must be the first step, because other programs will not be undertaken so long as so much of the market is pre-empted by institutional beds. Conversely, the closing of beds would no longer make it possible to avoid doing something about other services; the cop-out of sending people to nursing homes would have been removed, and people will be banging on the doors demanding help. Like all human institutions, government agencies respond best to stress, and when they have to do something about a problem, they generally do. Failure comes less from making mistakes than from not being forced to confront the problem directly at all. Closing nursing homes forces public agencies, and those private agencies concerned with the well-being of dependent old people, to do something. If funds are simultaneously made available for them to do sensible things, the odds that they will do them are pretty high.

Minimal and Maximal Programs

A maximalist program for reform of nursing home and long–term care services might look something like this:

1. A reduction of existing nursing-home capacity by one-third over a five-year period, with a target average occupancy of 75 percent in 1985 (with unused beds "stockpiled" to be put back into services as the over-seventy-five population and the number of extremely disabled grows). That reduction should be achieved by closing nursing homes with the lowest quality.
2. Conversion of 100,000 to 125,000 currently unused or under-used acute-care hospital beds to "extended-care facility" beds, admission to which would be contingent on expectation of death or discharge home within six months, and reimbursement for which would be on the basis of true incremental costs to the hospital (which should be in the range of current rates for high quality SNFs).
3. Creation of 250,000 or so additional units of congregate housing—in existing buildings to the extent possible.
4. A substantial expansion of services in the home, directed by local gatekeeping agencies, financed at least initially on a block-grant or capitation basis

with the funds saved from closing nursing home beds, combined with existing funds for categorical services. Those services should be provided on an ability-to-pay basis. There probably won't be enough to go around.

5. A redoubling of regulatory and other quality control mechanisms in nursing homes, abandoning the mythology of rehabilitation and concentrating on basic personal care, food, and protective services to ensure that an increasingly sicker nursing home population does not suffer the consequences of complete desertion by society.

If all this were to come to pass, the United States would have, with a few significant exceptions, a system much like that which has prevailed in parts of the United Kingdom for the last decade or more. The most significant difference is that, in Britain, the channeling function is performed by physicians.[24]

One of the advantages of this plan is that it can be accomplished a little bit at a time. With a little flexibility in Washington, individual states might attempt some variant of it by themselves or even give their local health systems agencies the power to try it in a more circumscribed area. Or Uncle Sam could encourage, without requiring, everyone to do it. Since the "market" for almost all services to the dependent elderly is overwhelmingly local, there is no requirement for rigid national uniformity, although some of the existing rigid uniformities in national programs, especially in Medicare, would have to be relaxed if localities were to attempt innovative programs. And some localities already are: in Holyoke, Massachusetts; Bristol-Plainview, Connecticut; Rochester, New York; Tuscon, Arizona; and San Francisco's Chinatown. And they, and their older residents, are doing pretty well. There is no single, indispensable element to any existing or proposed set of arrangements, save one: the supply of nursing home beds must be tightly controlled, and admissions to scarce beds must be limited to those for whom there simply aren't any other alternatives. Relative to that requirement, the exact balance between individuals receiving services in congregate dwelling units or in conventional housing, the details of gatekeeping agencies' operation, or the precise specification of size and shape for extended-care facilities just aren't very important.

Some Concluding Thoughts

As an inadvertent byproduct of public policy, the American nursing home, at least in its current profusion and variety, was a mistake. As an institution, it makes sense for no more than half of its residents. As an instrument of social policy, it illustrates the dangers of attempting to solve problems by indirection, buckpassing, and wishful thinking. Several years ago, gerontologist Elaine Brody described America's nursing homes as containing "a million Procrustean beds."[25] The only modification I would now make in that statement is to say "one million, three hundred thousand." Of course, if nursing homes did not exist, someone would have to invent them as institutions to care for the extremely and irreversibly senile—but *not* for the soon to die, or soon to recover, or the socially isolated.

It is difficult to be optimistic about the future of nursing home policy. The hardest thing in this political system is to reverse the continuing growth of a program buttressed by skillful and well-financed interest groups. But the growing numbers and political militancy of the elderly, combined with the growing restiveness of taxpayers and the prospects for moderate or nonexistent economic growth are, sooner or later, going to force something to give in the pattern of public expenditures for services to older citizens. There is no better place to start than nursing homes.

Not in Our Stars

"Your public servants serve you right"
—Adlai Stevenson

I T IS SAID that in the office of Senator Edward Kennedy (the most visible and perhaps most effective proponent of national health insurance) there hangs a poster bearing the message, "If you like the United States Postal Service, you'll love National Health Insurance." The story is often repeated because it reflects an attitude that is widely shared, not least among policymakers in Washington. If government cannot even deliver the mail, assigning it total control over the complex and vitally important system of medical care will lead to disaster.

The argument implicit in the poster ignores the extent to which postal service has deteriorated, or at least been perceived to have deteriorated, since it was "taken out of politics" and reorganized on a "business" basis in the Nixon administration. It ignores the extent to which the existing organization of health services may be totally inefficient, as well as the fact that the most compelling argument for something like national health insurance is one of equity, not efficiency: the moral unacceptability of a system in which citizens can be turned away from needed medical services because of inadequate financial means. But the poster meshes so nicely with prevailing political ideologies, eagerly reinforced by those who benefit most grandly from the status quo, that it effectively capsulizes the existing political stalemate on matters of health policy.

Opponents of government initiative might find nursing homes an even better example than the post office to support their case. Well over 90 percent of the mail does eventually get delivered; the proportion of nursing home residents receiving decent services is much smaller. While petty fraud and corruption undoubtedly persist in the postal service, it is necessary to go back to the Star Route cases of almost a century ago to find postal stealing of a magnitude comparable to that which has prevailed in the nursing home industry for a generation. The comparison could be extended indefinitely.

It is not enough, however, to simply label nursing home policy a failure. Doing so is too easy. The prevailing assumption, that public programs are bound to fail because governments are generally and generically incompetent, can become a form of self-fulfilling prophecy. (When reformers of the 1930s assumed that almshouses were so terrible because they were governmental, they barred Old Age Assistance payments to their residents and helped give rise to a whole new class of inadequate publicly supported facilities.) Yet so long as providing assistance to the most helpless members of society is left to governments—if for no other reason than the unwillingness or inability of other social institutions to do it—then giving up on government a priori means giving up on those people. If the concepts of social welfare, public interest, or common good have any meaning whatsoever, then giving up on government means giving up on the most plausible instrument for attaining them. As in Hobbes's time, the likeliest alternative is the war of each against all.

There are identifiable, relatively straightforward reasons why nursing home policy has failed: the difficulty of undoing past mistakes; dependence on the private sector; the culture of public welfare; problems in the federal system; the divergence between political time and policy time; the problem of fine tuning; the regulation of government; and human fallibility. There is no reason why the same mistakes must be repeated in the future. One result of the long-standing American mistrust of government has been a repeated inability to learn from either past failures—which are taken for granted, assumed to be the norm—or past successes, which are thought to be so extraordinary as to provide few useful lessons.

There is a demonstrable, if complex and tenuous, link between the behavior of an average voter on election day and the quality of care received by someone else's grandmother throughout the year, as there should be in a society that styles itself democratic. But demonstrating that proposition should not serve as a comforting excuse for self-congratulation. Rather, it represents the only means of preventing this book from being a counsel of despair. For if the problems of nursing homes are policy problems and if policy problems are political problems, and if the society is at all democratic, then the means to effect a solution exist. There is a prospect for redress. That prospect is political.

One, Two, Many Nursing Homes:
The Difficulty of Undoing Past Mistakes

Under certain sets of political and social conditions, governments find it harder to undo their mistakes than do most other social institutions, or most individuals. When the Ford Motor Company discontinued production of the Edsel, dealers felt some obligation to maintain parts inventories, but Edsel owners were soon left to scrounging from junkyards and trading with one another, and people (if there were any) who had set their hearts on owning an Edsel were immediately forced to turn elsewhere. Supermarkets or department stores losing money in inner-city locations can simply shut their doors. Corporations and individuals can file for bankruptcy, and an individual proprietor can, for all intents and purposes, walk away from his nursing home. But the state, once having assumed responsibility for overseeing the care of nursing home residents (or the mentally ill or mentally retarded) is stuck with them. When people have to turn to it for help, government, like the employers of Frost's hired man, has to take them in.

Under certain circumstances, once a public agency has assumed responsibility for dealing with a given problem, and in the course of attempting to deal with it has acquired a class of dependents, it cannot simply throw up its hands in despair and walk away. In order to cease supporting inadequate nursing homes, governments have to come up with something better; they cannot just stop supporting the nursing home population. It is not the unavailability of alternative programs, per se, that forestalls abandonment of a program everyone concedes to be inadequate, so much as the question of how the transition is to be made. A rational approach might well be to try something and, if it doesn't work, then try something else radically different. When incrementalism dominates the policy process, however, the characteristic response is to try something only very slightly different.

It is extraordinarily difficult to provide decent and humane long-

245

term care services to very old, very frail, often very senile, familyless indigent people. Given a problem of such difficulty, the prevailing school of policy analysis holds that the appropriate response is to lower expectations, to avoid the tendency of politicians to "overpromise," to recognize that a very limited success is the best than can be hoped for.[1] A more conservative view is that it is folly for governments to undertake tasks for which the prospect of success is so small. But in many instances, nursing homes being only one obvious case, there really is no choice as to whether or not government should be involved—it already is, and there is no way out. Lowering expectations and accepting a high degree of failure mean condemning hundreds of thousands of government nursing home clients to continued substandard services.

Lowering expectations also reinforces a vicious cycle, since it supports incrementalist tendencies to avoid radical policy change. If the most that can be expected is another form of expensive failure, and since a known problem is politically preferable to an unknown one, there seems little point in taking the risks of real policy experimentation. Public policies that deal unsuccessfully with complex problems like long-term care or inner-city elementary education or mass transit are perpetuated indefinitely because they are expected to fail and because innovating alternatives, it is presumed, will fail too.

Dissatisfaction with public performance breeds immobility. That ideological process is closely linked to a balance of political forces. A political system characterized by multiple independent veto powers is much less likely to remove benefits previously conferred than it is to confer new ones. No one is very happy with prevailing policies, which are themselves largely the product of past mistakes, but no one is able to do very much about them either. Incrementalism is thus both a policy style and a political outcome, and those two characteristics continually feed on one another.

It is possible to make a plausible argument that governments should never have gotten into the business of supporting nursing homes at all—that the ban on Old Age Assistance payments to residents of public institutions should have been extended to all institutions, while alternative arrangements, entirely divorced from income-maintenance programs, were provided for the disabled. Hindsight is always 20–20. But once mistakes are made, it is especially difficult for policymakers to undo them. Generically, this phenomenon might be described as the Waist Deep in the Big Muddy Problem; there are many domestic Vietnams, in which light is always receding from the end of the tunnel.

Private Uses of the Public Interest

The principal beneficiaries of past nursing home policy have been nursing home operators, especially those who got out when the getting was good, taking substantial windfall profits with them. However dissatisfied the industry may now appear to be with the twists and turns of government policy, that policy still remains the captive of industry pressures and activities.

Charles Lindblom has recently written of what he calls the "privileged position of business" in liberal-democratic, free-enterprise polities, which arises from the dependence of governments on private firms for the performance of important social tasks. According to Lindblom:

> Constitutional rules—especially the law of private property—specify that, although governments can forbid certain kinds of activity, they cannot command business to perform. They must induce rather than command. They must therefore offer benefits to businessmen in order to stimulate the required performance.[2]

The kinds of inducements governments have offered nursing home operators in the hope of eliciting the "required performance" have been discussed. Attempts to "forbid certain kinds of activity" have hinged on the extent to which regulators feared that excessive stringency might drive providers out of the business. If government has become stuck with taking care of the nursing home population, it has similarly become stuck with the nursing home industry. While nursing homes may be dependent on governments for most of their income, governments are dependent on nursing homes and their operators for the provision of service. The industry's strongest weapon is the threat of closing down. Government experiences great difficulty living with the nursing home industry, but can't live without it.

In Lindblom's analysis, the dependence of governments on private business for the provision of necessary public goods and services is only one component of the excessive power of business enterprise in the modern liberal state. The other is the disproportionate resources businesses can marshal in the role of private "citizens" seeking to influence government activity. The corporate executive is a citizen with all the First Amendment rights of political participation and because of his probable affluence, social status, and access to government officials is in a particularly good position to exercise them. But he is also the leader of a large organization with substantial resources of its own, which can itself participate in the political process—and which possesses, because of government's dependence on it, special entrée to government officials and the expectation that its concern will receive a sympathetic hearing.[3] This pattern is replicated in the nursing home arena. Nursing home interests devote considerable resources, in the form of time, money, and skilled talent, to influence the very government officials who are already dependent on them for the provision of services. Nursing home residents and their families, on the other hand, lack both the formal organization and the cash. From the perspective of government officials, moreover, residents are the problem, rather than an indispensable element of the solution.

Lindblom's analysis of the twofold sources of business power in public policy does not go far enough when applied to nursing homes. For in an industry in which so large a proportion of revenues comes from governments, the connection between the two components of influence is almost purely circular. Most of the dollars expended by the industry in pursuit of political influence are, at some slight remove, public dollars; every expansion of the industry resulting from a compound of political influence and other policy pressures further increases governmental dependence on the providers of service. Lindblom's analysis of the privileged position of business in the political system focuses almost exclusively on questions of macroeconomic policy—the great issues of unemployment, inflation, economic growth, regional prosperity. At the more microeconomic level of individual programs in single markets, that privileged position is not only stronger but more directly self-reinforcing.

Of course, both components of nursing home industry influence are rooted in the initial decision, made largely by accident, to arrange for the provision of nursing home services primarily through private, profit-seeking firms. While that decision probably cannot now be undone, its results should provide important perspective on the current penchant of governments to purchase goods and services from private firms, rather than provide them directly. This tendency encompasses everything from the hiring of private consultants to do an agency's long-range planning to the contracting out of municipal refuse collection, from management contracts for the operation of a municipal or county hospital to "turnkey" construction of public facilities. The temptation to "go outside" for the performance of these activities arises from the putatively superior efficiency and lower costs of private firms that often do prevail. But going outside is not without costs of its own. In the extreme case, and nursing homes are probably one, governments become highly dependent on private contractors, while those contractors are employing public funds to influence policy in directions favorable to their interests. Defense contractors provide the paradigmatic example, but it must be emphasized that even Boeing derives a smaller proportion of its total revenues from government than does a typical proprietary nursing home. As a rule of thumb, it might be suggested that the more a government agency is dependent on the provision of a specific good or service, the more likely "going outside" will produce excessive dependence on suppliers, and the less desirable it should be as a total strategy. A mixture of "inside" and "outside" may, however, be preferable to total provision from within government, if only to avoid promotion of an "inside" monopoly in the attempt to forestall development of an "outside" one.

There are two broad groups of private firms providing nursing home services to government-as-purchaser, and the difference in performance between them merits additional comment. On the whole, public agencies and their clients have been better served by nonprofit nursing homes than by profit-seeking ones, although in the great middle range of nursing home quality there is often not a dime's worth of difference between the two. Still, the contention is frequently made that public policy erred, not in its dependence on the private sector per se, but in its reliance on the private *profit-making* sector in an area in which the provision of intimate services to dependent individuals was involved. Governments should continue to go outside for nursing homes and other forms of long-term care, the argument goes, but should be more selective about who they go to. If it is too late to undo the damage caused by proprietary interests in the nursing home industry, there is still time to avoid repeating past mistakes in the area of home and home-health agencies.

It is clear that, in those areas in which governments are dependent on nonprofit firms for the provision of essential services, the problems that arise closely resemble those in for-profit industries. Hospitals are the clearest example. While voluntary, not for profit hospitals probably do a better job at rendering high-quality patient care than do most nursing homes, they are hardly much more responsive to governmental regulatory efforts and may be even less responsive to "inducements" incorporated in reimbursement systems. Nor does nonprofit status imply political chastity; the American Hospital Association is just as aggressive in protecting and promoting the political interests of its members as are any of the nursing home organizations. The "privileged position" of business applies, in many instances, to nonprofit businesses as well.

Moreover, precisely because they are profit-seeking, for-profit firms tend to be more responsive to economic inducements provided by governments in the hope of expanding the provision of services. Public policy largely succeeded in one of its major, even if misconceived, objectives—rapid and dramatic expansion in the availability of nursing home beds—by providing more-than-adequate, sometimes even excessive, inducements for the investment of private capital. Nonprofit organizations, whose objectives are more complex and more cross-pressured and which are probably less able to respond rapidly to anything, rose to the bait much more slowly. Indeed, nonprofit hospitals by and large failed to respond at all to repeated governmental efforts (first through the availability of Hill-Burton funds, then through the promotion of the extended-care facility idea) to get them into the long-term care business. In other sectors (kidney dialysis is one example, home-health agencies may soon become another), governments have turned to the for-profit sector only after they were unable to obtain an adequate supply of services from nonprofit institutions. Like most large formal organizations, nonprofit institutions exhibit substantial inertial momentum, which tends to keep them doing what they've been doing; unlike many for-profit organizations, they can often afford to.

The fact remains that public policy toward the provision of nursing home services has worked better, by and large, when implemented by nonprofit than by profit-seeking firms. The explanation lies in the greater, if still incomplete, congruence of motives. Nonprofit firms generally share at least some goals and attitudes with the government agencies seeking the provision of services, and that can be a more effective guarantor of "required performance" than any concatenation of economic incentives and regulatory commands. Whatever the enforcement mechanisms, laws work best when people would behave as the law commands them to even were there no law. Nonprofit institutions may be extremely balky instruments of public policy, but at least they generally straggle in the right direction.

The Culture of Welfare

In seeking to expand the provision of nursing home services, governments were largely concerned with delivering public assistance to the indigent. Nursing homes may, until recently, have been historically unique in that a for-profit industry thrived providing services to a welfare population. (In the last decade, day-care centers, health-maintenance organizations, kidney dialysis centers, and other industries or subindustries have also grown up in response to government-generated demand on behalf of public aid recipients. The unsatisfactoriness of their performance has mirrored the history of nursing homes.)

In most of public policy, Americans get what they pay for. Americans, or at least their elected representatives, are, in their attitudes toward welfare programs and their beneficiaries, grudging, stingy, and suspicious. As a proportion of gross national product, the United States still spends substantially less on social welfare than any other industrialized Western nation. But penny-wise is pound foolish. For instance, the unwillingness of government, acting through welfare agencies that administer Medicaid, to incur the marginally higher costs of excess capacity in the short run vitiates government bargaining power in the long run. Reluctance to spend adequately on administrative "overhead" may lead to a shortage of auditors, which in turn leads to expenditures many times the amount auditors would cost as facilities are reimbursed for inflated expenses. More generally, the absence of administrative controls on payments to providers played a central role in abetting the development of such a widespread pattern of stealing in the nursing home industry.

That is not to say that no efforts were made to control fraud in the Medicaid program. Extensive controls were instituted from the very outset, but they were directed at recipients, rather than providers. Some degree of harassment and humiliation has always been the price for receipt of welfare benefits in most jurisdictions in this country, and welfare agencies have been ever on the alert to deny Medicaid coverage to individuals who underreport income or family assets. Stealing by middle-class professionals was largely ignored until much later in the game.

The self-defeating ambivalence underlying many aspects of welfare policy is also reflected in the impact of Medicaid eligibility policies on the economic status of many middle-class and working-class families.

The drafters of Medicaid specifically sought to insulate middle-aged children from the prospect of financial catastrophe engendered by the need to institutionalize aged parents. Through the concept of "medical indigency," they also began to move in the direction of eligibility on the basis of need, rather than complete impoverishment. But generous definitions of medical indigency contributed to unexpectedly rapid increases in program costs and were soon barred by Congress, while the states, which retained substantial discretion over eligibility standards, rarely broke the old welfare molds. Thus the "spend-down" grew up. Middle-aged children are not forced to exhaust all their own resources in order to provide nursing home care for their parents, but they are forced to witness the destruction of their inheritances, for which their parents may have scrimped for a lifetime. Or else they break the law for the first time in their lives to effect covert transfers of their parents' assets. That is hardly as bad a dilemma as that which prevailed before Medicaid, but it remains demeaning, humiliating, and often tragic. Which is to say that it remains in keeping with the culture of welfare policy.

In general, nursing homes occupied predominately by Medicaid recipients are the worst nursing homes. Those facilities that can compete for the slightly more selective private patients do so; abysmal all-Medicaid nursing homes remain in existence because there is no political pressure to treat welfare recipients any better and because closing them would force welfare agencies to find something else to do with their clients. In many states, where invention of the ICF category was treated largely as an excuse to continue Medicaid certification of the least-satisfactory facilities, ICFs are almost purely Medicaid-dependent institutions, while the higher standards in SNFs are reserved for those who can put cash (or Medicare) on the barrelhead, at least at the time of admission. The very difference, both in standards and rates of payment, between Medicare and Medicaid speaks volumes on the treatment to which citizens are consigned once they fall into a welfare category.

Facilities to which the poor are committed tend to be poor facilities. One of the reasons government is so widely believed to be so entirely incompetent is the condition of public facilities for the poor—almshouses and hospitals in an earlier time, public housing and state institions for the mentally ill and mentally retarded in our own. The assumption is that those places are so bad because they are governmentally operated. The more accurate explanation is that they are bad because they are operated for the poor. Anyone who has ever been inside a public high school in an affluent suburb knows the conventional assumption can't be entirely correct; anyone who has visited a private nursing home occupied exclusively by Medicaid recipients will be convinced.

Critics of the nursing home industry have long emphasized the association between the awfulness of nursing homes and their relatively low political visibility combined with general societal indifference or hostility to the elderly. The evidence is decidedly mixed on attitudes toward the elderly, and political officials are increasingly cognizant of the power of the elderly as a voting bloc. It would be more accurate to say that the generally low quality of nursing home care and the apparent public indifference to it reflect attitudes toward recipients of public welfare and the institutions in which they live.

Political Space and Policy Space: Federalism

For all the easy acceptance of the notion that the United States has a unified national government, the financing and administration of public welfare more closely resemble the pattern of relationships between a medieval king and his barons. Or, to use a different analogy, economic historians speak of the rise of a national market in the American economy in the twentieth century, but there is as yet no "national market" in social policy. A displaced tenant farmer can drive his old Chevrolet from Mississippi to California and find standardized tires and replacement parts at every stop along the way, but he will be moving from one welfare system to another that is radically different in almost every important characteristic. The growth of corporate-chain ownership of nursing homes is related to the advantages accruing to a national corporation from operating in a number of states with different reimbursement, regulatory, and tax policies. The behavior of the chains may be likened to that of multinational corporations: charging particular costs, for accounting purposes, to facilities in those states that treat them most generously; manipulating income accounting to show the greatest nets in states with the lowest taxes; using legal and technical resources appropriate to the national level to do battle with small state bureaucracies equipped only to cope with smaller suppliers.

253

The absence of uniform national reimbursement and regulatory policies also plays a central role in nursing home availability. New nursing homes get built, not where the need is greatest, but where the potential return is highest. Since return is primarily a function of state reimbursement and regulatory policies, rather than "demand," there is almost no connection between the distribution of nursing homes and the distribution of people needing nursing home care. While other factors—most notably differing ethnic and religious patterns, which contribute to variations in the supply of nonprofit nursing homes—substantially affect the differences in availability, policy differences among the states are the primary cause.

State-dominated administration of nursing home programs also creates law-enforcement problems. Shady entrepreneurs are driven out of one jurisdiction only to reappear in another; licensing officials ruling on applications from facility operators are generally ignorant of information their colleagues in other states might possess. The patterns of nursing home ownership also strongly suggest that crooks, like capital, flow to those areas where the returns are highest.

The relationships between individual states and the national government have an even greater effect on the nursing home industry. Congress, in the intermittent periods in which it pays attention to nursing homes, is more protective of residents than of the industry's interests, and somewhat more willing to spend money on welfare programs of all kinds than are state legislatures (which are in general less professional, more easily influenced by industry interests, and more corrupt). But the federal administrators responsible for implementing congressional directives tread with great wariness on state prerogatives, because state officials are so willing to seek political redress in administrative quarrels. In doing so, they often receive help from congressmen who need assistance from local politicians to get reelected. In the complex trade-offs between quality of services, availability of beds, and program costs, the states, with a few exceptions, have been most willing to sacrifice quality, and they have, by and large, been able to get away with it.

Advocates of an expanded role for states and localities in the management of public programs contend that they are "closer to the people," and there is no gainsaying the repeated instances of indifference, unresponsiveness, or simple incompetence on the part of both the Congress and the executive branch in nursing home matters. But state governments are also closer to any number of private, narrowly defined interests, and their failure to protect the rights of the poor and the minorities to whom they are presumably closer has provided a major reason for taking power away from them and centralizing it in Washington.

State governments are forced to make harder choices than the federal government. The greater variety and diversity of national concerns, the superior revenue-raising power of the federal government, the looser fiscal constraints (including the ability to have a budget deficit), and the availability of the states as fall guys permit federal policymakers to finesse some of the more difficult trade-offs in public policy. They can choose both guns and butter, support open-ended, cost-generating mechanisms like those embodied in Medicare's reimbursement practices and come down more heavily on the side of quality in the quality-cost trade-off. To some extent, Congress is willfully irresponsible in its demands on the states, mandating difficult and conflicting requirements for which it knows the states will probably be unable to pay.

Recognition of the greater reluctance of state governments to be generous toward welfare recipients has been the keystone of the political strategy of those at the national level who are opposed to higher welfare expenditures or other measures to increase the well-being of those least well off. Since before the New Deal, those hostile to the interests of the poor have taken the position of: if you can't beat 'em, at least give lots of discretion to the states, where the balance of political forces is different. Kerr-Mills, the conservative alternative to Medicare, largely followed the pattern of other federal welfare programs in giving the states substantial discretion in nursing home policy. This suggests, again, the extent to which nursing home policy is colored more by attitudes toward welfare than by attitudes toward the elderly.

Policy Time vs. Political Time

The political process has a rhythm all its own, one that differs substantially from the needs of sound policymaking or the patterns of the private activities that governments seek to encourage, regulate, or control. The perspective of public officials, both appointive and elective, rarely extends past the next election—never for more than four years, and generally for less than two.

Given the inevitable lag between the time a phenomenon appears in society and the time its existence comes to be generally perceived, policymaking tends to be highly reactive and ex post facto, rather than anticipatory. Generals are always preparing to fight the last war; policymakers are always preoccupied with putting out today's fires, ignited from kindling that has been piling up for some time. The history of nursing home regulation is largely one of attempting to prevent in the future abuses discovered yesterday. Regulators are constantly confronted with faits accomplis, which they can rail against but rarely undo entirely. They build leaky sandbag walls, rather than damming the stream before it floods.

Conversely, it takes time for the effects of any new regulatory regime to emerge. Procedures must be established, new personnel hired, and then the industry must begin to figure out its responses. Because both regulatory and reimbursement reforms in nursing homes have been so closely tied to highly visible scandals, which are intrinsically short lived, the reform process tends to get short-circuited. Either administrative agencies are pilloried for not producing results more quickly, when results could not conceivably have begun to emerge, or, more likely, the enthusiasm for reform dies down just as its initial effects are beginning to be felt, so that while marginal improvements are attained, the momentum for still further change is lost. This phenomenon helps explain the apparent paradox that, while most regulatory mechanisms are thought to be highly unsatisfactory, the performance of the industry appears to have improved considerably, if very slowly, over time. Regulatory devices are judged ineffective, and hence discarded, before anyone has had time to figure out why they haven't worked, or even before they have had time to work.

Closely related to the divergence between the time it takes for regulatory initiatives to take effect and the much shorter cycles of political attention is the turnover rate among public officials. Anthony Downs has propounded a "Law of Inescapable Discontinuity," which holds that:

> High-level federal personnel change so fast that almost no major federal program is ever initially conceived of, drafted into legislation, shepherded through Congress and then carried out by the same officials.[4]

Downs's Law applies, in many instances, to state officials as well. Two corollaries may be drawn from Downs's Law that play an important role in nursing home policy. The first is the weakness of "institutional memory" in public agencies administering nursing home programs, which results in the repetition of past mistakes and constant reinventions of the wheel. The second is that, while public officials come and go, the industry abides. It has few permanent friends but a number of permanent interests. Not only do industry leaders, therefore, often have a better understanding of crucial issues, but they are also able to lie low for a while if a particularly unsympathetic official comes to power, waiting their turn for better times. Industry leaders have lived through regulatory crackdown after regulatory crackdown, reimbursement reform after reimbursement reform, and they can afford to be more patient than their counterparts in government. To Lindblom's dual sources of businesses' "privileged position" must be added another: superior staying power.

But the short time cycles of political rhythm do not work entirely to the industry's advantage. There are costs as well. Perhaps most important is the instability of government policies, the constant changing of ground rules, and the shifting of definitions. Businessmen value nothing so much as stability in the external environment. The businessman whose primary customer is government must learn to live with substantial turbulence and instability. If the nursing home industry has any justification at all in arguing for a profit premium on the basis of the risk of its investments, its strongest case lies in the propensity of government agencies to change their minds.

In December 1970, Ronald Reagan, then governor of California, unilaterally and without warning cut all Medicaid rates by a flat 10 percent. This action was quickly ruled invalid by the courts, but it was several months before payments were restored to their prior levels. In 1975, New York State froze all its Medicaid rates. In the past, they had always been adjusted annually to account for inflation. That decision is still being litigated. This capriciousness has certain advantages. In the examples cited, both California and New York did save some money, or at least postponed expenditures to later fiscal years, without apparent harmful effect on nursing home residents. But to the extent that instability encourages speculative activities while driving out more conservative entrepreneurs, its consequences are hardly desirable.

A final consequence of the short time perspective of politics is more narrowly tied to the budgetary process. Of all the things governments do without paying attention to their possible consequences more than a year or two in the future, budgeting is the most important. Public officials are reluctant to make relatively modest investments in the present even when there is promise of substantial savings in future fiscal years. This problem is particularly acute in welfare programs, with which officials would rather not have to deal at all, and especially so for Medicaid, the constantly spiraling costs of which have all but driven out the prospects for innovation. Uncontrollable costs arising from existing programs take precedence over controllable costs that might reduce "uncontrollables" at some point down the road. Reimbursement policies penalize nursing homes that operate at less than full capacity, invest in "human resources" through training programs or more careful recruitment policies, or seek greater managerial efficiency by sending their administrators back to school. Development of in-home "alternatives" to nursing home care is similarly frustrated. And, of greatest practical import, budget requests for additional and better-qualified inspectors and auditors are denied because all available funds are being eaten up by uncontrollable payments to substandard facilities.

Fine Tuning

Just as policymakers are often governed by unrealistically short time perspectives, so they often act as if they thought reality were substantially more malleable than it is. Ideas that seem perfectly plausible in abstract formulation may be impossible to translate into practical program activity. Laws that appear perfectly rational on their face turn out to be unenforceable in practice. Attempts to fine tune—to administer—a world that is grossly out of harmony are doomed to failure. The problem of fine tuning has traditionally been known, in the theory of public administration, as the problem of administrability. And the problem seems to have become more acute in recent years as a result of the increasing influence of academic policy analysts on legislative formulations and the increasing legislative distrust of executive agencies (which induces legislatures to delegate less and less discretion to administrators).

In nursing home policy, two ideas that in the abstract appear overwhelmingly seductive have produced only confusion and waste when governments have attempted to implement them. The first is that of providing "incentives" for quality and efficiency through sophisticated reimbursement schemes. The second is that of "levels of care."

In the case of "incentives" for quality, the assumptions of economic theory lead to the conclusion that if a nursing home operator can in-crease his annual revenue by \$25,000 by making a quality-enhancing investment of \$20,000, he will probably do so. Thus, nursing homes are given bonuses for high quality ratings or simply reimbursed on a cost-plus basis. But that syllogism will only work if the operator keeps honest books, and the state agency is capable of determining whether his books are honest; both the operator and the state know which ad-ditional expenditures will increase the quality of service, and the state is in a position to determine whether those expenditures have actually been made; the operator is certain that his investment will be reward-ed; the state doesn't run out of money in its Medicaid budget before the end of the fiscal year; the operator understands the reimbursement system; the operator himself knows how his income is tied to his out-go; and the state's definition and measurement of quality are suffi-ciently sophisticated that the operator can't raise the \$20,000 for qual-ity improvements by subtracting that much from some other area that is also critically related to quality. The problem with most reimburse-ment systems is that, to the extent providers fully understand them, they will invariably find a way to beat them; to the extent they can't beat them, it is because they don't understand them, and thus the "in-centives" they are supposed to contain can't possibly work. Besides, it takes time for incentive systems to have effect, and they are always be-ing changed.

If the logical of "levels of care" were to be carried to its extreme, ev-ery nursing home resident should be assessed at least once a month, and every time a resident's status changed more than marginally, he or she should be moved to a more "appropriate" level, for which the provider of service would be reimbursed at a different rate. That logic also assumes that there is little cost, either economic or human, in moving people from one place to another, and that there is always a correlation between a facility's capacity to provide a given range of services and its actually providing them.

Classical economic theory assumes that information is always per-fect and costless, that transactions are easy and costless, that people are always rational and simply motivated, and that nobody cheats. But ig-norance prevails, transactions are always costly and frequently involve compromises that alter the initial objectives of the parties to them, people are neither entirely rational nor without motivational conflict, and there are a lot of shifty characters out there. That is why adminis-tration remains a separate "science" (although it invariably partakes more of art).

The problem of fine tuning has prospective as well as retrospective importance for nursing home policy. Development of "gatekeeping" agencies, which would make possible dramatic expansion of in-home services as an alternative to institutionalization, has been delayed by the search for the perfect administrative design.

Legislators often display an inability to distinguish between the particular and the general, which leads to still further attempts to legislate the impossible. Policies, it is presumed, either work or don't work. "Evidence" that they don't work often consists of a handful of random incidents, anecdotes, or accidents. But nobody ever bats 1.000, and a program that bats .500 may be doing very well indeed. If, in a state with 300 nursing homes, a dozen are making windfall profits while another two or three dozen are providing abysmally poor quality, that should not constitute a priori evidence of the failure of a flat-rate reimbursement system, but legislators often behave as though it did. Findings that 25 percent of the residents of skilled nursing homes don't really "need" skilled care is taken as a prior proof of the need for intermediate care facilities, although simple random chance could well account for half that 25 percent.

In a normal statistical distribution, 5 percent of the cases will fall more than two standard deviations from the mean; to concentrate on the "tails" of the distribution distorts reality. Yet those tails often wag the dog of public policy. Regulatory standards are designed to eliminate the worst 5 percent of facilities, rather than upgrade the 90 percent in the middle. Utilization review committees halt one in three while paying no attention to the care received by the other two. Instead of fine tuning, policymakers might do better if they concentrated on finding the right channel.

Government as "Regulatee"

One place where fine tuning is carried to an extreme is in the management of government itself. A good, though only partial, excuse for the failure of government agencies responsible for implementing nursing home policy to perform more effectively is that those agencies are expected to do other things as well. Those other things include obeying civil service regulations and collective bargaining agreements, promoting affirmative action, not discriminating against any geographical areas or political subdivisions, keeping the public informed of what they are doing, providing employment, and, most importantly, observing the due process rights of all private citizens and firms they encounter. This is not to say that government agencies do those things any better than they regulate or reimburse nursing homes, only that they are expected to do them also.

James Q. Wilson and Patricia Rachal have recently argued that one shortcoming of the growing regulatory activities of the federal government is this inability of one government agency to regulate another.[5] They are probably right for the middle range, as in the example they suggest of the inability of the Environmental Protection Administration to affect the behavior of one of the nation's largest polluters, the Department of Defense, or in the inability federal officials have shown in closing some extremely bad county- or state-operated nursing homes. At the more microcosmic level of administration, regulatory agencies are constrained on matters of personnel, budgets, matériel, procedure, and the allocation of resources—the central components of management. And at the more macrocosmic level, those agencies are highly constrained, as has been seen, by legislatures and the courts.

A private firm buying services from a number of suppliers could be expected to provide bonuses or promotions to those purchasing agents who got the lowest prices for services of adequate quality; to pay no attention to the location, ethnic composition, or other characteristics of suppliers apart from their ability to deliver; to negotiate different deals with different suppliers, playing one off the other and occasionally threatening to go into the business itself; and to cut off cold any supplier who consistently underperformed. Medicaid agencies buying nursing home services can do none of these. They must obey civil service regulations for their own personnel; give special attention to the demands of rural communities, inner-cities, and ethnic minorities; avoid any hint of arbitrary or capricious behavior in dealing with private firms, and hold hearings before terminating a provider agreement.

Yet, as Herbert Kaufman has noted, one person's red tape is another's cherished and hard-won right.[6] Government, in fact, does a substantially better job of protecting employees' rights, hiring and promoting members of minority groups, keeping jobs in areas from which private industry has fled, being fair to those with whom it deals, and preventing stealing by its own employees, than just about any other institution in society. Nor should we expect any less.

This is not to condone red tape, the rigidity of civil service, the behavior of all civil service unions, or the incompetence of many government officials. All these considerations are less constraining than timid administrators would have us believe, and the ways in which government is regulated are only a few of the many causes for policy failure. But the post office is so inefficient at least in part because it must maintain an office in every village and dale, provide five classes of service, and pay high wages without being able to fire anyone— regulatory officials who would really like to punch recalcitrant nursing home operators in the nose have to observe all the formalities and cross all the t's because they know their decisions are subject to administrative hearings and judicial review. Madison feared excessive power more than government incapacity, and he was a skilled draftsman. The Madisonian tradition remains strong, even dominant.

Human Fallibility

As a final source of policy failure, it is necessary to include the limits of human beings. The world is very complicated, and everything is eventually connected to everything else, but most people can only think of a few things at a time, have short attention spans, are easily misled, and remember selectively. Collective bodies like legislatures are supposed to be able to overcome such difficulties, but modern legislatures have an enormous amount to do and are able to function at all only through a rigorous division of labor.

Sometimes bad policy is simply the product of mistaken judgment, erroneous information, the falseness of conventional wisdom, or reasoning from bad analogies. Such mistakes are not numerous in the history of nursing home policy, but the mistakes that have been made are all extremely important.

Most common has been the recurrent tendency to confuse nursing homes with hospitals—from the most basic aspects of physical construction to the fine points of reimbursement systems—when in fact they are profoundly different in the character of their residents, the kinds of services they are supposed to provide, and the way they are controlled and governed.

A central nursing station with patient rooms opening off both sides of a corridor makes considerable sense in an acute-care setting, where patients are constantly being wheeled in and out of their rooms on stretchers or trolleys, but is much less desirable in a place where people live; even the notion of a semiprivate room is more suited to nursing productivity in a hospital than privacy and autonomy in a place where the typical resident stays for a year and a half. And a capital reimbursement system designed to meet the needs of voluntary, community-based acute care-hospitals created a speculator's dream and a regulator's nightmare, as was seen in chapter 5, when extended to nursing home construction and acquisition.

A fundamental mistake in the logic of hospital reimbursement, the use of the average per diem room rate as the basis of all reimbursement, has had profound consequences for nursing home policy. It caused the widespread perception that having potential nursing home residents "backed up" in acute-care hospitals is extraordinarily costly, when in fact (given the excess capacity in the hospital industry) it is no more costly, over time, than putting them in nursing homes. Nothing has contributed more to the explosive growth of nursing homes than concern with those phantom hospital costs. That concern provided the primary rationale for extensive public subsidization, both direct and indirect, of nursing home construction and deterred public officials from closing substandard facilities because they believed the beds were so desperately "needed." The entire thrust of public policy has been generated by a simple confusion between average and marginal costs.

Another simple conceptual error that had disastrous consequences for nursing home policy was the failure of the drafters of the Social Security Act to recognize that the elderly residents of almshouses were not only poor but generally disabled, and that cash income alone would not meet their needs. The ban on payment of Old Age Assistance benefits to residents of public institutions and the simultaneous failure to provide programs for the disabled elderly remain the springs from which much else in nursing home policy has flowed. The authors of the Social Security Act were not indifferent to the needs of almshouse residents; they were deeply concerned. But preoccupied with other, more pressing matters and prey to the popular mythology, they simply failed to approach the problem correctly. After all, almshouse residents were only a small fraction of potential OAA beneficiaries and an even smaller fraction of the millions of citizens who could be expected to benefit from passage of the Social Security Act.

There lies the root of the problem. Most of those who have made policy for nursing homes throughout the last forty-five years have been neither callous nor uncaring, but they have had other, bigger things to worry about. No matter how the population pie is sliced, nursing home residents are always a minority of a minority. They are much less numerous, and much less clamorous, than others in need of health insurance benefits; much less numerous, and bearing less resemblance to popular stereotype, than the other recipients of public welfare; much less numerous than the noninstitutionalized elderly. They are hardly ever at the top of anyone's agenda. No one is paying attention, other than those who make a living from the status quo. The problem is not that nursing home residents are old or poor or without family or intrinsically hard to provide for, but that they are old *and* poor *and* without family *and* hard to care for. Everyone is terribly busy and has other things to do.

The Politics of Failure

It is the combination of the tendency of policymakers to make mistakes and their inability to undo them that creates policy failure. The problem is not so much that planners in 1935 or 1955 or 1965 were wrong, but that we are still living with their decisions. The causes of policy failure are, at root, political. They spring less from the nature of business enterprises or large formal organizations or the propensity of human beings to make mistakes than from the ways Americans have organized to govern themselves, and the attitudes they hold about government.

Undoing past mistakes is so difficult because the political system values stability and incremental innovation more than it does being right. Business enterprise has so privileged a position because the system was designed, in a world where the only kinds of property actually belonged to identifiable people, to set the rights of private property prior to those of governments, and now the same rights have been extended to the subsequently invented limited-liability, general-purpose corporation. Welfare politics is so self-defeating because politicians have only rarely identified sympathy and generosity toward the poor with their electoral self-interest. Federalism has become such a nightmare because influential citizens prefer corrupt and inefficient governments they can control locally to a less corrupt and less inefficient national government more responsive to the concerns of local minorities. Similarly, politicians tend to be so short-sighted at least in part because voters invariably appear more concerned with this year's taxes than some future state of affairs. Politicians try to fine tune complex programs because they fear they will be judged, not on program performance in the aggregate, but on particular scandals, embarrassments, and details. And government agencies are often hamstrung because the public is so afraid they will lie, steal, or act arbitrarily.

In the abstract, there is nothing wrong with any of these phenomena. In a democratic society, citizens should be able to constrain their governments in any way they want, and there is no evidence that Americans feel strong disagreement with the political attitudes underlying any of these causes of policy failure. If they all conduce to poor governmental performance, then that may simply be the price Americans pay for democratic self-government. People grumble all the time about the way their elected officials perform, but they keep reelecting them. While Americans believe that governments should do things, they don't much like to be governed—to pay taxes, to be told where they should go to receive health services or how they should invest their capital, to really have to obey the law when there is money to be made in ignoring it—and if that creates a serious contradiction, it is one that leads to a vague sense of resentment and alienation, and then to passive resignation rather than to rebellion.

The Failure of Politics

This is of little help to the lonely old lady trapped in a filthy and understaffed nursing home with nowhere else to go. It has become a cliché to argue that "we have met the enemy and he is us," as though every failure of public policy, every mistreatment of a public dependent, was the personal responsibility of every voter. In fact, matters are more complicated, and sympathy for that old lady, even if felt strongly by every citizen, would not be enough to substantially affect her well-being. As Thomas Schelling noted, if a six-year-old girl needs thousands of dollars for an operation that will prolong her life until Christmas, nickels and dimes will swamp the post office, but voters will not approve a one-cent sales tax increase to finance improvements in public hospitals that can save dozens of lives.[7] In mid-1978, public officials claimed that voters and politicians were sympathetic to the need for more stringent enforcement of nursing home regulations, but that the air was filled with talk of Proposition 13, and that cutting public expenditures had priority.

The enemy is us not because we are unsympathetic to people in need, although we are often uninterested, nor because there is disagreement on the appropriate ends of social action, although such disagreement often exists. But there are certain things that only governments can or will do, and we have denied government the means to do them. We don't like to pay taxes or have our private affairs regulated or invest very heavily in the future of the society as opposed to our personal futures. In the conflict between private rights and public authority, we tend to come down much more often than not on the side of private rights even when the old ladies in nursing homes fall between the stools.

These attitudes create an inescapable problem because there are private needs that can be met only by public action, and this is a society that has always valued the private much more than the public. For most of its citizens, who make their way in the world relatively comfortably on their own, with the help of families, friends, and social supports, a preference for private over public is simply rational, if somewhat self-interested. But when that which is public is weak, those who cannot make their way privately are out of luck. So they sit in their nursing homes, minds clouded by drugs, staring unfocusingly at daytime television, and soon, but not soon enough, they are dead.

NOTES

Chapter 1

1. Robert N. Butler, *Why Survive?: Being Old in America* (New York: Harper & Row, 1975), chap. 9.

2. Cf. Frank E. Moss and Val J. Halamandaris, *Too Old, Too Sick, Too Bad: Nursing Homes in America* (Germantown, Md.: Aspen Systems Press, 1977), p. xiv; also see pp. 12–14.

3. Speech by President Richard M. Nixon to American Association of Retired Persons/National Retired Teachers Association, Chicago, Ill., June 25, 1971.

4. U.S. Department of Health, Education, and Welfare, Public Health Service, Office of Nursing Home Affairs, *Long-Term Care Facility Improvement Study, Introductory Report* (Washington, D.C.: Government Printing Office, 1975), pp. 12, 15, 22–32; cf. Elaine M. Brody, "Environmental Factors in Dependency," in *Care of the Elderly: Meeting the Challenge of Dependency*, ed. A. N. Exton-Smith and J. Grimley Evans (New York: Grune and Stratton, 1977), pp. 84–85ff.

5. U.S. Department of Health, Education, and Welfare, Public Health Service, Office of Long-Term Care, *Physicians' Drug Prescribing Patterns in Skilled Nursing Facilities*, Long-Term Care Facility Improvement Campaign, Monograph No. 2 (Washington, D.C.: Government Printing Office, 1976); U.S. Congress, Senate, Special Committee on Aging, Subcommittee on Long-Term Care, *Nursing Home Care in the United States: Failure in Public Policy, Supporting Paper No. 2, Drugs in Nursing Homes: Misuse, High Costs, and Kickbacks*, 94th Cong., 1st sess., 1975; Butler, *Why Survive?*, p. 265.

6. U.S. Congress, Senate, Special Committee on Aging, Subcommittee on Long-Term Care, *Nursing Home Care in the United States: Failure in Public Policy, Introductory Report*, 93rd Cong., 2d sess., 1974, pp. 76–78.

7. U.S. Congress, Senate, Special Committee on Aging, Subcommittee on Long-Term Care, *Nursing Home Care in the United States: Failure in Public Policy, Supporting Paper No. 1, The Litany of Nursing Home Abuses and an Examination of the Roots of Controversy*, 93rd Cong., 2d sess., 1974, pp. 205–209.

8. For a retrospective summary of the New York scandals, see John L. Hess, "News Analysis: Nursing Homes Show Progress," *The New York Times*, 12 January 1976, p. 32; editorial, "Nursing Homes, One Year Later," *The New York Times*, 17 May 1977. For the major investigative results of the scandal, see New York State Moreland Act Commission on Nursing Homes and Residential Facilities, *Long-Term Care Regulation: Past Lapses and Future Prospects: A Summary Report*, New York: The Commission, April, 1976, and the three *Annual Reports* (1976, 1977, and 1978) of Special Prosecutor Charles J. Hynes (New York: Office of the Special Prosecutor).

9. U.S. Congress, House, Committee on Ways and Means, Subcommittee on Health, and Committee on Interstate and Foreign Commerce, Subcommittee on Health and the Environment, *Medicare-Medicaid Antifraud and Abuse Amendments. Joint Hearings on H.R.3. Serial 95–7*, 95th Cong., 1st sess., 3 and 7 March 1977, pp. 28–49; City Attorney Burt Pines, "Recommendations for New Legislation and Regulations Relating to Skilled Nursing Facilities, Community Care Facilities, Physicians and Other Health Care Professionals," mimeographed (Los Angeles, Calif.: Office of the City Attorney, 1976); U.S., Congress, House Committee on Interstate and Foreign Commerce, Subcommittee on Oversight and Investigations, *Nursing Home Abuses: Hearings, Serial 95-19*, 95th Cong., 1st sess., 15 and 16 March 1977, pp. 2–30, 160–200; cf. U.S. Congress, Senate, Special Committee on Aging, *Lack of Coordination Between Medicaid and Medicare at John J. Kane Hospital*, GAO Rept. no. HRD-77-44, 95th Cong., 1st sess., 6 May 1977; "A Program in Crisis,"

Report of the Ohio Nursing Home Commission to the Governor and Ohio General Assembly, Columbus, Ohio, June 1978; "Report of the Blue Ribbon Committee to Investigate the Nursing Home Industry in Connecticut," mimeographed (Hartford, December 1976); Minnesota State Legislature, Senate Select Committee on Nursing Homes/House Select Committee on Nursing Homes, "Final Report," mimeographed (January 1976); Wisconsin Department of Health and Social Services, Medicaid Management Study Team, "Final Report: Monitoring Quality of Nursing Home Care," and "Final Report: Nursing Home Reimbursement and Cost Reporting," mimeographed (1 June 1977); Michigan Legislature, Special Senate Committee to Investigate Nursing Homes, First and Second "Preliminary Reports," mimeographed (1977); U.S. Congress Senate, Subcommittee on Long-Term Care, *Medicare and Medicaid Frauds: Hearing*, Special Committee on Aging, 94th Cong., 1st sess., 13 November 1975, pp. 255–261, 275–286.

10. Subcommittee on Long-Term Care, *Failure in Public Policy, Supporting Paper No. 1*, pp. 165–204; AFL-CIO Executive Council, "Nursing Homes and the Nation's Elderly: America's Nursing Homes Profit in Human Misery" (statement and report adopted at Bal Harbour, Florida, 25 February 1977), pp. 10–12.

Chapter 2

1. J. Richard Elliott, Jr., "Long Bed Rest: Some Areas Have More Nursing Homes Than They Need," *Barron's*, 3 March 1969, p. 18.

2. American Health Care Association, *Long Term Care Facts* (Washington, D.C.: American Health Care Association, 1976), pp. 10–11.

3. U.S. Department of Health, Education, and Welfare, Public Health Service, Health Resources Administration, National Center for Health Statistics, Mark R. Meiners, *Selected Operating and Financial Characteristics of Nursing Homes, United States: 1973–74 National Nursing Home Survey*, Vital and Health Statistics, Series 13, no. 22 (Washington, D.C.: Government Printing Office, 1975), pp. 10–11.

4. Cf. U.S. Department of Health, Education, and Welfare, Public Health Service, Health Resources Administration, National Center for Health Statistics, *Health Resources Statistics, 1975* (Washington D.C.: Government Printing Office, 1976), p. 373.

5. Ibid.

6. American Health Care Association, *Long Term Care Facts*, pp. 10–11.

7. U.S. Department of Health, Education, and Welfare, Public Health Service, Health Resources Administration, National Center for Health Statistics, Jeannine Fox Sutton, *Utilization of Nursing Homes United States: National Nursing Home Survey August 1973–April 1974*, Vital and Health Statistics, Series 13, no. 28 (Washington, D.C.: Government Printing Office, 1977), p. 13.

8. Cf. U.S. Congress, Senate, Special Committee on Aging, Subcommittee on Long-Term Care, *Nursing Home Care in the United States: Failure in Public Policy, Introductory Report*, 93 Cong., 2d sess., 1974, p. 16.

9. Cf. Bernice L. Neugarten, "Age Groups in American Society and the Rise of the Young-Old," *The Annals* 415 (September 1974), pp. 187–198.

10. Sutton, *Utilization of Nursing Homes*, p. 24.

11. U.S. Department of Health, Education and Welfare, Public Health Service, Health Resources Administration, National Center for Health Statistics, Aurora Zappolo, *Characteristics, Social Contacts, and Activities of Nursing Home Residents*, Vital and Health Statistics, Series 13, no. 27 (Washington, D.C.: Government Printing Office, 1977), p. 6.

12. Ibid.

13. Elaine M. Brody, "Environmental Factors in Dependency," in *Care of the Elderly: Meeting the Challenge of Dependency*, ed. A. N. Exton-Smith and J. Grimley Evans (New York: Grune and Stratton, 1977), p. 92; Interview; Cf. U.S. Senate, Special Committee on Aging, Subcommittee on Long-Term Care, *Nursing Home Care in the United States: Failure in Public Policy, Introductory Report*, 93rd Cong., 2d sess., 1974, p. 16.

14. Subcommittee on Long-Term Care, *Failure in Public Policy, Introductory Report*, p. 17; unpublished data, National Center for Health Statistics.

Notes

15. U.S. Department of Health, Education, and Welfare, Public Health Service, Office of Nursing Home Affairs, *Long-Term Care Facility Improvement Study, Introductory Report* (Washington, D.C.: Government Printing Office, 1975), p. 30; unpublished data, National Center for Health Statistics.

16. Ibid.

17. Cf. U.S. Department of Health, Education, and Welfare, Public Health Service, Health Resources Administration, National Center for Health Statistics, *Health United States, 1975*, HEW Publication No. (HRA) 76–1232 (Rockville, MD.: HEW, 1976), Tables CD.IV.4 and CD.IV.7, pp. 557, 563.

18. Cf. Burton D. Dunlop, "Need for and Utilization of Long-Term Care Among Elderly Americans," *Journal of Chronic Diseases* 29 (February 1976), pp. 75–87; Stanley J. Brody, S. Walter Poulshock, and Carla F. Masciocchi, "The Family Caring Unit: A Major Consideration in the Long-Term Support System" (Paper delivered at 1977 Annual Meeting of the Gerontological Society, San Francisco, Calif.).

19. Brody, "Environmental Factors in Dependency," p. 91.

20. Cf. George L. Maddox, "Families as Context and Resource in Chronic Illness," in *Long-Term Care: A Handbook for Researchers, Planners, and Providers*, ed., Sylvia Sherwood (New York: Spectrum Publications, 1975), p. 340.

21. Zappolo, *Characteristics*, p. 6.

22. Ibid.

23. Dr. Andrew C. Fleck, Jr., personal communication.

24. U.S. Congress, Senate, Special Committee on Aging, Subcommittee on Long-Term Care, *Nursing Home Care in the United States: Failure in Public Policy, Supporting Paper No. 3: Doctors in Nursing Homes: The Shunned Responsibility*, 94th Cong., 1st sess., 1975, pp. 342–343.

25. U.S. Department of Health, Education, and Welfare, Public Health Service, Office of Long-Term Care, *Physicians' Drug Prescribing Patterns in Skilled Nursing Facilities*, Long-Term Care Facility Improvement Campaign, Monograph No. 2 (Washington, D.C.: Government Printing Office, 1976), pp. 13–14, 26–30.

26. Ibid., p. 8.

27. Cf. Subcommittee on Long-Term Care, *Failure in Public Policy, Supporting Paper No. 3*, p. 229.

28. Office of Nursing Home Affairs, *Facility Improvement Study, Introductory Report*, pp. 29–31.

29. Sutton, *Utilization*, pp. 15–16.

30. Ibid.

31. U.S. Congress, Senate, Special Committee on Aging, Subcommittee on Long-Term Care, *Nursing Home Care in the United States: Failure in Public Policy, Supporting Paper No. 4: Nurses in Nursing Homes, The Heavy Burden (The Reliance on Untrained and Unlicensed Personnel)*, 94th Cong., 1st sess., 1975, pp. 372–373, 381.

32. Sutton, *Utilization*, pp. 15–16.

33. U.S. Department of Labor, Bureau of Labor Statistics, *Industry Wage Survey: Nursing Homes and Related Facilities, May 1976* (Washington, D.C.: Government Printing Office, 1977).

34. Subcommittee on Long-Term Care, *Failure in Public Policy, Supporting Paper No. 4*, p. 362. Data cited was published in 1969.

35. Sutton, *Utilization*, p. 15; Bureau of Labor Statistics, Industry Wage Survey.

36. Sutton, *Utilization*, p. 15.

37. Bureau of Labor Statistics, *Industry Wage Survey*, p. 4.

38. Ibid., p. 2.

39. Robert M. Gibson and Charles R. Fisher, "National Health Expenditures, Fiscal Year 1977," *Social Security Bulletin* 41 (July 1978), p. 6.

40. Ibid., p. 7.

41. Ruth Bennett and Carl Eisdorfer, "The Institutional Environment and Behavior Change," in *Long-Term Care*, p. 406.

42. Barbara Bolling Manard, Ralph E. Woehle, and James M. Heilman, *Better Homes for the Old* (Lexington, Mass.: D.C. Heath and Co., Lexington Books, 1977), p. 22.

43. Ibid., p. 21.

44. Zappolo, *Characteristics*, pp. 11–13.

Chapter 3

1. Cf. Ethel McClure, *More Than a Roof: The Development of Minnesota Poor Farms and Homes for the Aged* (St. Paul: Minnesota Historical Society, 1968), pp. 20–38.

2. U.S. Bureau of Labor Statistics, Estelle M. Stewart, *The Cost of American Almshouses*, Bulletin No. 386 (Washington, D.C.: Government Printing Office, 1925), pp. 37–40.

3. Ibid.; interviews.

4. Steward, *Cost of American Almshouses*, p. 41.

5. Cf. U.S. Department of Commerce, Bureau of the Census, *Paupers in Almshouses: 1923* (Washington, D.C.: Government Printing Office, 1925), Table 61, p. 50.

6. Stewart, *Cost of American Almshouses*, p. 41.

7. Harry C. Evans, *The American Poor Farm and Its Inmates* (Des Moines, Iowa: Royal Order of the Moose, 1926).

8. Marjorie Shearon, "Economic Status of the Aged, " *Social Security Bulletin* 1 (March 1938), p. 6.

9. Cf. U.S. Bureau of Labor Statistics, *Care of Aged Persons in the United States*, Bulletin No. 489 (Washington, D.C.: Government Printing Office, 1929); and especially, McClure, *More Than a Roof*, chaps. 4, 7.

10. Shearon, "Economic Status of the Aged," pp. 6, 15.

11. Robert B. Stevens, ed., *Statutory History of the United States: Income Security* (New York: Chelsea House, 1972), pp. 73ff.; cf. Gilbert Steiner, *Social Insecurity: The Politics of Welfare* (Chicago: Rand McNally & Co., 1966), pp. 18ff.

12. 49 Stat. 620, Tit. I, 3(a)(1)(1935).

13. Stevens, *Statutory History*, pp. 73ff.; Steiner, *Social Insecurity*, pp. 18ff.

14. Cf. Stevens, *Statutory History*, pp. 275–289; Edwin B. Witte, *The Development of the Social Security Act* (Madison, Wisc.: University of Wisconsin Press, 1963), pp. 173–189.

15. "Almshouse Care and the Old-Age Assistance Program," *Social Security Bulletin* 1 (March 1938), pp. 42–43.

16. McClure, *More Than a Roof*, pp. 169–170; William C. Thomas, Jr., *Nursing Homes and Public Policy: Drift and Decision in New York State* (Ithaca, N.Y.: Cornell University Press, 1969), pp. 73–77.

17. Ibid.

18. This interpretation follows that in Glenn R. Markus, *Nursing Homes and the Congress: A Brief History of Developments and Issues*, rept. 72-224 ED (Washington, D.C.: Library of Congress, 1972).

19. Ibid., pp. 8–10; McClure, *More Than a Roof*, pp. 170–171, 190–191; Thomas, *Nursing Homes and Public Policy*, pp. 76–80.

20. Cf. Thomas, *Nursing Homes and Public Policy*, pp. 78–79.

21. McClure, *More Than a Roof*, pp. 172–184; Thomas, *Nursing Homes and Public Policy*, pp. 64–71.

22. Judith R. Lave and Lester B. Lave, *The Hospital Construction Act: An Evaluation of the Hill-Burton Program, 1948–1973*, Evaluative Studies 16 (Washington, D.C: American Enterprise Institute for Public Policy Research, 1974), pp. 7–15.

23. Stevens, *Statutory History*, pp. 422–430; Richard Harris, *A Sacred Trust* (New York: New American Library, 1966), pp. 30–53.

24. Stevens, *Statutory History*, pp. 246–253, 303–314, 320–323, 371–381.

25. Markus, *Nursing Homes and the Congress*, pp. 12–13; Thomas, *Nursing Homes and Public Policy*, pp. 94–99.

26. Markus, *Nursing Homes and the Congress*, pp. 14–15; Stevens, *Statutory History*, pp. 374–375.

27. Cf. Robert Stevens and Rosemary Stevens, *Welfare Medicine in America: A Case Study of Medicaid* (New York: The Free Press, 1974), p. 152.

28. Harris, *Sacred Trust*, pp. 54–57; Theodore R. Marmor, *The Politics of Medicare* (Chicago: Aldine Publishing Co., 1973), pp. 14–20.

29. Markus, *Nursing Homes and the Congress*, p. 24.

30. Ibid., pp. 15–21.

31. Ibid; Interviews.

32. Jerry Solon and Anna Mae Baney, "Inventory of Nursing Homes and Related Fa-

cilities," *Public Health Reports* 69 (December 1954), pp. 1122–1128. The other two categories were "personal care homes without nursing" and "sheltered homes."

33. Markus, *Nursing Homes and Congress*, p. 24.

34. Ibid., pp. 34–35.

35. These numbers are a guess because no actual counts were made between 1954 and 1963. Both numbers were rough linear interpolations between the two years. For 1954, see Solon and Baney, "Inventory"; for 1963, see American Health Care Association, *Long Term Care Facts* (Washington, D.C., American Health Care Association, 1976), p. 8.

36. Stevens and Stevens, *Welfare Medicine in America*, p. 34. The authors report that total nursing home vendor payments in fiscal 1960 were $47 million. A low estimate of $2,000 per patient per year would produce a figure of 23,000 beneficiaries at any one time. However, the same authors report, on the previous page, that Massachusetts had 14,000 vendor-payment recipients in nursing homes in 1960. This inconsistency should not be taken as evidence of poor work on the part of Stevens and Stevens, whose book is exemplary, but rather is characteristic of the problems of all nursing home data, especially for the pre-Medicare period.

37. Cf. Thomas, *Nursing Homes and Public Policy*, pp. 195–196; interviews.

38. Cf. Stevens and Stevens, *Welfare Medicine in America*, pp. 26, 27, 34.

39. Harris, *Sacred Trust*, pp. 99–109; Marmor, *Politics of Medicare*, p. 41; Stevens and Stevens, *Welfare Medicine in America*, p. 28.

40. Stevens and Stevens, *Welfare Medicine in America*, pp. 27–31.

41. Markus, *Nursing Homes and the Congress*, p. 58.

42. Stevens and Stevens, *Welfare Medicine in America*, pp. 29–34.

43. Ibid., p. 34.

44. Markus, *Nursing Homes and the Congress*, p. 46.

45. Cf. ibid., pp. 34–58; interviews.

46. U.S., Congress, Senate, Committee on Finance, *Medicare and Medicaid: Problems, Issues, and Alternatives*, 91st Cong., 2d sess., 1970, p. 91; interviews.

47. Stevens, *Statutory History*, p. 718.

48. Markus, *Nursing Homes and the Congress*, p. 50.

49. Stevens, *Statutory History*, p. 718.

50. Markus, *Nursing Homes and the Congress*, p. 41; interview.

51. Stevens, *Statutory History*, pp. 731, 759.

52. Cf. Markus, *Nursing Homes and the Congress*, pp. 39–41, 45, 47, 49–50, 60.

53. Cf. Marmor, *Politics of Medicare*, pp. 69–70, 80.

54. Cf. Markus, *Nursing Homes and the Congress*, pp. 45, 47, 58; Stevens and Stevens, *Welfare Medicine in America*, pp. 51, 66; interviews.

55. Judith M. Feder, *Medicare: The Politics of Federal Hospital Insurance* (Lexington, Mass. D.C. Heath & Co., Lexington Books, 1977), pp. 10ff.

56. Ibid., pp. 14–15.

57. Committee on Finance, *Medicare and Medicaid*, pp. 91–94; interview.

58. Committee on Finance, *Medicare and Medicaid*, p. 95.

59. Cf. Feder, *Medicare*, p. 16.

60. Committee on Finance, *Medicare and Medicaid*, pp. 91–95.

61. Ibid., p. 93.

62. Ibid., pp. 92–95.

63. For the least hysterical discussion, see the *Report of the National Advisory Commission on Health Manpower* (Washington, D.C.: Government Printing Office, 1967), vol. I, pp. 22–23.

64. Committee on Finance, *Medicare and Medicaid*, pp. 33–36.

65. Ibid.

66. Cf. Fred S. Hellinger, "Substitutability Among Different Types of Care Under Medicare," *Health Services Research* 12 (Spring 1977), pp. 11–18.

67. Cf. U.S. Senate, Committee on Aging, Subcommittee on Long-Term Care, *Nursing Home Care in the United States: Failure in Public Policy, Introductory Report*, 93rd Cong., 2d sess., 1974, pp. 30–31; interviews.

68. Markus, *Nursing Homes and the Congress*, pp. 79–85.

69. Cf. Subcommittee on Long-Term Care, *Failure in Public Policy, Introductory Report*, pp. 32–35, 113–116.

70. U.S. Department of Health, Education, and Welfare, Social Security Administration, *Social Security Bulletin Annual Statistical Supplement, 1975* (Washington, D.C.: Government Printing Office, 1977), Table 141, p. 164.

71. Stevens and Stevens, *Welfare Medicine in America*, pp. 75–81; Markus, *Nursing Homes and the Congress*, pp. 62–63.

72. Markus, *Nursing Homes and the Congress*, p. 72.

73. Ibid., pp. 63–68, 91–92.

74. U.S. Congress, Senate, Special Committee on Aging, Subcommittee on Long-Term Care, *Conditions and Problems in the Nation's Nursing Homes: Hearings*, 89th Cong., 1st sess., 1965.

75. Markus, *Nursing Homes and the Congress*, pp. 69–78; interviews.

76. Markus, *Nursing Homes and the Congress*, pp. 72–73; interviews.

77. Interviews.

78. Interviews.

79. Subcommittee on Long-Term Care, *Failure in Public Policy, Introductory Report*, p. 67; [Mal Schecter], "Default on Nursing Home Code," *Hospital Practice* (December 1969), pp. 14ff.

80. [Schecter], "Default," p. 19.

81. Ibid.

82. Ibid.; "Nursing-Home Standards Grow Feeble, Toothless," *Medical World News* (26 September 1969), pp. 24–25; cf. Subcommittee on Long-Term Care, *Failure in Public Policy, Introductory Report*, pp. 67–71; Markus, *Nursing Homes and the Congress*, pp. 92–103.

83. Markus, *Nursing Homes and the Congress*.

84. Interviews; Committee on Finance *Medicare and Medicaid*, pp. 97–98; Markus, *Nursing Homes and the Congress*, p. 109; Stevens and Stevens, *Welfare Medicine in America*, pp. 117–121.

85. Interviews.

86. Cf. U.S. Department of Health, Education, and Welfare, Disability Long-Term Care Study, Judith W. LaVor, "Intermediate Care Facilities: Expectations vs. Realities" (mimeograph), August 1974.

87. Committee on Finance, *Medicare and Medicaid*, pp. 97–98.

88. Ibid., pp. 99–104.

89. Markus, *Nursing Homes and the Congress*, pp. 111–116.

90. *Congressional Record*, August 3, 1970, p. H7620.

91. Cf. U.S. Congress, Senate, Special Committee on Aging, Subcommittee on Long-Term Care, *Nursing Home Care in the United States: Failure in Public Policy, Supporting Paper No. 5, The Continuing Chronicle of Nursing Home Fires*, 94th Cong., 1st sess., 1975, p. 459.

92. Cf. U.S. Congress, Senate, Special Committee on Aging, Subcommittee on Long-Term Care, *Nursing Home Care in the United States: Failure in Public Policy, Supporting Paper No. 3: Doctors in Nursing Homes: The Shunned Responsibility*, 94th Cong., 1st sess., 1975, pp. 338–340.

93. Cf. Claire Townsend, *Old Age: The Last Segregation* (New York: Grossman Publishers, 1971).

94. Interviews.

95. Interviews.

96. Subcommittee on Long-Term Care, *Failure in Public Policy, Introductory Report*, pp. 40–43, 149–155.

97. Interviews; Subcommittee on Long-Term Care, *Failure in Public Policy, Introductory report*, p. 104; internal HEW files.

98. Interviews.

99. For a general summary of the 1972 amendments, see Robert M. Ball, "Social Security Amendments of 1972: Summary and Legislative History," *Social Security Bulletin* 36 (March 1973), pp. 3–25.

100. Cf. U.S. Congress, Senate, Committee on Finance, *The Social Security Amendments of 1972: Report to Accompany H.R. 1* 92d Cong., 2d sess., S. Rept. 92-1230, pp. 281–282.

101. Ibid., pp. 314–315, 320–321.

102. Ibid., pp. 319, 320–323.

103. Ibid., pp. 287–288; interviews.

Notes

104. Cf. Richard P. Nathan, *The Plot That Failed: Nixon and the Administrative Presidency* (New York: John Wiley & Sons, 1975).

105. *Federal Register* 39 (17 January 1974), pt. III, pp. 2238–2257; revised at *Federal Register* 39 (3 October 1974), pt. II, pp. 35774–35778; *Federal Register* 39 (19 January 1974), pt. II, pp. 2219–2237.

106. *Federal Register* 41 (1 July 1976), pt. V, pp. 27300–27308.

107. Robert M. Gibson and Marjorie Smith Mueller, "National Health Expenditures, Fiscal Year 1976," *Social Security Bulletin* 40, (April 1977), pp. 10–13.

108. Mary Adelaide Mendelson, *Tender Loving Greed: How the Incredibly Lucrative Nursing Home "Industry" Is Exploiting America's Old People and Defrauding Us All* (New York: Alfred A. Knopf, 1974); interviews.

Chapter 4

1. I am indebted to Professor Marilyn Field, formerly of the Maxwell School, Syracuse University, for clarifying this point for me.

2. First expressed in Charles L. Schultze, *The Politics and Economics of Public Spending* (Washington, D.C.: The Brookings Institution, 1968), pp. 103ff.; most fully formulated in Charles L. Schultze, *The Public Use of Private Interest* (Washington, D.C.: The Brookings Institution, 1977).

3. Robert M. Gibson and Charles D. Fisher, "National Health Expenditures, Fiscal Year 1977," *Social Security Bulletin* 41 (July 1978): 6, 11.

4. The estimate was derived as follows. It was assumed that the average Medicaid recipient had social security or other public pension benefits of $200 a month and that private charges exceeded Medicaid rates by 30 percent, on average. Since total expenditures, Medicaid expenditures, and total residents were known, it was then possible to solve a series of simultaneous equations for x-number of Medicaid recipients. It should be emphasized that both assumptions are relatively conservative, so the 75 percent figure is similarly conservatively low.

5. After the calculations described in note 6 were completed, this figure was derived by multiplying the number of Medicaid recipients multiplied by $2,400 ($200 a month X 12 months), and dividing that number by the total private share reported by Gibson and Mueller.

6. Wolf and Company, CPAS, comps., *How Medicaid Pays for Long Term Care: A Survey of State Medicaid Payment Methods for Nursing Homes* (Washington, D.C.: American Health Care Association, 1978), pp. 55.1–55.6.

7. U.S. Department of Health, Education, and Welfare, Health Care Financing Administration, Medicaid Bureau, Institute for Medicaid Management, *Data on the Medicaid Program: Eligibility, Services, Expenditures Fiscal Years 1966–1977* (Washington, D.C.: Institute for Medicaid Management, 1977), pp. 42–43.

8. Institute for Medicaid Management, *Data on the Medicaid Program*, pp. 44–45, 62; Gibson and Fisher, "National Health Expenditures," pp. 9, 11.

9. Cf. Bruce Spitz and John Holahan, *Modifying Medicaid Eligibility and Benefits*, Publication 986-13 (Washington, D.C.: The Urban Institute, 1977), pp. 6–7, 19.

10. Cf. William Pollak, "Long Term Care Facility Reimbursement," in John Holahan, Bruce Spitz, William Pollak, and Judith Feder, *Altering Medicaid Provider Reimbursement Methods*, Publication 986-14 (Washington, D.C.: The Urban Institute, 1977), pp. 103–104.

11. *American Hospital Association Guide to the Health Care Field*, 1977 ed. (Chicago: American Hospital Association, 1977), p. 8.

12. This statement is subject to the implicit *ceteris paribus* modifier. For some preliminary empirical evidence on its validity, see U.S., Department of Health, Education, and Welfare, Health Care Financing Administration, Office of Policy, Planning, and Research, *An Evaluation of an Experiment to Provide Long-Term Care in Rural Hospitals in Utah*, vol. 1, Summary Report, Health Insurance Studies: Contract Research Series (Rockville,

Md.: Department of Health, Education, and Welfare, 1978). In public utilities, this is known as the problem of peak-load marginal cost. It is relatively cheap to provide more power at night, when generators are functioning at a fraction of their capacity, but much more expensive to respond to increased demand at peak hours, since doing so requires building new generators.

13. Cf. U.S. Department of Health, Education, and Welfare, Health Resources Administration, National Center for Health Services Research, Applied Management Sciences, *Report on Systems of Reimbursement for Long-Term Care (LTC) Services,* Final Report vol. 3: Background Materials (Silver Spring, Md.: Applied Management Sciences, 1976), pp. 3.121–3.125; Institute for Medicaid Management, *Data on the Medicaid Program,* pp. 20–21; interviews.

14. Cf. New York State Moreland Act Commission on Nursing Homes and Residential Facilities, *Reimbursing Operating Costs: Dollars Without Sense,* Rept. no. 5, Appendix B., "History of Reimbursement for Proprietary Nursing Homes" (New York: The Commission, 1976).

15. U.S. Department of Labor, Bureau of Labor Statistics, *Industry Wage Survey: Nursing Homes and Related Facilities,* May 1976, Bulletin 1964 (Washington, D.C.: Government Printing Office, 1977), pp. 7–8, 43–49.

16. Moreland Commission, *Dollars Without Sense,* pp. 2–5.

17. Applied Management Sciences, *Systems of Reimbursement for Long-Term Care,* pp. 3.11–3.13; interviews.

18. Interviews.

19. *Federal Register* 41 (July 1, 1976), pt. V. pp. 27300–27308.

20. Cf. Alfred E. Kahn, *The Economics of Regulation: Principles and Institutions,* vol. 1, *Economic Principles* (New York: John Wiley & Sons, 1970), pp. 35ff.; interviews.

21. Notably *American Health Care Ass'n v. Califano,* Civil Action No. 77–0250, (D.D.C.).

22. *Federal Register* 43 (February 6, 1978), pp. 4861–4864.

23. Interviews.

24. Cf. David Shulman and Ruth Galanter, "Reorganizing the Nursing Industry: A Proposal," *Milbank Memorial Fund Quarterly/Health and Society* 54 (Spring 1976): 129–143.

25. This idea was suggested to me by Maurice May, Executive Director of the Hebrew Gerontological Center for Aged, Roslindale, Massachusetts.

Chapter 5

1. Interviews.

2. Interviews.

3. Interviews; cf. Mary Adelaide Mendelson, *Tender Loving Greed: How the Incredibly Lucrative Nursing Home "Industry" Is Exploiting America's Old People and Defrauding Us All* (New York: Alfred A. Knopf, 1974) pp. 56–58, 78; Ethel McClure, *More Than A Roof: The Development of Minnesota Poor Farms and Homes for the Aged* (St. Paul, Minn.: Minnesota Historical Society, 1968), p. 190.

4. McClure, *More Than a Roof,* pp. 199, 215.

5. Interviews.

6. Cf. Mendelson, *Tender Loving Greed,* pp. 103, 202; interviews.

7. Interviews.

8. Cf. Janet Kline, *Federal Financial Support for the Construction of Nursing Homes,* Report #70–119 ED (Washington, D.C.: Library of Congress, 1970), pp. 7–14.

9. Ibid., pp. 22–32.

10. Data supplied by the Federal Housing Administration, personal communications.

11. Cf. Henry J. Aaron, *Shelters and Subsidies: Who Benefits from Federal Housing Policies?* (Washington, D.C.: The Brookings Institution, 1972), pp. 80–90.

12. Interviews.

13. Cf. Feder, *Medicare,* pp. 57–59, 64–70.

14. The exception was in New York. In 1968, Article 28–A was added to the New York

Notes

State Health Code, permitting the state to issue moral-obligation bonds to provide mortgages for the construction of nonprofit nursing homes. The program was one of many such "moral-obligation"-financed undertakings of the Rockefeller administration and appears to have been generated as part of a broader strategy to issue government paper for every conceivable socially acceptable enterprise. To date, Article 28–A has financed eighty-nine projects with a total of 17,000 beds through mortgage loans of $570 million. It has been widely criticized for the expense of the projects it has supported: construction costs under 28–A have been 50 to 100 percent higher than those for proprietary facilities constructed in the same period. There is considerable dispute as to how much of the additional cost is attributable to superior facilities and how much to sheer wastefulness. To the extent that costs under 28–A were unnecessarily high, the state has been trapped coming and going. Not only has it subsidized inflated mortgages but, under cost-based reimbursement, has paid similarly inflated depreciation costs under Medicaid.

While Article 28–A has had a massive impact on the capital plant of New York nursing homes, from another perspective its impact has been surprisingly small. For the voluntary sector in New York is no larger proportionately than it is in many other states that had no program similar to 28–A. Had the program not existed, it is highly likely that voluntary nursing homes and their sponsors in New York State would have found financing as their counterparts in other states did. In that sense, New York simply served as an intermediary between lenders and borrowers, shifting part of the cost to the public expense and insulating the lenders. Cf. New York State Department of Health, Division of Health Facilities Development, Bureau of Health Facility Finances, "Summary of Status of Mortgage Loan Projects as of December 31, 1976," New York State Moreland Act Commission on Nursing Homes and Residential Facilities, *Reimbursement of Nursing Home Property Costs: Pruning the Money Tree* (New York: The Commission, 1976), pp. 120– 123.

15. Ibid., pp. 120–123; David Shulman and Ruth Galanter, "Reorganizing the Nursing Home Industry: A Proposal," *Milbank Memorial Fund Quarterly: Health and Society* 54 (Spring 1976): 129–143.

16. Interviews.

17. Moreland Commission, *Pruning the Money Tree;* Mendelson, *Tender Loving Greed*, pp. 101–122; interviews.

18. Gerald M. Calvario, Assistant to the President, Thrift Associations Service Corporation, New York, September 23, 1977, personal communication.

19. Interviews.

20. Los Angeles County Board of Supervisors, "Los Angeles County Nursing Home Study," 1976, mimeographed.

21. Maria R. Traska, "Nursing Home Survey: Proprietary Chains Operated 20% More Beds in 1977," *Modern Healthcare* (June 1978): 38–43.

22. J. Richard Elliott, Jr., "Unhealthy Growth?: Nursing Home Building Is Expanding at a Feverish Pace," *Barron's,* February 10, 1969, pp. 3ff.

23. Derived from ibid., pp. 3ff., and J. Richard Elliott, Jr., "Long Bed Rest: Some Areas Have More Nursing Homes Than They Need," *Barron's,* March 3, 1969, pp. 3ff.

24. J. Richard Elliott, Jr., "No Tired Blood: Nursing Home Operators Are Long on Enthusiasm, Short on Experience," *Barron's,* March 24, 1969, p. 3.

25. Derived from *Moody's Industrial Manual; Moody's OTC Industrial Manual; Standard and Poor's Industry Surveys;* annual reports and SEC Form 10–Ks of nursing home chains.

26. Cf. "Hillhaven Is Purchasing Merit's Nursing Homes," *Modern Healthcare* (August 1977): 17–10.

27. "National Medical Enterprises Purchases $7.5 Million of Hillhaven Corp. Preferred Stock and Debentures," National Medical Enterprises, Inc., press release, May 5, 1978.

28. *Moody's Industrial Manual.* (New York: Moody's Investor Service, 1977).

29. *Moody's Industrial OTC Manual.* (New York: Moody's Investor Service, 1977).

30. Derived from annual reports and SEC Form 10–Ks of relevant nursing home chains.

31. Interviews.

32. Interviews.

33. Cf. Temporary State Commission on Living Costs and the Economy, *Report on Nursing Homes and Health Related Facilities in New York State* (Albany, N.Y.: The Commission, 1975); AFL–CIO Executive Council, "Nursing Homes and the Nation's Elderly: America's Nursing Homes Profit in Human Misery," statement and report adopted at Bal Harbour, Florida, February 25, 1977.

34. Cf. Leonard E. Gottesman, "Nursing Home Performance as Related to Resident Traits, Ownership, Size, and Source of Payment," *American Journal of Public Health* 64 (March 1974): 269–276; Sharon Winn, "Analysis of Selected Characteristics of a Matched Sample of Nonprofit and Proprietary Nursing Homes in the State of Washington," *Medical Care* 12 (March 1974): 221–228; Samuel Levey et al., "Nursing Homes in Massachusetts: Industry in Transition," *American Journal of Public Health* 65 (January 1975): 66–71; R. Hopkins Holmberg and Nancy N. Anderson, "Implications of Ownership for Nursing Home Care," *Medical Care* 6 (July–August 1968): 300–307.

35. Cf. Amitai Etzioni and Pamela Doty, "Profit in Not-for-Profit Corporations: The Example of Health Care," *Political Science Quarterly* 91 (Fall 1976): 433–453.

36. William J. Bicknell and Diana Chapman Walsh, "Certificate-of-Need: The Massachusetts Experience," *New England Journal of Medicine* 292 (May 15, 1975): 1054–1061; David S. Salkever and Thomas W. Bice, "The Impact of Certificate-of-Need Controls on Hospital Investment," *Milbank Memorial Fund Quarterly: Health and Society* 54 (Spring 1976): 185–214.

37. Interviews.

38. The discussion that follows is heavily indebted to Shulman and Galanter, "Reforming the Nursing Home Industry."

39. Harold Stein, "The Disposal of the Aluminum Plants," in *Public Administration and Policy Development*, ed. Stein (New York: Harcourt, Brace & Co., 1952), pp. 313–361.

40. I have been playing this tune for some time. The fullest statement is "Why Non-Profits Go Broke," *The Public Interest* 42 (Winter 1976): 86–101; for the specific case of higher education, see "Buildings and Budgets: The Overinvestment Crisis," *Change* (December–January 1978–79): 36–40.

Chapter 6

1. 20 Code of Federal Regulations (hereafter referred to as C.F.R.) no. 405.127 (1976).

2. 45 C.F.R. no. 249.10 (1976).

3. These studies are well-summarized in U.S., Congress, Congressional Budget Office, *Long-Term Care for the Elderly and Disabled*, Budget Issue Paper Appendix B (Washington, D.C.: Congressional Budget Office, 1977), pp. 55–58.

4. Cf. U.S. Department of Health, Education, and Welfare, Health Resources Administration, National Center for Health Services Research, Ian R. Lawson, "Title XIX Reimbursement in Long-Term Care," in Applied Management Sciences, *Report on Systems of Reimbursement for Long-Term Care (LTC) Services, Final Report*, vol. 2: *Proceedings of Conferences* (Silver Spring, Md.: Applied Management Sciences 1976), pp. 9.3–9.5.

5. Cf. 45 C.F.R. no. 249.10(b)(4) (1976); 45 C.F.R. no. 249.10(b)(15) (1976); 20 C.F.R. no. 405, Subpart K (1976); and 45 C.F.R. no. 249.12 (1976).

6. U.S. Department of Health, Education, and Welfare, Health Services Administration, Public Health Service, Bureau of Quality Assurance, Community Research Applications, Inc., *Excerpt Summary of a National Study of Levels of Care in Intermediate Care Facilities (ICFs)*, esp. Appendix A (Rockville, Md.: Department of Health, Education, and Welfare, 1976).

7. Ibid.

8. Cf. Charles H. Brooks and John A. Hoffman, "Type of Ownership and Medicaid Use of Nursing Care Beds," *Journal of Community Health* 3 (Spring 1978); 236–244.

9. 45 C.F.R. no. 250.18–19 (1976).

10. *Social Security Act* (49 Stat. 620, as amended), Title XI, pt. B.

Notes

11. Esther Hing and Aurora Zappolo, "A Comparison of Nursing Home Residents and Discharges from the 1977 National Nursing Home Survey: United States," *Advance Data* 29 (May 17, 1978): 7.

12. Cf. Richard T. Smith and Frederick N. Brand, "Effects of Enforced Relocation on Life Adjustment in a Nursing Home," *International Journal of Aging and Human Development* 6 (1975): 249–259.

13. Stanislav V. Kasl, "Physical and Mental Health Effects of Involuntary Relocation and Institutionalization on the Elderly—A Review," *American Journal of Public Health* 62 (March 1972): esp. p. 379 and references cited therein.

14. Mary Adelaide Mendelson, *Tender Loving Greed: How the Incredibly Lucrative Nursing Home "Industry" Is Exploiting America's Old People and Defrauding Us All* (New York: Alfred A. Knopf, 1974), pp. 8, 42.

15. Cf. New York State Moreland Act Commission on Nursing Homes and Residential Facilities, *Assessment and Placement: Anything Goes* (New York: The Commission, 1976), pp. 3–13.

16. Cf. U.S. Department of Health, Education, and Welfare, Public Health Service, Office of Long-Term Care, *Five Years of Accomplishments of the Office of Long-Term Care, 1971-1976* (Rockville, Md.: Public Health Service, 1976), pp. 25–26; interviews.

17. New York State Department of Health, "Hospital Procedures for Completing and Using the Long-Term Care Placement Form (DMS-1) and Application of New York State Health Department Numerical Standards," Hospital Memorandum 77–9, January 31, 1977.

Chapter 7

1. This taxonomy follows closely on that of Otto A. Davis and Morton I. Kamien, "Externalities, Information and Alternative Collective Action," in *Public Expenditures and Policy Analysis*, ed. Robert H. Haveman and Julius Margolis (Chicago: Markham Publishers, 1970), pp. 74–95.

2. *Social Security Act* (49 Stat. 620, as amended), Sec. 1861 (3)(i); Sec. 1902.

3. 405 C.F.R., Subpart K (1976).

4. 45 C.F.R. no. 249.12 (1976).

5. 20 C.F.R. no. 405.1134(e) (1976); 45 C.F.R. no. 249.12(a)(6)(i)(a) (1976).

6. 20 C.F.R. no. 405.1134(g) (1976); cf. 45 C.F.R. no. 249.12(a)(6)(vii) (1976).

7. 20 C.F.R. no. 405.1125(d)(1976); 45 C.F.R. no. 249.12(a)(7)(i), but there is no nighttime snack requirement in ICFs.

8. 20 C.F.R. no. 405.1125(e) (1976); there is no federal ICF analogue, but most states have similar language for ICFs.

9. Robert N. Brown, "An Appraisal of the Nursing Home Enforcement Process," *Arizona Law Review* (1975): 320.

10. Cf. 20 C.F.R. no. 405.1121(k) (1976); cf. 45 C.F.R. no. 249.12(a)(1)(B) (1976), which is less restrictive.

11. Cf. Robert L. Kane and Rosalie A. Kane, "Care of the Aged: Old Problems in Need of New Solutions," *Science* 200 (May 1978): 918; Hirsch S. Ruchlin, "A New Strategy for Regulating Long-Term Care Facilities," *Journal of Health Politics, Policy, and Law* 2 (Summer 1977): 190–211.

12. Minnesota State Legislature, Senate Select Committee on Nursing Homes/House Select Committee on Nursing Homes, "Final Report," mimeographed, January 1976, p. 6, and memo on "Scheduling of Nursing Home Inspections," Appendix.

13. Cf. Lowell E. Bellin, "Local Health Departments: A Prescription Against Obsolescence," in *Health Services: The Local Perspective* vol. 32 *Proceedings of the Academy of Political Science*, ed. Arthur Levin (New York: The Academy, 1977), p. 44.

14. Jerome H. Skolnick, "Social Control in the Adversary System," *Journal of Conflict Resolution* II (March 1967): 52–63.

15. Cf. New York State Moreland Act Commission on Nursing Home and Residential Facilities, *Regulating Nursing Home Care: The Paper Tigers* Rept. no. 1. (New York: The Commission, 1975), p. 9; Interviews.

16. A leading case is the appositely named *Shady Acres Nursing Home v. Canary*, 39 Ohio App. 2nd 47 (1973). More generally, see Brown, "An Appraisal."

17. Edith Evans Asbury, "Bergman Resumes Nursing Home Role," *The New York Times*, June 11, 1977, p. 1; "Bergman Denies He Wants to Stay as an Operator of Nursing Homes," *New York Times*, 13 June 1977, p. 24. For the sequel, see David Bird, "Guilty Owners Face Nursing-Home Curb," *The New York Times*, July 9, 1977, p. 30.

18. National Association of Attorneys General, *Enforcing Quality of Care in Nursing Homes* (Raleigh, N.C.: The Association, 1978), pp. 34–36.

19. Frank P. Grad, "Upgrading Health Facilities: Medical Receiverships as an Alternative to License Revocation," *University of Colorado Law Review* 42 (1971), pp. 419–436; National Association of Attorneys General, *Enforcing Quality*, pp. 45–49; "Receivership and Nursing Homes," *Nursing Home Law Letter* 14 (31 October 1977).

20. Cf. Brown, "An Appraisal," pp. 346–348, who has a different view on the possible uses of tort liability.

21. Ronald Sullivan, "Rise in Reports of Abuse of Elderly Patients Spurred by New Law," *New York Times*, 30 May 1978, p. B7.

22. Cf. Alfred E. Kahn, *The Economics of Regulation: Principles and Institutions*, vol. 2, *Institutional Issues* (New York: John Wiley & Sons, 1971), passim.

23. Jane Lockwood Barney, "Community Presences as a Key to Quality of Life in Nursing Homes," *American Journal of Public Health* 64 (March 1974): 265–268.

Chapter 8

1. Cf. Comptroller General of the United States, "Improvements Needed in the Managing and Monitoring of Patients' Funds Maintained by Skilled Nursing Facilities and Intermediate Care Facilities," Rept. no. MWD–76–102 (Washington, D.C.: General Accounting Office, 1976); Deputy Attorney General Charles J. Hynes, "Protecting Patients' Personal Funds Failures and Needed Improvements" (New York: Office of the Special Prosecutor for Nursing Homes, Health, and Social Services, 1977).

2. Interview.

3. Public Law No. 95–142, no. 21, 91 Stat. 1175 *et. seq.*

4. Elizabeth Hanford Dole, "An Investigation into the Business of Caring for the Elderly" (address before the 1978 Indiana Governor's Conference on Aging, South Bend, Indiana, October 24, 1978).

5. Public Law No. 95–142, no. 4, 91 Stat. 1175 *et. seq.*

6. Cf. U.S. Senate, Special Committee on Aging, Subcommittee on Long-Term Care, *Nursing Home Care in the United States: Failure in Public Policy, Supporting Paper No. 3: Doctors in Nursing Homes: The Shunned Responsibility*, 94th Cong., 1st sess., 1975, pp. 331–338.

7. U.S. Senate, Special Committee on Aging, Subcommittee on Long-Term Care, *Nursing Home Care in the United States: Failure in Public Policy, Supporting Paper No. 2: Drugs in Nursing Homes: Misuse, High Costs, and Kickbacks*, 94th Cong., 1st sess., 1975, pp. 284ff.

8. Interviews.

9. Charles J. Hynes, Deputy Attorney General for Nursing Homes, Health, and Social Services, *Third Annual Report* (New York: Office of the Special Prosecutor, 1978), pp. 14–15.

10. Ibid., p. 20.

11. Ibid., pp. 15–18.

12. Subcommittee on Long-Term Care, *Failure in Public Policy, Supporting Paper No. 2*.

13. Cf. David Caplovitz, *The Poor Pay More: Consumer Practices of Low-Income Families*, 2d ed. (New York: The Free Press, 1967), chap. 10 *et passim*; on victimization from violent crime, James Q. Wilson, *Thinking About Crime* (New York: Vintage Books, 1977), p. 38.

14. Cf. Edwin H. Sutherland, "White Collar Criminality," *White-Collar Crime: Offenses*

Notes

in *Business, Politics, and the Professions*, ed. Gilbert Geis and Robert F. Meier, rev. ed. (New York: The Free Press, 1977), pp. 44–45.

15. Ibid., p. 48.

16. Wilson, *Thinking About Crime*, pp. 149–151ff.

17. Interviews.

18. Pub. L. No. 95–142, nos. 4, 21, 7, 91 Stat. 1175 *et. seq.*

19. Pub. L. No. 95–142, nos. 9, 17, 91 Stat. 1175 *et. seq.*

20. See Hynes's testimony in U.S. Congress, House Committee on Ways and Means, Subcommittee on Health, and Committee on Interstate and Foreign Commerce, Subcommittee on Health and the Environment, *Medicare-Medicaid Antifraud and Abuse Amendments, Joint Hearings on H.R. 3*, 95th Cong., 1st sess., Serial 95-7, 1977, pp. 53–55.

21. Pub. L. No. 95–142, nos. 19, 10, 21, 8, 3, 15, 4, 91 Stat. 1175 *et seq.*

22. James L. Sundquist, *Politics and Policy: The Eisenhower, Kennedy, and Johnson Years* (Washington: The Brookings Institution, 1968), p. 481.

Chapter 9

1. Cf. Wendell Rawls, Jr., "O'Neill's Business Dealings Raise Questions of Conflict and Candor," *New York Times*, 9 April, 1978, p. 1.

2. Cf. Mary Adelaide Mendelson and David Hapgood, "The Political Economy of Nursing Homes," The *Annals* 415 (September 1974): 95.

3. Cf. *Washington Report on Long-Term Care*, December 23, 1977, p. 4.

4. Cf. *Federal Register* 43 (February 6, 1978), pp. 4861–4864.

5. Henry J. Pratt, *The Gray Lobby* (Chicago: University of Chicago Press, 1976), pp. 88–89.

6. Cf. Francis E. Rourke, *Bureaucracy, Politics, and Public Policy*, 2d ed. (Boston: Little, Brown, & Co., 1976), pp. 42–58; Theodore J. Lowi, *The End of Liberalism: Ideology, Policy, and the Crisis of Public Authority* (New York: W. W. Norton & Co., 1969), pp. 102–124.

7. Samuel H. Beer, "The Adoption of General Revenue Sharing: A Case Study in Public Sector Politics," 24 *Public Policy* (Spring, 1976): 127–195.

8. Cf. David E. Rogers and Robert J. Blendon, "The Academic Medical Center: A Stressed American Institution," *New England Journal of Medicine* 298 (27 April, 1978): pp. 940–950.

Chapter 10

1. Derived from U.S. Congress, Congressional Budget Office, *Long-Term Care: Actuarial Cost Estimates* (Washington, D.C.: Government Printing Office 1977), Table 5, p. 20; see also U.S., Congress, Congressional Budget Office, *Long-Term Care for Elderly and Disabled* (Washington, D.C.: Government Printing Office, 1977).

2. Cf. Herman B. Brotman, "Population Projections, Part I. Tomorrow's Older Population," *The Gerontologist* 17, no. 3, (1977): 203–209.

3. Cf. Ernest M. Gruenberg, "The Failures of Success. *Milbank Fund Quarterly: Health and Society* 55 (Winter 1977): esp. 7–9.

4. Congressional Budget Office, *Long-Term Care for the Elderly and Disabled*, p. 43; Congressional Budget Office, *Actuarial Cost Estimates*, pp. 69–100.

5. U.S. Department of Health, Education, and Welfare, Health Care Financing Administration, "Notice of Public Meetings: New Directions for Skilled Nursing and Intermediate Care Facilities," June 1, 1978.

6. Ken Fireman, "Nursing Home Law Toughens the Rules," *Detroit Free Press*, 19 November, 1978, p. 3A.

7. I am indebted to Professor Robert Morris of Brandeis University for this paragraph.

8. Cf. Comptroller General of the United States, "Home Health—The Need for a National Policy to Better Provide for the Elderly" (Washington, D.C.: General Accounting Office, 1977).

9. Ibid., pp. 9–22.

10. For examples of this process already in motion, see U.S. Congress, House, Select Committee on Aging, *The National Crisis in Adult Care Homes*, 95th Cong., 1st sess., 1977, pp. 29, 31. 37.

11. Congressional Budget Office, *Actuarial Cost Estimates*, p. 54.

12. Esther Hing and Aurora Zappolo, "A Comparison of Nursing Home Residents and Discharges from the 1977 National Nursing Home Survey; United States," *Advance Data* 29 (17 May, 1978): 6.

13. Cf. Harold J. Wershow, "Comment: Reality Orientation for Gerontologists, Some Thoughts About Senility," *The Gerontologist* 17 (Summer 1977): 297–302.

14. Hing and Zappolo, "Nursing Home Residents and Discharges," p. 5.

15. A public relations campaign in this vein was launched in 1977 by the Washington Federal Savings and Loan Association of New York City, which, as holder of the mortgage of Bernard Bergman's unlicenseable Danube nursing home, had a very direct stake in the issue. See the statement by George A. Mooney, Chairman of the Washington Federal Savings and Loan Association of New York City, entitled, "State Actions Peril Future Financing of Nursing Homes by Banking Institutions," issued as a press release February 14, 1977, which subsequently appeared in *The American Banker*.

16. Congressional Budget Office, *Actuarial Cost Estimates*, pp. 49–69.

17. Institute of Medicine, National Academy of Sciences, *A Policy Statement: Controlling the Supply of Hospital Beds* (Washington, D.C.: National Academy of Sciences, 1976); "National Guidelines for Health Planning," *Federal Register* 42 (23 September, 1977); 48503; and *Federal Register* 43 (20 January, 1978): 3056–3060, 3064–3065.

18. For empirical evidence, see note 13 to chapter 4.

19. Funds to encourage hospitals to "convert" excess acute-care beds to long-term care were authorized in the Health Planning Amendments of 1978, which died in the House Rules Committee at the end of the 95th Congress, but which are widely expected to pass in 1979.

20. Elaine M. Brody, "Environmental Factors in Dependency," in *Care of the Elderly: Meeting the Challenge of Dependency*, eds. A. N. Exton-Smith and J. Grimley Evans (New York: Grune & Stratton, 1977), pp. 84–87.

21. Credit for this notion belongs to Professor Robert Morris of Brandeis University.

22. Cf. Harold S. Luft, "HMOs and Medical Costs: The Rhetoric and the Evidence," *New England Journal of Medicine* 298 (15 June, 1978): 1336–1343.

23. Cf. Wershow, "Reality Orientation for Gerontologists."

24. Cf. Ian R. Lawson, "Community-Based Medical Care in Three Settings," in *Topias and Utopias in Health: Policy Studies*, eds. Stanley R. Ingman and Anthony E. Thomas (The Hague: Mouton Publishers, 1972), pp. 373–392.

25. Elaine M. Brody, "A Million Procrustean Beds," *The Gerontologist* 13 (Winter 1973): 430–435.

Chapter 11

1. Cf. Daniel P. Moynihan, *Coping: Essays on the Practice of Government* (New York: Random House, 1973), Introduction and passim; Aaron Wildavsky, *The Revolt Against the Masses, And Other Essays on Politics and Public Policy* (New York: Basic Books, 1971), esp. pt. 2; or any random selection in *The American Commonwealth—1976*, a special issue of *The Public Interest* 41 (Fall 1975).

2. Charles E. Lindblom, *Politics and Markets: The World's Political-Economic Systems* (New York: Basic Books, 1977), p. 173.

3. Ibid., pp. 189ff.

Notes

4. Anthony Downs, "The Successes and Failures of Federal Housing Policy," in *The Great Society. Lessons for the Future*, eds. Eli Ginzberg and Robert M. Solow (New York: Basic Books, 1974), pp. 134–135.

5. James Q. Wilson and Patricia Rachal, "Can the Government Regulate Itself?" *The Public Interest* 46 (Winter 1977): 3–14.

6. Herbert Kaufman, *Red Tape: Its Origins, Uses, and Abuses* (Washington, D.C.: The Brookings Institution, 1977), pp. 4ff.

7. T. C. Schelling, "The Life You Save May Be Your Own," in *Problems In Public Expenditures Analysis*, ed. Samuel B. Chase, Jr. (Washington, D.C.: The Brookings Institution, 1968), p. 129.

BIBLIOGRAPHICAL NOTE

The useful published material on nursing homes and related issues is remarkably scanty, of questionable quality, and often difficult to find. This book is heavily based on interviews and my own visits to nursing homes and government agencies. What follows is a very selective listing, comprising only those materials that I found to be of some real interest or utility.

General Material

The basic, indispensable source on nursing homes and public policy is the series of reports issued by the Subcommittee on Long-Term Care of the U.S. Senate Special Committee on Aging under the general title of *Nursing Home Care in the United States: Failure in Public Policy* over the period 1974–1976 (Washington, D.C.: Government Printing Office). *Failure in Public Policy* consists of an *Introductory Report* and seven "supporting papers," of which the most useful are *Drugs in Nursing Homes* (no. 2), *Nurses in Nursing Homes* (no. 4), and the report on the impact on nursing homes of the discharge of elderly patients from state mental hospitals (no. 6). While the subcommittee's reports are uneven, often badly organized, and frequently stronger on argument than evidence, they remain fundamental documents. Senator Frank Moss, chairman of the subcommittee at the time *Failure in Public Policy* was produced, and Val J. Halamandaris, its principal staff official, collected and digested much of the subcommittee's reports into a volume issued by Aspen Systems Press under the title of *Too Old, Too Sick, Too Bad: Nursing Homes in America* (1977).

Two other books are also useful, though limited in their focus. Perhaps the most politically important book ever written about nursing homes in America is Mary Adelaide Mendelson's *Tender Loving Greed: How the Incredibly Lucrative Nursing Home "Industry" Is Exploiting America's Old People and Defrauding Us All* (New York: Alfred A. Knopf, 1974; paperback edition, Vintage Books, 1975), which is particularly good in tracing the careers of some of the industry's more notorious charlatans. *Old Age: The Last Segregation* (New York: Grossman, 1971) is the result of a Ralph Nader-sponsored investigation undertaken by high school students at Miss Porter's School in Connecticut, with Claire Townsend as the project director. The students took "undercover" jobs as aides and assistants in a variety of nursing homes, and their diaries of their experiences contain some of the best first-hand reporting on the inadequacies of nursing home care.

Useful for their description of nursing homes and their residents are two studies produced by a team of researchers at the University of Virginia: Barbara Bolling Manard, Carey Steven Kirt, and Dirk W. L. van Gils, *Old-Age Institutions* (Lexington, Mass.: Lexington Books, 1975), and Barbara Bolling Manard, Ralph E. Woehle, and James M. Heilman, *Better Homes for the Old* (Lexington, Mass.: Lexington Books, 1977). For a cross-national comparison, Ian R. Lawson's "Community-Based Medical Care in Three Settings," in *Topias and Utopias in Health: Policy Studies*, edited by Stanley R. Ingman and Anthony E. Thomas (The Hague: Mouton Publishers, 1972), is highly provocative.

Sylvia Sherwood, editor, *Long-Term Care: A Handbook for Researchers, Planners, and Providers* (New York: Spectrum, 1975), is highly uneven and often dated, but a useful source-book. Sherwood's "Introduction" and the chapters by George L. Maddox, "Families as Context and Resource in Chronic Illness," and Ruth Bennett and Carl Eisdorfer,

Bibliographical Note

"The Institutional Environment and Behavior Change," are especially good. Somewhat more technical, broader in focus, and more current is A. N. Exton-Smith and J. Grimley Evans, editors, *Care of the Elderly: Meeting the Challenge of Dependency* (New York: Grune & Stratton, 1977), which contains the proceedings of an Anglo-American conference held in Washington in 1976.

Often full of valuable insight or detail are the reports of investigative bodies at the state or local level—most useful are those on management of state responsibilities in reimbursement, inspection, and standard-setting. The landmark here is clearly the seven volumes, the last of which is a summary, issued by the New York State Moreland Act Commission on Nursing Homes and Residential Facilities between October 1975 and February 1976. While uneven in quality and often surprisingly short-sighted, the best volumes—those on property-cost reimbursement and assessment and placement—are basic documents for anyone who would understand the nursing home industry.

Exemplary, if less detailed, is the *Interim Report* of the Ohio Nursing Home Commission, entitled *A Program in Crisis* (Columbus, Ohio, June 1978). Older, but comprehensive, is the Maryland *Report of the Governor's Commission on Nursing Homes* (Annapolis 1973). Also useful are the *Report of the Blue Ribbon Committee to Investigate the Nursing Home Industry in Connecticut* (Hartford, December 1976), the *Final Report of the Medicaid Management Study Team, Wisconsin Department of Health and Social Services* (Madison, June 1, 1977), and the *First* and *Second Preliminary Reports*, Special Senate Committee to Investigate Nursing Homes, Michigan Legislature (Lansing, 1977).

The primary source of statistical data on nursing homes and their residents is the National Nursing Home Survey conducted triennially by the National Center for Health Statistics, results of which are reported in the Center's *Vital and Health Statistics* series, generally several years after data collection. Most of the data used in this book come from the 1973–74 survey, especially as reported in Mark R. Meiners, *Selected Operating and Financial Characteristics of Nursing Homes, United States: 1973–1974 National Nursing Home Survey, Vital and Health Statistics*, Series 13, no. 22 (Washington, D.C.: Government Printing Office, 1975); Aurora Zappolo, *Characteristics, Social Contacts, and Activities of Nursing Home Residents, Vital and Health Statistics* Series 13, no. 27 (Washington, D.C.: Government Printing Office, 1977); and Jeannine Fox Sutton, *Utilization of Nursing Homes, United States: National Nursing Home Survey, August 1973–April 1974, Vital and Health Statistics* Series 13, no. 28 (Washington, D.C.: Government Printing Office, 1977). The first publication of data from the 1977 survey was "A Comparison of Nursing Home Residents and Discharges from the 1977 National Nursing Home Survey: United States," by Esther Hing and Aurora Zappolo, in *Advance Data*, put out by the Vital and Health Statistics Service of the National Center for Health Statistics, May 17, 1978.

Particularly useful for diagnostic medical and staffing data, but limited to skilled nursing facilities, is the report of the Office of Nursing Home Affairs entitled, *Long-Term Care Facility Improvement Study: Introductory Report* (Washington, D.C.: Government Printing Office, 1975). The "Facility Improvement Project" also published the best study of drug-prescribing patterns in skilled nursing facilities, *Physicians' Drug Prescribing Patterns in Skilled Nursing Facilities* (Washington, D.C.: Government Printing Office, 1976).

The standard reference on health-care expenditures is the report published each year in the *Social Security Bulletin*. The latest version is Robert M. Gibson and Charles R. Fisher, "National Health Expenditures, Fiscal Year 1977," *Social Security Bulletin* 41 (July 1978): 3–20—although much of the nursing home data contained therein is based on the National Center for Health Statistics' nursing home surveys. On employee wages in nursing homes, see U.S. Department of Labor, Bureau of Labor Statistics, *Industry Wage Survey: Nursing Homes and Related Facilities, May 1976* (Washington, D.C.: Government Printing Office, 1977). Data on chronic illness in the elderly from the National Health Interview Survey can be found in another publication from the National Center for Health Statistics, *Health United States*, 1975 (Rockville, Md.: Department of Health, Education, and Welfare, 1976). The best comparison between the institutionalized and non-institutionalized elderly is Burton D. Dunlop, "Need for and Utilization of Long-Term Care Among Elderly Americans," *Journal of Chronic Diseases* 29 (February 1976): 75–87. For British data, and some very useful observations, see R. W. Canvin and N. G. Pearson, editors, *Needs of the Elderly for Health and Welfare Services* (Exeter, England: Institute of Biometry and Community Medicine, University of Exeter, 1973). Less data-rich, but conceptually important, is *A Policy Statement: The Elderly and Functional Dependency* (Washington, D.C.: National Academy of Sciences, Institute of Medicine, 1977).

The best introduction to the generic problems of the elderly is Robert N. Butler, *Why Survive?: Being Old in America* (New York: Harper & Row, 1975). More detailed discussions of critical demographic and political issues can be found in *Political Consequences of Aging, The Annals* 415 (September 1974). Robert Binstock and Ethel Shanas, editors, *The Handbook of Aging and the Social Sciences* (New York: Van Nostrand Reinhold, 1976), is comprehensive and indispensable.

In the category of "miscellaneous" is Robert J. Kastenbaum and S. E. Candy, "The 4% Fallacy: A Methodological and Empirical Critique of Extended Care Facility Population Statistics," *Journal of Aging and Human Development* 4 (Winter 1973): 15–22; Harold J. Wershow, "Comment: Reality Orientation for Gerontologists, Some Thoughts About Senility," *The Gerontologist* 17 (Summer 1977): 297–302; Ernest M. Gruenberg, "The Failures of Success," *Milbank Memorial Fund Quarterly: Health and Society* 55 (Winter 1977): 3–24; and "Medical Care of the Elderly, Report of the Working Party of the Royal College of Physicians of London," *The Lancet* (May 21, 1977); pp. 1092–1095.

History

Four works are essential to understanding the history of public policy toward nursing homes. Glenn R. Markus, *Nursing Homes and the Congress: A Brief History of Developments and Issues* (Washington, D.C.: Library of Congress, 1972), provides the most comprehensive legislative history. There are two studies tracing the history of nursing homes in individual states, both very well done. William C. Thomas, Jr., *Nursing Homes and Public Policy: Drift and Decision in New York State* (Ithaca: Cornell University Press, 1969), although it ends with the enactment of Medicaid, is particularly informative on vacillation between support of and opposition to proprietary facilities. Ethel McClure, *More Than a Roof: The Development of Minnesota Poor Farms and Homes for the Aged* (St. Paul: Minnesota Historical Society, 1968), peters out in the mid–1950s but is an extraordinarily good book, especially in its description of the poor-farm system and in its exploration of the role of denominational charitable organizations. The other indispensable work is Robert Stevens and Rosemary Stevens, *Welfare Medicine in America: A Case Study of Medicaid* (New York: The Free Press, 1974), considered something of a classic. Robert Stevens also edited *Statutory History of the United States: Income Security* (New York: Chelsea House, 1970), a useful compendium of public documents.

A good general, introductory history of American social welfare is Walter I. Trattner, *From Poor Law to Welfare State: A History of Social Welfare in America* (New York: The Free Press, 1974). The standard history of the passage of the Social Security Act is Roy Lubove, *The Struggle for Social Security* (Cambridge: Harvard University Press, 1968). Edwin E. Witte, *The Development of the Social Security Act* (Madison: University of Wisconsin Press, 1962), provides an insider's view. On the subsequent politics of welfare, Gilbert Steiner, *Social Insecurity: The Politics of Welfare* (Chicago: Rand, McNally, 1966), is superb.

The best history of Medicare is still Richard Harris, *A Sacred Trust* (New York: New American Library, 1966). Theodore R. Marmor, *The Politics of Medicare* (Chicago: Aldine, 1973), is useful. Other sources on Medicare include Max J. Skidmore, *Medicare and the American Rhetoric of Reconciliation* (University, Ala.: University of Alabama Press, 1970); Eugene Feingold, *Medicare: Policy and Politics* (San Francisco: Chandler, 1966); and Peter A. Corning, *The Evolution of Medicare . . . from Idea to Law,* Social Security Administration, Office of Research and Statistics, Research Report No. 29 (Washington, D.C.: Government Printing Office, 1969).

On the implementation of Medicare, two items are crucial: Judith M. Feder, *Medicare: The Politics of Federal Hospital Insurance* (Lexington, Mass.: Lexington Books, 1977); and

Bibliographical Note

U.S., Senate, Committee on Finance, *Medicare and Medicaid: Problems, Issues, and Alternatives* (Washington, D.C.: Government Printing Office, 1970). Also see Robert M. Ball, "Social Security Amendments of 1972 Summary and Legislative History," *Social Security Bulletin* 36 (March 1973); 3–25.

Reimbursement and Financing

There does not yet exist a sound, readily accessible text on the principles of hospital reimbursement. The federal administration of Medicaid was, until the past several years, particularly negligent in the ways in which it collected, collated, and made available information from the states, each of which functioned as a quasi-autonomous duchy reporting to a federal regional office rather than to Washington. Thus, as late as 1978, the only comprehensive survey of state reimbursement systems under the new "reasonable cost-related" requirements was one compiled for the American Health Care Association by a private consulting firm. Federal officials eager for a quick survey of differing state policies relied on that document.

The few exceptions to this state of affairs appear all the more useful. On Medicaid, the single really useful compilation of relatively current data is superb: U.S., Department of Health, Education, and Welfare, Health Care Financing Administration, Medicaid Bureau, Institute for Medicaid Management, *Data on the Medicaid Program: Eligibility, Services, Expenditures Fiscal Years 1966–1967* (Washington, D.C.: Institute for Medicaid Management, 1977). William Pollak, "Long-Term Care Facility Reimbursement," in John Holahan, Bruce Spitz, William Pollak, and Judith Feder, *Altering Medicaid Provider Reimbursement Methods*, Publication 986-14 (Washington, D.C.: The Urban Institute, 1977), is similarly invaluable. Preliminary versions of a series of case studies of prospective reimbursement in seven states, by Bruce Spitz and Jane Weeks of the Urban Institute, was of enormous help. It should be published shortly.

In addition to the report of the Moreland Act Commission on property reimbursement and Feder's analysis of Medicare reimbursement principles, cited earlier, other bits and pieces can be gleaned from Sylvia Law, *Blue Cross: What Went Wrong?* (New Haven: Yale University Press, 1974), especially on Medicare reimbursement administration and the retroactive denial of extended-care facility claims; Karen Davis, "Hospital Cost and the Medicare Program," *Social Security Bulletin* 36 (August 1973): 18–36; and Michael Zubkoff, editor, *Health: A Victim or Cause of Inflation?* (New York: Prodist, 1976), especially the chapter on "Inflation in the Health Industry" by Stuart H. Altman and Joseph Eichenholz.

Howard J. Berman and Lewis E. Weeks, *The Financial Management of Hospitals*, 3rd ed. (Ann Arbor, Mich.: Health Administration Press, 1976), is the standard text. On prospective reimbursement, see William L. Dowling's "Prospective Reimbursement of Hospitals," *Inquiry* II (September 1974): 163–180; and Katherine G. Bauer's "Hospital Rate Setting—This Way to Salvation?" *Milbank Memorial Fund Quarterly: Health and Society* 55 (Winter 1977): 117–158.

On capital financing, the most useful items are the Moreland Commission's volume, *Pruning the Money Tree* (New York: The Commission 1967), Markus's legislative history, and David Shulman and Ruth Galanter, "Reorganizing the Nursing Home Industry: A Proposal," *Milbank Memorial Fund Quarterly: Health and Society* 54 (Spring 1976): 129–143. Janet Kline, *Federal Financial Support for the Construction of Nursing Homes* (Washington, D.C.: Library of Congress, 1972), is elementary but straightforward.

On nursing home chains, the best source of information remains the four articles written by J. Richard Elliott, Jr., for *Barron's* at the height of the stock market boom in early 1969. They are: "Unhealthy Growth?: Nursing Home Building Is Expanding at a Feverish Pace" (10 February, 1969); "Long Bed Rest: Some Areas Have More Nursing Homes Than They Need" (3 March, 1969); "Wards of the State?: Healthy Growth in Nursing Homes Calls for Intensive Care" (17 March, 1969); and "No Tired Blood: Nursing Home Operators Are Long on Enthusiasm, Short on Experience" (24 March, 1969).

Such economic theory as there is on the behavior of not-for-profit firms can be found in Burton A. Weisbrod, *The Voluntary Non-Profit Sector: An Economic Analysis* (Lexington, Mass.: Lexington Books, 1977); Joseph P. Newhouse, "Toward a Theory of Non-Profit Institutions: An Economic Model of a Hospital," *American Economic Review* 60 (March 1970): 64–73; Maw Lin Lee, "A Conspicuous Production Theory of Hospital Behavior," *Southern Economic Journal* 38 (July 1971): 48–59; and Mark Pauly and Michael Redisch, "The Not-for-Profit Hospital as a Physician's Cooperative," *American Economic Review* 63 (March 1973): 87–99. Also recommended is my "Why Non-Profits Go Broke," *The Public Interest* (Winter 1976), pp. 86–101.

On "certificate-of-need," see Eugene J. Rubel, "Implementing the National Health Planning and Resources Development Act of 1974," *Public Health Reports* 91 (January–February 1976): 3–8; Samuel V. Stiles, "Regulatory and Review Functions Created by the Act," *Public Health Reports* 91 (January–February 1976) pp. 24–28; William J. Bicknell and Diana Chapman Walsh, "Certificate-of-Need: The Massachusetts Experience," *New England Journal of Medicine* 292 (May 15, 1975): 1054–1061; and David S. Salkever and Thomas W. Bice, "The Impact of Certificate-of-Need Controls on Hospital Investment," *Milbank Memorial Fund Quarterly: Health and Society* 54 (Spring 1976): 185–214.

Placement, Assessment, and Quality of Care

The classic studies on "inappropriate" placement include T. Franklin Williams et al., "Appropriate Placement of the Chronically Ill and Aged: A Successful Approach by Evaluation," *Journal of American Medical Association* 226 (10 December, 1973): 1332–1335; James G. Zimmer, "Characteristics of Patients and Care Provided in Health-Related and Skilled Nursing Facilities," *Medical Care* 13 (December 1975): 992–1010; John W. Davis and Marilyn J. Gibbin, "An Areawide Examination of Nursing Home Use, Misuse and Nonuse," *American Journal of Public Health* 61 (June 1971): 1146–1155; and Robert L. Berg, Francis E. Browning, John G. Hill, and Walter Wenkert, "Assessing the Health Care Needs of the Aged," *Health Services Research* 5 (Spring 1970): 36–59; the percentages of "inappropriate" placements in these studies run from 13 to 74 percent.

Ellen W. Jones, Paul M. Densen, and Barbara J. McNitt, *An Approach to the Assessment of Long-Term Care, Final Report* (Harvard Center for Community Health and Medical Care, mimeograph, 13 December, 1976), presents the most comprehensive attack on problems of patient classification and tying classification to quality measures; the work it summarizes and reports provides much of the basis for the new invisible federal PACE initiative. A good introduction to quality evaluation in medical care is Institute of Medicine, *Advancing the Quality of Health Care: Key Issues and Fundamental Principles* (Washington, D.C.: National Academy of Sciences, 1974); a particularly effective argument for "outcome" measures is contained in Robert H. Brook et al., *Quality of Medical Care Assessment Using Outcome Measures: An Overview of the Method* (Santa Monica, Calif.: The Rand Corporation, 1976).

On the intermediate-care facility category and "levels-of-care" controversy, the more useful items include Judith W. LaVor, "Intermediate Care Facilities: Expectations vs. Realities" (U.S. Department of Health, Education, and Welfare, mimeograph, 1974); the Moreland Act Commission's volume on *Assessment and Placement: Anything Goes* (New York: The Commission, 1976); Community Research Applications, Inc., *Excerpt Summary of a National Study of Levels of Care in Intermediate Care Facilities (ICFs)* (U.S. Department of Health, Education, and Welfare, Bureau of Quality Assurance, 1976); Ian R. Lawson, "Title XIX Reimbursement in Long-Term Care," in Applied Management Sciences, *Report on Systems of Reimbursement for Long-Term Care (LTC) Services, Final Report*, vol. 2 (Silver Spring, Md.: Applied Management Sciences, 1976); and Charles H. Brooks and John A. Hoffman, "Type of Ownership and Medicaid Use of Nursing Home Beds" *Journal of Community Health* 3 (Spring 1978): 236–244.

Bibliographical Note

On quality regulation, the most useful sources were the state investigations cited previously and interviews. Also helpful were Robert N. Brown, "An Appraisal of the Nursing Home Enforcement Process," *Arizona Law Review* 17 (1975); National Association of Attorneys General, Committee on the Office of Attorney General, *Enforcing Quality of Care in Nursing Homes* (Raleigh, N.C.: The Association, 1978); and Hirsch S. Ruchlin, "A New Strategy for Regulating Long-Term Care Facilities," *Journal of Health Politics, Policy, and Law* 2 (Summer 1977): 190–211. The current debate over government regulation is largely dominated by the position expressed in Charles L. Schultze, *The Public Use of Private Interest* (Washington, D.C.: The Brookings Institution, 1977), which I hope chapter 7 demonstrates to be largely irrelevant, if not simply wrong, and the American Enterprise Institute's polemical journal *Regulation*.

Where to Go and How to Get There

For those seeking a general introduction to "alternatives" to nursing home care, most important is the Congressional Budget Office Study entitled *Long-Term Care for the Elderly and Disabled* (Washington, D.C.: Congressional Budget Office, 1977), and its technical supporting document, *Long-Term Care: Actuarial Cost Estimates* (Washington, D.C.: Congressional Budget Office, 1977). Less technical are Robert Morris, *Alternatives to Nursing Home Care: A Proposal*, prepared for use by the U.S., Senate, Special Committee on Aging (Washington, D.C.: Government Printing Office, 1971), and Robert L. Kane and Rosalie A. Kane, "Care of the Aged: Old Problems in Need of New Solutions," *Science* 200 (May 17, 1978): 913–918.

The best, though very limited, recent study of the elderly in politics is Henry J. Pratt, *The Gray Lobby* (Chicago: University of Chicago Press, 1976); a bit more dated, but still perhaps the best single study written on the politics of the elderly, is Robert H. Binstock, "Interest-Group Liberalism and the Politics of Aging," pt. 1 *Gerontologist* 12 (Autumn 1972): 265–280. The only published article I was able to locate on nursing home politics per se is Mary Adelaide Mendelson and David Hapgood, "The Political Economy of Nursing Homes," *The Annals* 415 (September 1974): 95–105, which is incisive but brief. Robert Hudson has written extensively on the Administration on Aging and its political dynamics; see, for example, Hudson and Martha Veley, "Federal Funding and State Planning: The Case of State Units on Aging," *The Gerontologist* 14 (April 1974): 122–128. It seems appropriate to end with Linda Horn and Elma Griesel, *Nursing Homes: A Citizen's Action Guide* (Boston: Beacon Press, 1977); its authors will only be pleased if its listing of consumer groups and their triumphs becomes quickly dated.

APPENDIX

The primary "methodology" employed in this study consisted of my asking questions of people who knew more about the subject than I. Because there is so much variation in nursing home policy from state to state, I selected a sample of eight states in which to conduct field research: New York, California, Ohio, Minnesota, Oklahoma, Connecticut, New Jersey, and Arizona. In each state, I sought to speak to: state officials; industry representatives, from both proprietary and voluntary sectors; members of special investigative bodies; consumer advocates; employee representatives; and other knowledgeable people.

I also sought to collect whatever documents of any relevance to nursing homes were available, many of which are not generally made public. I also talked to leading officials and experts in Washington, and anywhere else I could find them. Finally, I made it a point to go to as many nursing homes as I could and to talk to the people who worked and lived in them.

Without the openness and generosity of the almost 200 people listed below, this book would not have been possible, although none of them are responsible in any way for my interpretations or conclusions.

Most of the people on this list participated in formal interviews, but the information gained from many others came in more casual encounters at meetings or conferences, or just from discussions among friends or research colleagues. To apply the term "interviews" to all those listed would thus be erroneous, but everyone on the list helped.

In all such discussions, I promised confidentiality—explicitly or implicitly. With a few exceptions, statements and information from interviews are, therefore, not attributed in the text.

The organizational affiliations listed are those that prevailed at the time of my encounters with those on the list.

Dr. Faye G. Abdellah
Office of Long-Term Care, DHEW
Rockville, Maryland

Mr. Ben Abramovice
Home for Jewish Parents
Oakland, California

Dr. Stuart Altman
Brandeis University
Waltham, Massachusetts

Mr. Steve Anderman
New York Department of Health
Albany, New York

Dr. Nancy Anderson
The University of Minnesota
Minneapolis, Minnesota

Ms. Pat Anderson
Ebenezer Ridges
Burnsville, Minnesota

Ms. Louise Ansak
On Lok
San Francisco, California

Professor Eugene Bardach
University of California-Berkeley
Berkeley, California

Mr. Berkeley Bennett
The Bennett Group
Washington, D.C.

Mr. Morton C. Berkowitz
Office of Long-Term Care, DHEW
New York, New York

Hon. Peter A.A. Berle
Commission of Environmental
  Conservation
New York, New York

Mr. Steven Blader
Office of Public Interest Advocacy
Trenton, New Jersey

Mr. Harry F. Blair
Office of the Special Prosecutor
New York, New York

Mr. Edward Bohan
Office of the Special Prosecutor
New York, New York

Ms. Jeanne Bost
Connecticut Dept. of Aging
Hartford, Connecticut

Mr. Jack Boyd
Oklahoma Health Planning Commission
Oklahoma City, Oklahoma

Mr. Howard Bram
Menorah Park Hebrew Home for the
  Aged
Beachwood, Ohio

Ms. Mary Bremhorst
The Beatitudes Campus of Care
Phoenix, Arizona

Dr. Robert Burmeister
American College of Nursing Home
  Administrators
Washington, D.C.

Dr. Robert N. Butler
National Institute on Aging
Bethesda, Maryland

Mr. Del Callaway
California Association of Health Facilities
Sacramento, California

Dr. Marie Callender
Connecticut Health Plan
Bridgeport, Connecticut

Mr. David Carboni
The University of Bridgeport
Bridgeport, Connecticut

Mr. Charles Chowmet
Citizens for Better Care
Detroit, Michigan

Dean Wilbur J. Cohen
The University of Michigan
Ann Arbor, Michigan

Ms. Nancy Coleman
National Health Law Center
Washington, D.C.

Mr. Jay Constantine
Committee on Finance
U.S. Senate
Washington, D.C.

Mr. David Crowley
American Association of Homes for the
  Aged
Washington, D.C.

Mr. Nelson Cruikshank
Federal Council on Aging
Washington, D.C.

Mr. Walt Davis
Retail Clerks International Assoc.
Washington, D.C.

Mr. Wayne Davis
Westminster Terrace
Columbus, Ohio

Mr. Charles Delbaum
Cleveland Legal Aid Society
Cleveland, Ohio

Mr. Harvey Demsky
Office of Long Term Care, DHEW
New York, New York

Mr. Milt Dezube
Medical Services Administration, DHEW
Washington, D.C.

Dr. Burton Dunlop
The Urban Institute
Washington, D.C.

Mr. Dennis Dunne
California Dept. of Health
Sacramento, California

Dr. Gerald Eggert
Monroe County Long-Term Care Program
Rochester, New York

Ms. Mary Erlanger
Connecticut Department of Aging
Hartford, Connecticut

Rev. Msgr. Charles J. Fahey
Catholic Charities of Syracuse
Syracuse, New York

Mr. Ben Fatheree
Oklahoma Dept. of Institutions
Social and Rehabilitative Services
Oklahoma City, Oklahoma

Dr. Andrew Fleck
New York State Department of Health
Albany, New York

Mr. Frank Frantz
Mott-MacDonald Associates
Washington, D.C.

Ms. Eleanor Friedenberg
Division of Long-Term Care, DHEW
Rockville, Maryland

Ms. Ruth Galanter
National Health Law Project
Santa Monica, California

Mrs. Florence Galkin
Community Action & Resources for The
  Elderly
New York, New York

Prof. Victor Garlin
California Health Facilities Commission
Sacramento, California

Mr. John Geagan
Service Employees International Union
Washington, D.C.

Mr. Frank Gebauer
Mid-Ohio Health Systems Agency
Columbus, Ohio

Ms. Barbara E. Geddes
Ohio Commission on Aging
Columbus, Ohio

Mr. Joseph Gentlecore
Ohio Health Care Association
Columbus, Ohio

Dr. Joseph Gibboney
Ohio Association of Philanthropic Homes
  for the Aged
Columbus, Ohio

Dr. Erik Gjullin
American College of Nursing Home
  Administrators
Washington, D.C.

Mr. Donald H. Goldberg
Hebrew Home and Hospital
Hartford, Connecticut

Dr. Solomon Goldberg
New Jersey Department of Health
Trenton, New Jersey

Mrs. Rose Goldstein
Jewish Home and Hospital
Bronx, New York

Mr. Richard Grant
Washington Federal Savings & Loan
New York, New York

Mr. Jim Green
Minnesota Association of Health Care
  Facilities
Bloomington, Minnesota

Dr. George Greenberg
Office of the Assistant Secretary for
  Planning and Evaluation, DHEW
Washington, D.C.

Dr. Gerald Grob
Rutgers University
New Brunswick, New Jersey

Ms. Kathryn Haller
Office of Legal Services
Columbus, Ohio

Mr. Louis J. Halpryn
Connecticut Association of Health Care
  Facilities
Manchester, Connecticut

Mr. Alfred D. Hammes
Arizona Department of Health Services
Phoenix, Arizona

Dr. Charlene Harrington
California Department of Health
Sacramento, California

Ms. Adele Hart
Menorah Park Hebrew Home for the
  Aged
Beachwood, Ohio

Ms. Cathy Hawes
Ohio Nursing Home Commission
Columbus, Ohio

Mr. Charles Hawkins
Bethesda, Maryland

Appendix

Mr. Fred Hebeler
New Jersey Department of Health
Trenton, New Jersey

Mr. John Hess
The New York Times
New York, New York

Mr. Joe Hodgson
Triage, Inc.
Bristol, Connecticut

Mr. Hillel Hoffman
Office of the Special Prosecutor
New York, New York

Mr. Jim Horton
Service Employees International Union
Cleveland, Ohio

Mr. Marvin Hrubes
Retail Clerks International Association
Washington, D.C.

Hon. Charles J. Hynes
Special Prosecutor for Nursing Homes
New York, New York

Dr. Stanley Ingman
Univeristy of Connecticut
Hartford, Connecticut

Professor Robert Kagan
University of California-Berkeley
Berkeley, California

Mr. Paul A. Kershner
Andrus Gerontology Center
University of Southern California
Los Angeles, California

Mr. Roger King
California State Senate
Sacramento, California

Mr. Jerry Klein
Service Employees International Union
San Francisco, California

Mr. Ernest Kramer
Minnesota Department of Health
Minneapolis, Minnesota

Mrs. Daphne Krause
Minneapolis Age and Opportunity Center
Minneapolis, Minnesota

Ms. Polly Kuehl
The Ebenezer Society
Minneapolis, Minnesota

Mr. Laurence F. Lane
American Association of Homes for the
Aging
Washington, D.C.

Mr. Lawrence Larson
Isabella Geriatric Center
New York, New York

Mr. Benjamin Latt
Division of Long-Term Care, DHEW
Rockville, Maryland

Mrs. Judy LaVor
Office of the Assistant Secretary for
Planning and Evaluation, DHEW
Washington, D.C.

Dr. Ian Lawson
Danbury Hospital
Danbury, Connecticut

Mrs. Gerta Leshin
Isabella Geriatric Center
New York, New York

Dr. Bertha Levy
Oklahoma Department of Institutions
Social and Rehabilitative Services
Oklahoma City, Oklahoma

Dr. Richard A. Leibes
Services Employees International Union
San Francisco, California

Mr. Mike Loughman
Office of the Attorney General
Columbus, Ohio

Mr. Jack MacDonald
National Council of Health
Care Services
Washington, D.C.

Mr. Andy Martin
Service Employees International Union
Cleveland, Ohio

Mr. Maurice May
Hebrew Gerontological Center for Aged
Boston, Massachusetts

Dr. Walter McClure
InterStudy
Excelsior, Minnesota

Mrs. Mary Adelaide Mendelson
Cleveland, Ohio

Mr. Donald Meyers
Peter Rogatz and Donald Meyers
Associates, Inc.
Roslyn Heights, New York

Mr. Dwight B. Mezo
Retail Clerks International Association
Minneapolis, Minnesota

Mrs. Dulcy Miller
White Plains Geriatric Center
White Plains, New York

Mr. A. Luther Molberg
The Ebenezer Society
Minneapolis, Minnesota

Mr. Tom Moore
San Francisco, California

Professor Robert Morris
Brandeis University
Waltham, Massachusetts

Mr. Jerry Murphy
New Jersey Medicaid Program
Trenton, New Jersey

Ms. Mary Brugger Murphy
National Association of Counties
Washington, D.C.

Mr. Hal G. Norris
Arizona Department of Health Services
Phoenix, Arizona

Mr. Herman Owens
Retail Clerks International Association
Minneapolis, Minnesota

Ms. Pam Parker & officers
Nursing Home Residents Advisory
    Council
Minneapolis, Minnesota

Ms. Lu Pearman
Minneapolis, Minnesota

Mr. Arthur Penn
Office of the Public Advocate
Trenton, New Jersey

Mr. Leo Perlis
AFL-CIO
Washington, D.C.

Dr. Eric A. Plaut
Commissioner of Mental Health
Hartford, Connecticut

Ms. Joan Quinn
Triage
Bristol, Connecticut

Mr. Ronald Ramstead
Southland Geriatric Center
Norwalk, California

Mr. William Ratchford
Connecticut Commissioner on Aging
Hartford, Connecticut

Mr. John Regan
California Association of Homes
    for the Aged
Sacramento, California

Dr. Richard A. Rettig
The Rand Corporation
Washington, D.C.

Mr. Jerome J. Richgels
Retail Clerks International Association
St. Paul, Minnesota

Mr. Jim Rischl
Ohio Office of the Attorney General
Columbus, Ohio

Dr. Joe O. Rogers
Oklahoma Nursing Home Association
Oklahoma City, Oklahoma

Dr. Bill Scanlon
The Urban Institute
Washington, D.C.

Ms. Jane Schoenbrun
Office of Congressman Donald Fraser
Washington, D.C.

Mr. Stuart Schmid
Office of the Assistant Secretary for
    Planning & Evaluation, DHEW
Washington, D.C.

Dr. David Schulman
University of California-Riverside
Riverside, California

Dr. Arthur Schwartz
Andrus Gerontology Center
University of Southern California
Los Angeles, California

Appendix

Mr. Robert Schwartz
Office of the Special Prosecutor
New York, New York

Mrs. Annabel Seidman
National Council of Senior Citizens
Washington, D.C.

Mr. Bert Seidman
AFL-CIO
Washington, D.C.

Ms. Jeanne Setness
The Ebenezer Society
Minneapolis, Minnesota

Ms. Mildred Shapiro
New York State Health Planning
    Commission
Albany, New York

Mr. Bill Smith
California Department of Health
Sacramento, California

Ms. Cathy Smith
Central Arizona Health Systems Agency
Phoenix, Arizona

Mr. Marall Smith
Service Employees International Union
San Francisco, California

Mr. Bruce Spitz
The Urban Institute
Washington, D.C.

Rev. John Steinhaus
California Lutheran Homes
Norwalk, California

Mr. Jack Stewart
Oklahoma Department of Institutions
Social and Rehabilitative Services
Oklahoma City, Oklahoma

Ms. Mary Sughrue
Office of the Special Prosecutor
New York, New York

Ms. Elizabeth Taylor
The Federal Trade Commission
Seattle, Washington

Mr. Clarence Teng
Samaritan Health Services
Phoenix, Arizona

Mr. Bruce D. Thevenot
American Health Care Association
Washington, D.C.

Dr. Paul Thompson
Columbia University
New York, New York

Ms. Joan Tracyzk
The Ebenezer Society
Minneapolis, Minnesota

Mr. Charles Turner, III
Mid-Ohio Health Systems Agency
Columbus, Ohio

Ms. Eldora Vaitkus
Arizona Department of Health Services
Phoenix, Arizona

Ms. Joan Van Nostrand
National Center for Health Statistics,
    DHEW
Rockville, Md.

Mr. David A. Wagner
New Jersey Department of Health
Trenton, New Jersey

Ms. Jacqueline Walker
Connecticut Nursing Home Ombudsman
Hartford, Connecticut

Mr. Richard Waltz
Ohio Attorney General's Office
Columbus, Ohio

Mr. F. John Walzer, Jr.
New Jersey Nursing Home Ombudsman
Trenton, New Jersey

Ms. Jane Weeks
The Urban Institute
Washington, D.C.

Mr. Chuck Weisen
Minneapolis Age & Opportunity Center
Minneapolis, Minnesota

Mrs. Anne Weiss
Jewish Home and Hospital
Bronx, New York

Dr. Wes Whittlesey
Oklahoma Dept. of Institutions
Social and Rehabilitative Services
Oklahoma City, Oklahoma

Dr. Stanley Wisneiski
Service Employees International Union
Washington, D.C.

Hon. Dennis Wojtanowski
Ohio House of Representatives
Columbus, Ohio

Mr. Charles T. Wood
Massachusetts Eye and Ear Hospital
Boston, Massachusetts

Ms. Cathy Worley
Ohio Nursing Home Commission
Columbus, Ohio

Mr. Howard Worley
California Association of Health Care
  Facilities
Sacramento, California

Mr. J. Albin Yokie
American College of Nursing Home
  Administrators
Washington, D.C.

Mr. Don Yost
Arizona Department of Health Services
Phoenix, Arizona

INDEX

295

Index

Butler, Robert N., 284

California: availability of beds in, 12; budgetary restraints in, 203; construction in, 218; levels of care in, 137; lobbying in, 194; MAA and, 47; Medicaid expenditures in, 73; Medicaid rate cuts in, 257; proprietary vs. voluntary homes in, 125; publicity as enforcement tool in, 166; rate commission in, 95; reimbursement policy in, 82, 88–89, 100; sale of nursing homes in, 112; scandal in, 4; total industry capacity in, 129
Callender, Marie, 66
Campaign contributions, 196–97
Candy, S.E., 284
Canvin, R. W., 283
Capacity reduction, reform through, 224–27
Capital finance fraud, 180
Capital formation, 102, 104
Carter, Jimmy, 211
Cash assistance, eligibility for, 75–76
Catholic nursing homes, 194
Ceilings on costs, 87–89; profile-generated, 89–91
Central Arizona Health Systems Agency, 169
Certificate-of-need laws, 127–28; control of bed supply through, 218
Chains, corporate: lobbying for, 193; national corporation advantages of, 253; ownership of proprietary homes by, 117–22
Charitable contributions, 178, 187
Charitable homes for aged, 35; OAA and, 38
Children of nursing home residents, 13–14
Chronic illness, 14–15
Citizens for Better Care (Detroit), 200
Civil receivership, 148, 165, 214
Civil Rights Act (1964), 53
Civil service regulations, 261
Classical market theory, 92
Clothing, 25
CNA (financial conglomerate), 120
Code of Federal Regulations, 150, 152
Cohen, Wilbur, 41, 44, 48, 51, 58, 60
Collective bargaining agreements, 261
Colorado, director of public welfare in, 62
Committee on Economic Security, 36–37
Committee for National Health Insurance, 198
Common-carrier requirements, 95
Community involvement, 213–14
Community Research Applications, Inc., 286

Competitive bidding, 97
Complaints, inspections in response to, 160
Conditions of participation, 147; for SNFs, 149–51
Congregate housing, 230–33
Congress, 30; Great Society, 189; health policies of, 40–42; HEW inspector general created by, 188; ICFs and, 63–64; influence of lobbyists for elderly in, 198; intergovernmental politics and, 204, 205, 254–55; investigation of theft by, 174; Medicaid and, 58; Medicaid and Medicare enacted by, 48; Medicaid eligibility policies of, 252; Medicaid fraud and, 179; regulatory process and, 173; social legislation in, 51; social security benefits and, 232
Congressional Budget Office (CBO), 210–11, 220, 227, 233, 287
Connecticut: construction in, 218; criminal activity in, 185; flat-rate reimbursement in, 82, 100; HMO demonstration project in, 236; investigation in, 4; Medicaid expenditures in, 73; quality of nursing homes in, 101; rate commission in, 95; total industry capacity in, 129
Constituency-building, 199
Construction and financing, 102–33; of congregate housing, 231; by corporate chains, 117–22; depreciation and, 109–10; FHA mortgages for, 107–8; limitations on, 104; limitations on profits from, 218; during 1950s, 105–7; during postwar economic boom, 105; proposed role of government in, 130–33; regulatory mechanisms and, 127–29; SBA loans for, 107–8; speculation and, 110–17
Consultants, 154
Consumer fraud, 178
Consumer representatives, 214
Contributions, tax-deductible, 178, 187
Convalescent homes, 37–38
Corning, Peter A., 284
Corporate chains, 117–22
Corruption: political, 174, 185; see also Criminal activity
Cost-related reimbursement, 86–95; depreciation and, 109; fraud involving, 179–80; inflation and, 218–19; lobbying for, 197; for Medicare, 79–80; postponement of implementation of, 69, 204; profits generated under, 115, 117; under Public Law 92–603, 68; reform through, 212; for SNFs, 82
Cost-sharing for home services, 235
Costs, 23–24; confusion between average

296

Index

Gatekeeping agencies, 218, 234–37; design for, 260
General Revenue-Sharing Act (1972), 204
Generic programs for aging, 208
Georgia: availability of beds in, 9, 12; levels of care in, 137; MAA and, 46
"Ghettoization" of elderly, 231
Gibbin, Marilyn J., 286
Gibson, Robert M., 283
GI bill, 105
Government agencies, regulation of, 262
Graft, 196–97
Grants-in-aid: for Medicaid, 75; in OAA program, 35, 36
Great Depression, 31
Griesel, Elma, 287
Grooming, 25
Groupings, 87–88; profiles by, 91
Gruenberg, Ernest M., 284
Guidelines, 150

Haircutting, 25
Halamandaris, Val J., 282
Haldeman, H. R., 69
Hapgood, David, 287
Harris, Richard, 284
Health Care Financing Administration, 199
Health, Education and Welfare, Department of (HEW), 285; administration of Medicaid by, 58, 60; administration of Medicare by, 52–57; auditing technology in, 182; constituency of, 199; creation of, 42; Freedom of Information action against, 166; guidelines for planning agencies issued by, 128; home services and, 216; ICFs and, 64; intergovernmental politics and, 204, 205; lobbying and, 195, 197; Moss amendments and, 60–62; during Nixon administration, 65–67; office of inspector general created by, 188; proposed consolidation of ICF and SNF standards by, 146; Public Law 92–603 and, 68; reimbursement systems and, 87, 88, 90, 91; revision of standards by, 211; Social Security Act and, 36–37; supervision of certification by, 157, 158, 160
Health Maintenance Organizations (HMOs), 236
Health Planning Amendments (1978), 280
Health programs, public, 31, 32; postwar, 39–41
Hearing impairment, 15
Heart disease, 14, 15
Heilman, James M., 282
Hess, John, 202
Hill, John G., 286
Hill-Burton Act (1946), 39–40, 250; amend-

ments to, 42–45, 49; construction funds available through, 107
Hillhaven, Inc., 119, 120
Hing, Esther, 283
Hispanics, 14; employed as aides, 21
Hoffman, John A., 286
Holahan, John, 285
Holiday Inn, 118
Hollander (owner), 105
Holyoke, Mass.: innovative program in, 241; public nursing homes in, 126
Home health and help services, 145, 215–18; administrative design for, 260; need for expansion of, 211, 215–16; strategy for, 234–37
Hoover, Herbert, 199
Horn, Linda, 287
Hospital Practice (magazine), 166
Hospital Survey and Construction Act (1946), 39–40
Hospitals: certificate-of-need laws and, 128; confusion of nursing homes with, in policymaking, 262–63; construction of, 105; depreciation and reimbursement of, 109; federal aid to, 39–41; growth in, 131; Hill-Burton construction funds for, 107; inflation in rates charged by, 48; Medicaid payments to, 52; Medicare and, 53, 54; political influence of, 206–8; privileged position of, 249–50; rate-setting commissions for, 95; reforms and, 227–29; reimbursement of, 79–83; transfer agreements with, 60; utilization of, extended-care facilities and, 56, 229; utilization review in, 142
House of Representatives: Committee on Aging of, 205; Committee on Interstate and Foreign Commerce, Health Subcommittee of, 205; Miller amendment in, 64; Rules Committee of, 280n; Ways and Means Committee of, 46, 50, 64, 205
Housing, congregate, 230–33
H.R.3, 188–89, 205, 212
Hudson, Robert, 287
Human fallibility, 262–64
Hynes, Charles J., 188
Hypertension, 18

Ideological legitimacy, 196
Illinois: Medicaid expenditures in, 73; scandal in, 4
Imagery, political, 201–2
Immigrant self-help organizatons, 35
Incentives: administrability problem of, 258–59; reimbursement systems and, 92–94, 99–101; as response to "market failure," 148; for voluntary homes, 123
Income of residents, 14
Incontinence, 14

Index